Dental Biomechanics

Dental Biomechanics

Edited by

Arturo N Natali

Centre of Mechanics of Biological Materials,
University of Padova, Italy

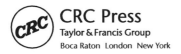

CRC Press
Taylor & Francis Group
Boca Raton London New York

CRC Press is an imprint of the
Taylor & Francis Group, an **informa** business
A TAYLOR & FRANCIS BOOK

CRC Press
Taylor & Francis Group
6000 Broken Sound Parkway NW, Suite 300
Boca Raton, FL 33487-2742

First issued in paperback 2019

© 2003 by Taylor & Francis Group, LLC
CRC Press is an imprint of Taylor & Francis Group, an Informa business

Typeset in Times by
Integra Software Services Pvt. Ltd, Pondicherry, India

Integra Software Services Pvt. Ltd, Pondicherry, India

ISBN-13: 978-0-415-30666-9 (hbk)
ISBN-13: 978-0-367-39525-4 (pbk)

British Library Cataloguing in Publication Data
A catalogue record for this book is available from the British Library

Library of Congress Cataloging in Publication Data
Dental biomechanics / edited by Arturo Natali.
  p. cm.
 Includes bibliographical references and index.
 ISBN 0-415-30666-3 (hardback: alk. paper)
 1. Dentistry, Operative. 2. Dental materials. 3. Biomechanics.
 4. Human mechanics.
 [DNLM: 1. Biomechanics. 2. Dental Implants. 3. Materials Testing.
 4. Osseointegration. 5. Periodontal Ligament. 6. Tomography, X-Ray.
 WU 640 D4132 2003] I. Natali, Arturo.

 RK501.5 .D466 2003
 617. 6'05—dc21   2002151289

Visit the Taylor & Francis Web site at
http://www.taylorandfrancis.com

and the CRC Press Web site at
http://www.crcpress.com

Contents

3. Computer tomography for virtual models in dental imaging   35

AN NATALI, MM VIOLA

4. Computer-aided, pre-surgical analysis for oral rehabilitation   52

H VAN OOSTERWYCK, J VANDER SLOTEN, J DUYCK, J VAN CLEYNENBREUGEL,
B PUERS, I NAERT

7. Testing the reliability of dental implant devices   111

M SONCINI, RP PIETRABISSA, AN NATALI, PG PAVAN, KR WILLIAMS

8. On the mechanics of superelastic orthodontic appliances   132

FA AURICCHIO, VC CACCIAFESTA, LP PETRINI, RP PIETRABISSA

Preface

. . .

Thus my plan here is not to teach the method that everyone must follow in order to guide his reason, but merely to explain how I have tried to guide my own.

Those who set themselves up to instruct others must think they are better than those whom they instruct, and if they misguide them in the slightest they can be held responsible.

But, since I am proposing this work merely as a history or, if you prefer, a fable – in which, among a number of examples that may be imitated, there may also be many others where it would be reasonable not to follow them – I hope it will be useful for some readers without being harmful to others, and that everyone will be grateful for my frankness.

. . .

. . . I hope that those who use only their pure natural reason will be better judges of my views than those who trust only ancient books. For those who combine common sense and study – and I hope that they alone will be my judges . . .

. . .

I would say only that I decided to use the time that remains to me in life for nothing else except trying to acquire a knowledge of nature, from which one could draw some more reliable rules for medicine than those we have had up to now.

René Descartes, "Discourse on method"

I consider it essential to question my dedication to research and, once I am in the midst of it, to reflect on the outstanding privilege of treating the mechanics of biological tissues. I like to consider the approach to be taken on, aiming at the integration of all of the knowledge and competencies that are a part of the research. The significant complexity of biomechanical processes is the manifestation of a superior formulation. Nevertheless, problems that may at first appear insurmountable, can be successfully interpreted by means of an attentive and humble approach that can lead towards the definition of a realistic final configuration. The functional response of biological tissues is, in and of itself, a fundamental reference, which can then be used to access the mechanics within the biological phenomena being dealt with.

The strong desire to reach a solution, or the reduced potentiality of the resources adopted for the investigation, should not lead to inadmissible approximations. On the contrary, regardless of how they have been chosen, they must be evaluated for the implication they have on the reliability of the final result, and should represent a cautious passage towards a more complete interpretation. A comparison of the results deriving from subsequent models, whose accuracy has been improved by taking the characterising aspects into account, will tell us how appropriately the investigation has been carried out. These models will be milestones, which confirm that the right course has been taken.

With this in mind, the mechanics written in biological phenomena should be read leaving aside the fear of facing their enormous complexity; however, at the same time the researcher must also be guided by the precaution taught by experience. The researcher should not be tempted by immediate results, even if they are attractive, rather than seeking deeper insight into the subject at hand. To carry out research in this way, an ethical approach must be taken, coupling biology and mechanics by using the most updated methodology. Mechanics, physics and chemistry are strictly related to clinical practice for the evaluation of the operational reliability of the results obtained.

I intend to report part of the experience and results deriving from many years of activity, in research and education, regarding dental biomechanics. When presenting this work, I am faced with problems pertaining to form and depth with regards to different aspects of bioengineering, which must be treated while remaining compatible with clinical knowledge. The difference in the methods in these cultural areas makes it difficult to propose a unitary presentation of the problems dealt with. Nevertheless, great effort must be made to overcome this discrepancy, with the aim of arriving at a fruitful confrontation and moving towards a unitary definition.

The cooperation efforts between bioengineers and clinicians have proved to be a challenge. It is necessary to be realistic and consider the significant difficulties inherent in this situation. As Renè Descart stated, "If artisans cannot implement immediately the invention I explained, I do no think that, for that reason, it can be said to be defective. Since skill and practice are required to construct and adjust the machines that I described, even though no detail is omitted, I would be just as surprised if they succeeded on their first attempt as if someone were able to learn to play the lute very well in a single day, when they are provided with only a good tablature".

I hope that the final results of this challenge, rather than displease both engineers and clinicians, promote the substantial integration of interest and engagement in facing sophisticated biomechanical problems.

The structure of this work is based on the intention of describing a sequence of events that, in a general sense, should characterise the biomechanical analysis in the dental area. First of all, the mechanics of hard and soft biological tissues, namely the bone and periodontal ligament, is given. Following this characterisation of materials, the geometric configuration of the anatomical site is defined, using tomographic techniques, along with a description of pre-surgical procedures. A significant portion is devoted to the definition of the materials used in dental practice, with regard to both implantology and orthodontics, considering specific manufacturing techniques as well. In the same way, the clinical aspects are reported because of their relevance to practice in implantology and orthodontics. The numerical approach to the biomechanical analysis of dental problems is presented in order to describe the potentialities offered by numerical simulation. A summary of the mechanics of materials, in terms of basic formulation, is reported, as a fundamental reference for approaching the biomechanical aspects treated.

The outstanding complexity of biomechanical phenomena expresses a level of optimisation that seems inaccessible for our knowledge, and is source of wonder and respect. The careful consideration of the magnificence of this reality should move anyone involved in this investigation to humility, and to great dedication. Even if this involvement pertains to the definition a small portion of a problem, it could nonetheless represent a great achievement. To be aware of our own position within the field of knowledge constitutes a preliminary requirement for knowledge itself.

A discussion on method and knowledge becomes a unique task, passing through the ethics of the person, with the aim of achieving a common end. If my work could serve the purpose of a better integration of researchers and teachers who differ because of their scientific education, I hope it could also serve the purpose of helping create better understanding among the people themselves.

I would like to thank everyone that helped me to give substance to these thoughts. For this, I give my profession of gratitude.

Arturo N Natali

Contributors

S Abati
University of Milan, Milan, Italy

C Aparicio
Technical University of Catalonia, Barcelona

FA Auricchio
University of Pavia, Pavia, Italy

F Bonollo
University of Padua, Padua, Italy

VC Cacciafesta
University of Pavia, Pavia, Italy

J Casals
Technical University of Catalonia, Barcelona, Spain

M Chiapasco
University of Milan, Milan, Italy

J Duyck
Catholic University of Leuven, Haverlee, Belgium

E Fernández
Technical University of Catalonia, Barcelona, Spain

G Garattini
University of Milan, Milan, Italy

FJ Gil
Technical University of Catalonia, Barcelona, Spain

MP Ginebra
Technical University of Catalonia, Barcelona, Spain

RT Hart
Tulane University, New Orleans, United States of America

H Ishikawa
Fukuoka Dental College, Fukuoka, Japan

I Knets
Riga Technical University, Riga, Latvia

JM Manero
Technical University of Catalonia, Barcelona, Spain

MC Meazzini
University of Milan, Milan, Italy

EM Meroi
IUAV, Venice, Italy

I Naert
Catholic University of Leuven, Haverlee, Belgium

AN Natali
University of Padua, Padua, Italy

M Navarro
Technical University of Catalonia, Barcelona, Spain

M Nilsson
Technical University of Catalonia, Barcelona, Spain

M Nishihira
Akita University, Akita, Japan

PG Pavan
University of Padua, Padua, Italy

LP Petrini
University of Pavia, Pavia, Italy

RP Pietrabissa
Polytechnic of Milan, Milan, Italy

JA Planell
Technical University of Catalonia, Barcelona, Spain

B Puers
Catholic University of Leuven, Haverlee, Belgium

D Rodriguez
Technical University of Catalonia, Barcelona, Spain

E Romeo
University of Milan, Milan, Italy

S Sarda
Technical University of Catalonia, Barcelona, Spain

Y Sato
Hokkaido University, Sapporo, Japan

M Soncini
Polytechnic of Milan, Milan, Italy

J Van Cleynenbreugel
Catholic University of Leuven, Haverlee, Belgium

H Van Oosterwyck
Catholic University of Leuven, Haverlee, Belgium

J Vander Sloten
Catholic University of Leuven, Haverlee, Belgium

MM Viola
University of Padua, Padua, Italy

G Vogel
University of Milan, Milan, Italy

KR Williams
University of Wales, Cardiff, United Kingdom

K Yamamoto
Hokkaido University, Sapporo, Japan

1 Mechanics of bone tissue

AN Natali, RT Hart, PG Pavan, I Knets

1.1 INTRODUCTION

The present chapter deals with the mechanics of hard tissues, namely cortical bone and trabecular bone. The chapter presents various aspects of experimental activities that have been developed for the investigation of the mechanical responses of bone tissue. Tissue properties depend on the environmental conditions of the tissue, including hydration, age of specimen, etc., as well as on mechanical loading conditions, such as the rate of loading, duration of loading, etc.

It is probably superfluous to underline that experimental testing in the field of biological tissues, in particular with regard to bone tissue, requires a sophisticated approach. In fact, the limited dimensions and acquisition procedures of vitro specimens make it difficult to interpret experimental results. Moreover, the mechanical characteristics of the tissue depend on many factors, such as temperature and moisture during testing, because bone specimens are subject to the degradation caused by environmental and biochemical conditions.

Experimental testing of bone is carried out in order to get a deeper knowledge of the mechanics of bone and also to create a database to be used to perform numerical analyses of biomechanical problems (Natali and Meroi, 1989).

Numerical methods, especially the finite element method, provide powerful tools for simulating and predicting the mechanical behaviour of biological tissues. They make it possible to obtain a detailed representation of many different factors that affect the biomechanical behaviour of bone: mechanical properties, shape, loading configuration, and boundary conditions. In order to control the validity of numerical techniques, numerical results and experimental data must be compared to ensure that the models represent the real behaviour of biological structures. The results obtained validated the finite element method as a fundamental approach to investigating phenomena such as implant bone interaction or even the remodelling of bone. These *in vivo* responses, including bone reaction to orthodontic procedures or to dental implant practice, are aspects of bone behaviour that are particularly pertinent to dental biomechanics.

The study of bone, a unique living structural material, requires an interdisciplinary approach to understand and quantify bone functions and adaptations. Bone's functional adaptation to mechanical loading implies the interpretation of a physiological control process. Essential components for this process include sensors for detecting mechanical response and transducers to convert these measurements to cellular response. The cellular response leads to gradual changes in bone shape and/or material properties, and once the structure has adapted, the feedback signal is diminished and further changes to shape and properties are stopped.

In order to make progress in understanding the complex response of living bone, the material and structural properties must first be quantified.

1.2 BONE

Bone is classified as a hard tissue, a definition that includes all calcified tissues. To adequately describe bone, a hierarchic scale must be identified in order to study its functional activity and properties. In fact, the macroscopic behaviour of bone is the reflection of a complex micro system relating to functions that determine the evolution of bone itself over time (Cowin, 1989). At the macroscopic level, namely for a large sample of material, bone strongly depends on the sample location and orientation as well as on specimen status and environmental factors.

At tissue level scale, bone has two distinct structures called cortical bone and trabecular bone. Cortical bone is the hard outer shell-like region of a bone and can further be classified as either primary or secondary. Primary cortical bone is made up of highly organized lamellar sheets, while secondary cortical bone is made up of sheets that are disrupted by the tunnelling of osteons centred around a Haversian canal. Trabecular bone, also called cancellous or spongy bone, is composed of calcified tissue, which forms a porous continuum.

Bone can be described as a complex of activities of three main types of cells: osteoblasts, osteoclasts and osteocytes. Osteoblasts are the cells responsible for new tissue production. Osteoclasts are related to the resorption of bone. Osteocytes are cells that are present in compietely formed bone.

Mineralised microfibrils of collagen are recognised to be the components at an ultra-structural level. Their dimension is of the order of 3–5 μm. At a molecular level, three left handed helical peptide chains coiled into a triple helix form the tropocollagen molecule. These molecular structures have a dimension in the range of 1.5–280 nm (Katz, 1995)

Bone tissue is continuously renewed via a complex but well coordinated sequence of activities that results first in the replacement of primary bone by secondary (osteonal) bone tissue, followed by continual renewal of the secondary bone. Bone surfaces, including not only periosteal and endocortical surfaces, but also intracortical Haversian and trabecular surfaces, are the sites for cellular activity. The bone renewal process, called remodelling, depends on a vascular supply not only for oxygen and the exchange of nutrients and minerals, but also because the pre-osteoclasts, originating in the marrow, are present in the circulation before differentiating into active osteoclasts. The multi-nucleated osteoclasts adhere to bone surfaces with a characteristic ruffled border. This allows for the creation of a (permeable) sealed microenvironment where resorption occurs, bone mineral is dissolved and the collagen and other proteins are digested (Jee, 2001).

The local coupling of bone resorption followed by new bone formation during remodelling is not yet fully understood. However, it is known that bone renewal takes place as discrete packets of cortical or trabecular bone are destroyed and replaced by a group of osteoclasts and osteoblasts referred to as a BMU (Basic Multicellular Unit). As recently described by Jee (Jee, 2001), the BMU cycle includes six consecutive stages, resting, activation, resorption, reversal, formation, mineralization, that result in the coordinated removal of bone and the construction of a new structural bone unit, either an osteon or a trabecular packet (hemiosteon). Even if the key signals for each of these steps are not fully understood, the local mechanical environment and the local chemical environment (including hormones and growth factors) are both known to be important. In addition, since the renewal process is not perfect, only about 95 per cent of the removed bone is replaced (Jee, 2001), the bone structure becomes increasingly compromised over time.

Bone can also be stimulated to change its shape and size, a process called either modelling or net remodelling. Most modelling occurs during growth with changes in bone shape and size. However, even after maturity, bone may be stimulated by altering mechanical loading or by different agents that affects change of shape and/or material properties.

1.3 EXPERIMENTAL TESTING AND RESULTS

In spite of the fact that an official codification of experimental testing procedures has not been fully defined, the preparation of specimens follows an almost standard procedure. The main problem is to obtain *in vitro* specimens that should have, as far as possible, the same characteristics of the tissue *in vivo*, especially with regard to bone hydration (Ashman, 1989). Freezing specimens is probably the most common process used to maintain the original water content in bone. Furthermore, freezing has a marginal influence on bone mechanical properties.

The method of testing traditional engineering materials is also adopted for bone, paying attention to the small dimension of the specimens taken from *in vivo* bones (Reilly et al., 1974). Samples of the cortical portion of bone are usually about 5/5/15 mm, with square or circular cross section. The samples of cancellous bone have similar dimensions but are usually potted in acrylic at the ends.

Several tissue characteristics are highlighted in the following description of experimental testing results for cortical and trabecular bone.

1.3.1 Anisotropic characteristics of bone tissue

The anisotropic stiffness properties of cortical bone are revealed by simply loading the specimens in different directions. Values of the elastic parameters are found, depending on the loading direction, as reported in Table 1.1. In addition, the strength of bone depends on the loading direction and differs depending on compression or tension loads. Table 1.2 shows values which are usually assumed for yield and ultimate stress. They are obtained by applying axial loading and torsional loading to cortical bone specimens taken from human femur (Cowin et al., 1989). The maximum value of the yield stress is found for compression

Table 1.1 Average elastic constants for mandibular corpus in different zones

	Inferior	*Lingual*	*Buccal*
E_1 [GPa]	10.63	10.85	11.04
E_2 [GPa]	12.51	16.39	15.94
E_3 [GPa]	19.75	18.52	18.06
G_{12} [GPa]	3.89	4.59	4.31
G_{13} [GPa]	4.85	5.45	5.2
G_{23} [GPa]	5.84	6.49	6.45
ν_{12}	0.313	0.138	0.138
ν_{13}	0.246	0.338	0.322
ν_{23}	0.226	0.332	0.294
ν_{21}	0.368	0.178	0.257
ν_{31}	0.465	0.572	0.518
ν_{32}	0.356	0.357	0.326

Table 1.2 Yield and ultimate stress values for human cortical bone

	Yield stress	*Ultimate stress*
σ_0^+ [MPa]	115	133
σ_0^- [MPa]	182	195
σ_{90}^+ [MPa]	-	51
σ_{90}^- [MPa]	121	133
τ [MPa]	54	69

along the main axis of a long bone and is about 180 MPa. Tensile yield stress along the same material axis is approximately 120 MPa. Yielding under torsional loading in the plane normal to the main axis of bone is close to 55 MPa.

It is also important to outline the influence of combined loading configurations, which better characterize the *in vivo* conditions, on bone response. The anisotropic characteristics of trabecular bone are mostly related to the architecture of the trabecular network

1.3.2 Time dependent response

Bone shows a time dependent behaviour described as viscoelastic in certain conditions. Typical viscoelastic behaviour, such as strain that continues to increase over time in response to a constant applied load, is called creep. This type of time dependent behaviour of long bone is depicted in Figure 1.1, as a function of stress induced on the long axis, normalized with respect to ultimate stress. The graph refers to cortical bone specimens loaded with a constant axial force applied in the first 200 minutes and then monitored for another 200 minutes after its removal. The initial application of loading shows an elastic response of bone. The axial strain is continuously measured and increases over time during the application of load showing an active creep process. The rate of strain depends on the magnitude of loading. After removal of the loading, the strain decreases, tending toward zero, evidence of passive creep behaviour.

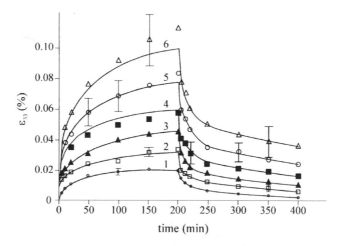

Figure 1.1 Active and passive creep as a function of the stress level normalised to ultimate stress: σ_{33}/σ_{33u}: 0.2 (1); 0.3 (2); 0.4 (3); 0.5 (4); 0.6 (5); 0.7 (6).

Residual (non-zero) strains are found for larger loads as a consequence of inelastic phenomena that induce degradation on the micro-structure of the bone tissue, as permanent deformation caused by non-recoverable material damage.

1.3.3 Bone hydration

The mechanical response of bone is sensitive to its liquid content. In Figure 1.2 quasi-static tensile tests with a low strain rate of 10^{-5} s^{-1} are reported. Note how the behaviour of dried and hydrated samples is similar in the initial elastic strain range, showing that the liquid content has no relevant effects on the initial values of bone stiffness. Hydrated specimens with a 10.5 per cent water content (Figure 1.2 (b)) show more ductile behaviour with a larger strain at failure, while brittle failure is typical of samples with a low liquid content (Figure 1.2 (a)).

The mechanical response of bone is sensitive to the rate of loading. Increased stiffness is a result of higher rates of loading, as clearly depicted in Figure 1.3. The difference in stiffness is accentuated for specimens with larger liquid content (Figure 1.3 (b)). Experimental results show that bone reaches failure at higher values of strain if the water content is greater.

1.3.4 Influence of specimen location and age

The mechanical properties of bone typically depend on the type of bone, e.g. tibia, femur, etc., and, for a given type of bone, on the location of the specimen considered.

Figure 1.4 shows the relationship between the elastic modulus and the bone region in a cross section of a human tibia. The pattern of the elastic modulus in different regions can modify with age, confirming that aging is an additional factor influencing the properties of bone.

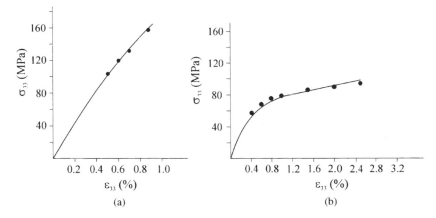

Figure 1.2 Stress-strain curve at 2.5 per cent (a) and 10.5 per cent (b) moisture level for 10^{-5} s^{-1} strain rate.

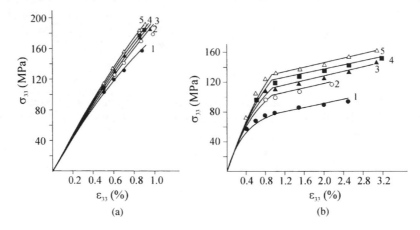

Figure 1.3 Stress-strain curves at different moisture levels of 2.5 per cent (a) and 10.5 per cent (b) and strain rates: 10^{-5} (1); 10^{-4} (2); 10^{-3} (3); 10^{-2} (4); 10^{-1} (5).

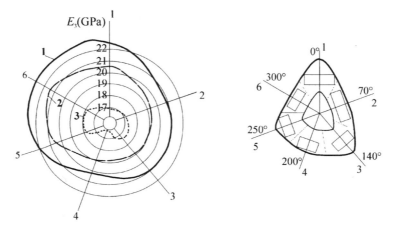

Figure 1.4 Values of elastic modulus in different positions within a tibia cross-section for different ages: 25–34 years (1); 35–59 (2); 60–95 (3).

1.3.5 Fatigue strength

The tendency to failure induced by a progressive material degradation, due to the development of micro cracks, is called fatigue. This phenomenon is related to the application of a cyclic load, even with limited stress magnitudes below the elastic limit. Fatigue phenomena are found in bone specimens (Carter et al., 1981) that show a decrease in strength and stiffness with an increase in the number of load cycles applied (Figure 1.5). The results are spread over a large range and depend on multiple aspects, including values of maximum and minimum strain, mean stress and strain and primarily on the cyclic strain pattern. Recent results should focus additional attention on the testing procedures, in particular the type of stress configuration induced.

Effective *in vivo* behaviour of bone, that in normal conditions does not experience fatigue failure, suggests that the remodelling process of bone induced by cyclic loading can be considered an antagonistic factor in the damage process.

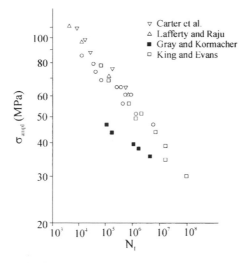

Figure 1.5 Fatigue data obtained by different authors for *in vitro* bone specimens under alternated loading cycles.

1.3.6 Trabecular bone: mechanical properties

As in other porous materials, the mechanical response of trabecular bone depends on its structural density, considered as the mass of bone in the specimen volume. Tensile uni-axial tests on cancellous bone specimens show a strong correlation between the structural density and the elastic modulus, as seen in Figure 1.6. Data pertaining to compressive and tensile load are reported.

The predictable results are that the elastic modulus is a function of the structural density of bone (Kuhn et al., 1987; Ashman and Rho, 1988), and is also a predictor of axial strength. The different mechanical responses in tensile and compressive loading are typical behaviour

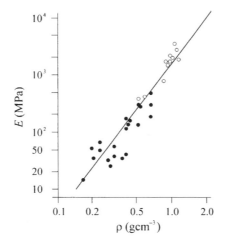

Figure 1.6 Correlation of density and elastic modulus in tension (filled circles) and compression (empty circles) for cancellous bone.

of trabecular bone (Ford and Keaveny, 1996). It is important to point out that the elastic modulus of individual trabeculae may be different than that of cortical bone. The difficulty in properly defining the mechanical characteristics of an individual trabecula is significant, and leads to uncertainties in the results, as reported in the Table 1.3.

The complexity of experimental tests does not refer only to the investigation of the characteristics of a singular trabecula, but in general to the use of samples of cancellous bone. Furthermore, it represents the principal source of indeterminacy.

1.3.7 Analysis using the ultrasound technique

Ultrasound analysis is currently employed to determine the mechanical characteristics of bone, both for cortical and trabecular specimens. The measure is based on the relationship between the velocity of propagation of ultrasonic waves in a specimen and the stiffness of the specimen. An advantage of ultrasound techniques is the non-invasive approach that allows the application of experimental testing *in vivo*. Information given by ultrasound techniques on cancellous bone pertains to both the density and organisation of the trabeculae, resulting in a fundamental task for defining the macroscopic mechanical parameters (Gluer et al., 1993; Langton et al., 1996). Anisotropy in the spatial distribution of trabeculae causes different ultrasonic velocity values depending on the different directions considered (Nicholson et al., 1994). Consequently, the evaluation of the velocity of wave propagation and broadband attenuation should be considered in order to estimate both the bone density and the configuration of the trabecular network. Figure 1.7 shows a typical example of the structural configuration of cancellous bone for the calcaneous and vertebra, pointing out the fact that the arrangements are very different.

The different correlations between the ultrasound parameters and the material characteristics of bone must be defined. Good relationships can be found between the velocity of ultrasound waves and broadband ultrasound attenuation and the mechanics of trabecular bone.

Table 1.3 Elastic modulus of individual trabecula of cancellous bone. Comparison of different experimental data

Source	Type of bone	Estimate of trabeculae elastic modulus
Wolff	Human	17 to 20 GPa (wet)
	bovine	18 to 22 GPa (wet)
Pugh et al.	Human, Distal femur	modulus of trabecula is less than that of compact bone
Townsend et al.	Human, Proximal tibia	11.38 GPa (wet)
		14.13 GPa (dry)
Ashman and Rho	Bovine femur	10.90 ± 1.60 GPa (wet)
	human femur	12.7 ± 2.0 GPa (wet)
Runkle and Pugh	Human, Distal femur	8.69 ± 3.17 GPa (dry)
Mente and Lewis	Dried human femur fresh human tibia	5.3 ± 2.6 GPa
Khun et al.	Fresh frozen human tibia	3.17 ± 1.5 GPa
Williams and Lewis	Human, proximal tibia	1.30 GPa
Rice et al.	Bovine	1.17 GPa
Ryan and Williams	Fresh bovine femur	0.76 ± 0.39 GPa
Rice et al.	Human	0.61 GPa

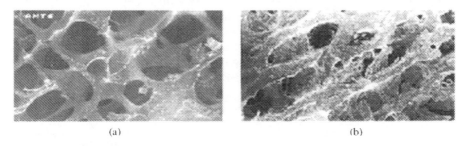

(a)   (b)

Figure 1.7 Structural arrangement of trabecular bone in first lumbar (a) vertebra and calcaneus (b).

However, the correlation between ultrasound parameters and material characteristics depends on the structural configuration of bone and its constitutive properties.

Figure 1.8 shows the correlation between velocity and density for two different types of trabecular bone pertaining to vertebra and calcaneus. Even if the qualitative correlation between density or geometry of the bone structure and its elastic properties has been investigated, further efforts seem to be necessary in order to get precise relationships for quantitative estimates (Trebacz and Natali, 1999).

1.4 CONSTITUTIVE MODELS FOR BONE

1.4.1 Linear elastic models

Bone is a heterogeneous material and presents distinct anisotropic properties. As described above, experimental determination of mechanical properties depends on multiple factors including age, sex, metabolic and hormonal functions, physical activity of subject, etc., and also on the specific region considered such as the femur or jaw. With reference to the strength properties of bone, the deformation rate during loading and the level of moisture have a significant influence, as previously reported. All these aspects must be taken into

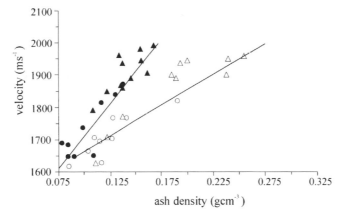

Figure 1.8 Influence of the trabecular configuration on the velocity of the ultrasound signal for males (triangles) and females (circles). Samples, from first lumbar vertebra are indicated with filled symbols; samples from calcaneus with empty symbols.

account to evaluate their mutual influence. However, in many cases related to operational practice, a linear elastic law, which has an acceptable margin of accuracy up to a reasonable value of loading, can be assumed. Hence, the assumption of a linear relation between stress and strain is an acceptable approximation to the real behaviour, but keeping in mind the limits of applicability. With regard to general anisotropic materials, the relation between the components of stress tensor σ_{ij} and the components of strain tensor ε_{kl} is given by:

$$\sigma_{ij} = D_{ijkl}\varepsilon_{kl} \tag{1}$$

A general restriction based on physical laws of balance defines the number of independent constants as 21 because of the symmetry $D_{ijkl} = D_{klij}$ and $D_{ijkl} = D_{jilk}$. Furthermore, if a full symmetry of the material can be assumed, ignoring anisotropic effects, there are just two independent material constants. When a material is recognised to be isotropic, defining mechanical parameters through experimental testing becomes reasonably simple. An example is the use of uni-axial tensile tests, which make it possible to evaluate the elastic modulus as well as the lateral contraction coefficient of the specimen. When the material shows a higher degree of asymmetry, as in the case of cortical bone, it is necessary to perform more experimental tests in order to define all the independent elastic constants. Orthotropic materials need nine independent constants to be defined. However, if there is a unique plane of symmetry, as is the case for transversely isotropic materials, there are only five independent material constants. In particular, in the cortical portion of bones, such as femur, tibia or mandible, the symmetry is usually described as orthotropic or as transversally isotropic. Average elastic constants of cortical bone in the mandible are reported in Table 1.1, with reference to different zones, while Table 1.3 shows data pertaining to the elastic properties of trabecular bone tissue as a function of the type of bone. The constants reported in Table 1.1 can be interpreted using the following relation between stress and strain, reported with regards to an orthotropic material and distinguishing direct and shear components:

$$\begin{Bmatrix} \sigma_{11} \\ \sigma_{22} \\ \sigma_{33} \end{Bmatrix} = \begin{bmatrix} \dfrac{1}{E_1} & -\dfrac{v_{12}}{E_2} & -\dfrac{v_{13}}{E_3} \\ -\dfrac{v_{21}}{E_1} & \dfrac{1}{E_2} & -\dfrac{v_{23}}{E_3} \\ -\dfrac{v_{31}}{E_1} & -\dfrac{v_{32}}{E_2} & \dfrac{1}{E_3} \end{bmatrix} \begin{Bmatrix} \varepsilon_{11} \\ \varepsilon_{22} \\ \varepsilon_{33} \end{Bmatrix} \tag{2}$$

$$\begin{Bmatrix} \sigma_{12} \\ \sigma_{23} \\ \sigma_{31} \end{Bmatrix} = \begin{bmatrix} \dfrac{1}{G_{12}} & 0 & 0 \\ 0 & \dfrac{1}{G_{23}} & 0 \\ 0 & 0 & \dfrac{1}{G_{31}} \end{bmatrix} \begin{Bmatrix} \varepsilon_{12} \\ \varepsilon_{23} \\ \varepsilon_{31} \end{Bmatrix} \tag{3}$$

where E_i represents Young's moduli, G_{ij} the shear moduli and v_{ij} Poisson's ratios.

1.4.2 Structural properties

At a macroscopic level, bone shows a strong anisotropic response. For cortical bone the macroscopic anisotropy is determined by the microstructure, while for cancellous bone the anisotropic response mostly depends on the structural arrangements of the trabecular network, as shown in Figure 1.7.

Carter made a correlation between the structure of bone and its mechanical behaviour (Carter and Hayes, 1977). He correlated the density of bone to the elastic modulus and the rate of strain for a compressive loading of the specimen, as:

$$E = 3790 \dot{\varepsilon}^{0.06} \rho^3 \tag{4}$$

The elastic modulus E is expressed in MPa, the density ρ in g/cm^3 and the strain rate in s^{-1}. The previous relation was found for bovine and human bone. The specimens used by Carter included both cortical and trabecular bone tissues, hence relation (4) is a combination of their mechanical contributions. Because the microstructural arrangement of cortical bone and trabecular bone are different, one can expect that a different relation is found using only cortical or trabecular specimens. The investigation of samples of cancellous bone determined a square relationship between elasticity modulus and density (Rice et al., 1988).

Many efforts have been spent in defining a relation between density and the strength properties of bone. Again Carter found a correlation between density and the compressive strength in cancellous bone:

$$\sigma^- = 68 \dot{\varepsilon}^{0.06} \rho^2 \tag{5}$$

Note how the strain rate has a slight influence on the elastic modulus and on the compressive strength if compared to the influence of bone density. Relations (4) and (5) should be related to the specific testing direction and to the type of loading induced. For cancellous bone, both the elastic modulus and the strength demonstrate a quadratic dependence on structural density; hence, they are linearly proportional to one another.

As mentioned above, the properties of bone in different directions of the material are related to local bone architecture (Turner, 1997; Whitehouse, 1974). For cancellous bone, a quantitative description of the trabecular architecture can be based on the mean intercept length (MIL). An example in two dimensions is shown in Figure 1.9.

Figure 1.9 (a) shows the trabecular structure and Figure 1.9 (b) shows the structure with a series of parallel lines, with a specified angle θ, shown superimposed on the image. The number of transitions between bone and void along a specific line is defined as the number of intercepts, while the intercept length is the length of the line divided by the number of bone-void transitions. It is possible to measure a mean intercept length for every sheaf of parallel lines. Hence, the mean intercept length is a function of the angle of the sheaf and can be plotted in a polar diagram for all the possible values of the angle θ. In a three dimensional space an ellipsoid is found that represents the anisotropic configuration of the tissue. The mean intercept length, as a geometric measure of the architecture, forms the basis for the definition of the ellipsoid, whose mathematical description is a second rank tensor, called fabric tensor, as proposed by Cowin (Cowin et al., 1989). The ellipsoid, including the orientation of its axes, is related to the anisotropy characteristics of the trabecular bone (Odgaard et al., 1997), and provides a quantitative basis for material properties that can take the local trabecular architecture into account.

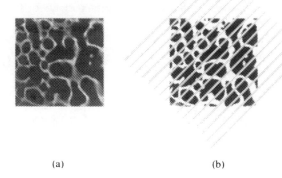

(a)   (b)

Figure 1.9 Trabecular structure (a) and graphical representation of mean intercept length (b).

1.4.3 Limit state of bone

Much effort has been spent trying to evaluate the behaviour of bone at the limit of the elastic field due to the interest in the applications that operate at these limits, such as the interaction between a dental implant thread and the surrounding tissue. Bone shows a plastic behaviour that in some aspects appears very similar to the inelastic behaviour of other materials, as shown, for example, by the stress strain curve represented in Figure 1.3 (b) for a uni-axial test on a human cortical bone sample. The elastic portion is often followed by a plastic portion that leads to ductile behaviour up to the point of failure.

Basically *in vivo* stress states are caused by multi-axial loading configurations. A suitable criterion must be introduced in order to define the limits of the strength surface. An adequate criterion to define the multi-axial limit state of bone is given by Hill's potential function. This can be considered as an extension of the Von Mises plastic criterion and can be written as:

$$f(\sigma_{ij}) = \left[A(\sigma_{11} - \sigma_{22})^2 + B(\sigma_{22} - \sigma_{33})^2 + C(\sigma_{33} - \sigma_{11})^2 + \right.$$
$$\left. + 2D\sigma_{12}^2 + 2E\sigma_{23}^2 + 2F\sigma_{31}^2 \right]^{\frac{1}{2}} \leq 1 \tag{6}$$

Constants A,B,C,D,E,F are established on the basis of experimental tests which evaluate the yield response for different loading modes.

The Tsai Wu function (Tsai and Wu, 1971; Wu, 1972) is another important criterion adopted to describe the elastic limit or the failure limit of cortical bone. The criterion is written using a second order polynomial function in the stress components as:

$$f(\sigma_{ij}) = a_1\sigma_{11} + a_2\sigma_{22} + a_3\sigma_{33} + a_4\sigma_{11}^2 + a_5\sigma_{22}^2 + a_6\sigma_{33}^2 +$$
$$+ a_7\sigma_{12}^2 + a_8\sigma_{13}^2 + a_9\sigma_{23}^2 + a_{10}\sigma_{11}\sigma_{22} + a_{11}\sigma_{11}\sigma_{33} + \tag{7}$$
$$+ a_{12}\sigma_{22}\sigma_{33} \leq 1$$

where again constants a_i are deduced by experimental tests at the plastic limit and at the failure limit.

Figure 1.10 shows a comparison of the limit surfaces obtained from the two criteria compared with the experimental yield stress values, evaluated on cortical bone specimens. Bi-axial stress states are induced by the simultaneous application of axial and torsional forces. Equation (7) gives good results when applied to bi-axial stress states, although they may fail to adequately describe tri-axial stress states.

This is due to the fact that the criterion is actually extended to the three axial states on the basis of bi-axial data. Alternative criteria have been proposed in order to overcome this limitation in describing multi axial strength. These criteria are based on the modification of the Kelvin modes method (Arramon et al., 2000).

The complexity of experimental activity is the main impediment to establishing a complete definition of a phenomenological model that should provide a constitutive model for bone that adequately accounts for the limit conditions.

1.5 ROLE OF MECHANICS IN ADAPTATION

In addition to the need to establish models and experimentally determined parameters that can adequately account for the passive behaviour of bone, there is a need to further develop models to account for the living behaviour of bone, including adaptation to mechanical forces. Current models and simulation techniques have been reviewed (Hart, 2001) which highlight the objectives, applications and limitations of several models.

Models used to describe functional adaptation may be classified as phenomenological or mechanistic. Phenomenological models try to describe cause and effect, e.g. changed mechanical loading leading to changed bone architecture, without examining the (biological) mechanisms. Therefore, they make it possible to conveniently test the outcomes and consequences of different hypotheses regarding bone adaptation. They may be useful in eliminating assumptions that cannot match experimental or clinical results and observations, e.g. only compressive static loading leads to bone formation, and may also stimulate further investigations, e.g. strain rates and spatial gradients may regulate adaptation.

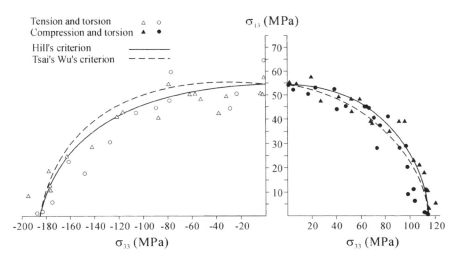

Figure 1.10 Yield stress for human femur under combined axial and torsional loading. Comparison between experimental data and estimated values, using different strength criteria.

On the other hand, mechanistic models start with a set of measurable biological parameters, e.g. bone cell activities, distributions, and/or mechanical parameters, e.g. evidence of bone fatigue damage. Mechanistic models offer the promise of not only extending the descriptive and predictive capabilities of phenomenological models, but may also offer insights into the manipulation of bone response and development of pharmacological therapeutic agents. Both types of models are still being actively developed and tested and fundamental questions about their utility and validity discussed (Currey, 1995; Huiskes, 1995).

1.5.1 Phenomenological models

Cowin and co-workers

Cowin and co-workers developed a phenomenological theory of adaptive elasticity (Cowin, 1981) that has been implemented in finite element, beam theory, and boundary element codes (Hart et al., 1984a; Cowin et al., 1985; Sadegh et al., 1993). The theory assumes that the net remodeling process is driven by an error signal. The error signal is assumed to be based on the difference between the mechanical state in its "remodeling equilibrium" configuration, a hypothesized quiescent state with no net remodeling), and the current mechanical state, following a change such as a changed mechanical load or the implantation of a prosthesis. Adaptive elasticity has been distinguished in three parts: the shape change of cortical bone, as net surface remodeling, the density changes of cortical bone, as net internal remodeling, and trabecular responses that include changes in the density and orientation of continuum representations of trabecular bone tissue.

Cowin and Van Buskirk (Cowin and Van Buskirk, 1979) proposed the following equation for net surface remodeling:

$$U = C_{ij}(Q) \left[\varepsilon_{ij}(Q) - \varepsilon_{ij}^0(Q) \right] \tag{8}$$

where U is the velocity of the bone's external surface at point Q, change in position over time, Q_{ij} the remodeling rate parameters, $\varepsilon_{ij}(Q)$ strain at point Q, and $\varepsilon_{ij}^0(Q)$ remodeling equilibrium strain at point Q.

For net internal remodeling, Cowin and Hegedus (Cowin and Hegedus, 1976) proposed:

$$\dot{e} = a(e) + tr\,[A(e)\varepsilon] \tag{9}$$

where $\dot{e}$ is the rate of change in solid portion of bone, A a remodeling rate parameter, and ε the strain tensor.

To implement the idea that trabecular bone tissue changes its orientation based on the direction of the principle stresses, known in the literature as the trajectoral theory of trabecular orientation, Cowin (Cowin, 1986) developed an extension for the theory for net internal remodeling. In addition to equations for describing changes in the density of the trabecular bone, equations were developed to describe changing the predominant orientation of the struts of trabecular bone. A second rank tensor, called the fabric tensor, was defined based on a stereological measure known as the mean intercept length (Figure 1.9). The trabecular elastic material properties, **D**, and the fabric tensor, **H**, were written as a function of the solid volume fraction, v, and the stress, **T**, was written as a function of all three: **T** = **T** (v, **E**, **H**). The mathematical expression of the trajectoral theory (Cowin et al., 1986) as the commutative multiplication property of the relevant tensors is: $\mathbf{T}*\mathbf{H}* = \mathbf{H}*\mathbf{T}*$, $\mathbf{T}*\mathbf{E}* = \mathbf{E}*\mathbf{T}*$ and $\mathbf{H}*\mathbf{E}* = \mathbf{E}*\mathbf{H}*$, where the asterisk indicates a remodeling equilibrium value. The geometric representation of a second rank tensor is an ellipsoid with orientation of the axes giving the principal directions while normalised length of the axes is proportional to the eigenvalues. This means the primary axes of the ellipsoid representing stress, strain, and fabric are all aligned. Based on this insight, Cowin (Cowin et al., 1992) wrote a series of rate equations for the evolution of the fabric tensor re-orientation back to the remodeling equilibrium configuration simultaneously with the change in density. Although this formulation, based on a continuum description of trabecular bone, can describe the predominant orientation and density of trabecular bone, it cannot describe changes in individual trabecular struts or at the interface with an implant.

Huiskes and co-workers

An error-driven approach similar to Cowin's was developed by Huiskes et al. (Huiskes et al., 1987). There are, however, two primary differences: the strain energy density, $U = 1/2 \, E_{ij}T_{ij}$, is assumed to be the mechanical stimulus that regulates adaptation. The model allows for a threshold that must be overcome to start the adaptive response, called a lazy zone or a dead zone.

The rate equation is written as:

$$\frac{dX}{dt} = \begin{cases} C_x[U - (1 + s)U_n] & U > (1 + s)U_n \\ 0 & U_n < U < (1 + s)U_n \\ C_x[U - (1 - s)U_n] & U < (1 + s)U_n \end{cases} \tag{10}$$

where X is the surface growth, C_x the remodeling rate coefficient, $2s$ the width of the "lazy zone", and U_n a homeostatic strain energy density.

Beaupré, Orr and Carter

In the model proposed by Beaupré, Orr, and Carter (Beaupré et al., 1990) the key measure of mechanical usage is a daily tissue level stress stimulus defined as $\varphi_b = (\Sigma_i n_i \sigma_{bi}^m)^{1/m}$ where n_i is the number of cycles of load type i, σ_{bi} a bone tissue level stress, and m an empirical constant, summed over the course of one day. Then:

$$\frac{dr}{dt} = \begin{cases} C(\varphi b - \varphi_{bAS}) + c \cdot w & \varphi_\beta - \varphi_{bAS} < -w \\ 0 & -w \le \varphi_\beta - \varphi_{bAS} \le w \\ C(\varphi b - \varphi_{bAS}) - c \cdot w & \varphi_\beta - \varphi_{bAS} > w \end{cases} \tag{11}$$

Mattheck

A different phenomenological approach was developed by Mattheck (Mattheck and Huber-Betzer, 1991) based on the observation that "…good mechanical design is characterized by a homogeneous stress distribution at its surface." Adaptation is implemented computationally by iteratively changing the boundary to eliminate notch stress as measured by the Von Mises equivalent stress.

The governing equation is:

$$\dot{\varepsilon}_n = k(\sigma_M - \sigma_{ref})$$

(12)

where $\dot{\varepsilon}_n$ is defined as the volumetric swelling rate and σ_M is the Von Mises equivalent stress.

1.5.2 Mechanistic models

The main advantage of developing mechanistic approaches for bone adaptation comes from successful link between mechanical and biological causes and effects. Unfortunately, these models are complex and there is still uncertainty about which of the many mechanical and biological parameters are most important to measure and track.

McNamara, Prendergast and Taylor

McNamara et al., (McNamara et al., 1992) developed adaptation simulations based on the hypothesis that net bone adaptation is activated by accumulated damage. They assume that even at RE (Remodeling Equilibrium), there is some damage and that the rate of repair is associated with the damage rate.

Mathematically, at *RE*, $\dot{\omega}_{eff} = 0$ and $\dot{\omega} = \omega_{RE}$, where ω_{eff} is the effective damage, ω the current rate of damage production, and ω_{RE} the rate of damage production at *RE*. Then:

$$\frac{dX}{dt} = C \cdot \omega_{eff}$$

(13)

Davy, Hart and Heiple

Davy, Hart and Heiple developed a model based on observable cellular measures (Davy and Hart, 1983; Hart et al., 1984b). According to the work of Martin (Martin et al., 1972), the net remodeling is based on the balance between competing cellular activities and numbers, with a rate equation written as:

$$\dot{d} = \lambda_b a_b n_b - \lambda_c a_c n_c$$

(14)

where, λ is the surface area fraction available, a a measure of cellular activity, n a measure of cellular number, and the subscripts b or c refer to osteoblasts and osteoclasts, respectively. Each of these parameters, λ, a, and n, can not only be observed experimentally, but can be cast mathematically as functions of multiple factors that are know to influence them: mechanical usage, genetics, and hormonal and chemical environments. The theory has recently been used to make *a priori* predictions of experimentally induced net surface remodeling with encouraging results (Oden et al., 1995). However, there are many uncertainties and assumptions to examine before these notions can be well enough developed to lead to operational practice.

Increasingly sophisticated computational methods and simulation theories hold the promise of being able to predict bone response to a variety of changed loading conditions, including changes in the proximity of medical devices, mostly orthopaedic implants. These simulation techniques can be adapted for use with dental applications, including orthodontic correction and tooth replacement. However, the role of the periodontal ligament and the rich supply of cells at this natural interface between tooth and bone will require substantial modifications to adaptation models, both phenomenological and mechanistic. This is an area ripe for further experimental, theoretical, and computational studies that can blend mechanics and cell-tissue physiology to improve the outcomes of clinical practice.

1.6 CONCLUSIONS

This chapter has presented a short report on the mechanical properties of cortical and trabecular bone by discussing the experimental activity that has been developed. The main aspects of the constitutive models were presented in light of the consolidated theories pertaining to the mechanics of materials. Though the chapter is intended as a preliminary introduction to bone mechanics, the main topics were treated covering a large field of analysis. Theoretical formulations within the mechanics of materials offers the possibility of describing the behaviour of bone in many different conditions by using constitutive models, namely the mathematical relations between stress and strain. The reliability of numerical approaches to bone mechanics problems depends strongly on the appropriate definition of the mechanical characteristics required for a specific model, which are obtained by experimental analysis. It is important to adapt the characteristics of the analysis according to the accuracy of the expected results. Experimental activity is particularly challenging because of the very difficult operational conditions. The activity described in this chapter is aimed also at the possibility of developing numerical simulations of bone mechanical response by using the finite element method. For example, the interaction between endosseous implants and bone is particularly suited for numerical simulations and useful in evaluating the limit state of these systems or their adaptive behaviour over time.

The study of experimental and theoretical aspects pertaining to bone mechanics represents an essential basis for the study of dental biomechanics in a broad sense.

REFERENCES

Y.P. Arramon, M.M. Mehrabadi, D.W. Martin, S.C. Cowin, A multi-dimensional anisotropic strength criterion based on Kelvin modes, Int. J. Solids and Struct., Vol. 37, pp. 2915–2935, 2000.

R.B. Ashman, J.Y. Rho, Elastic moduli of trabecular bone material, J. Biomech., Vol. 21, pp. 177, 1988.

R.B. Ashman, Experimental Techniques, Bone Mechanics, S.C. Cowin, Boca Raton, CRC Press, Inc., pp. 75–96, 1989.

G.S. Beaupré, T.E. Orr, D.R. Carter, An approach for time-dependent bone modeling and remodeling – theoretical development, J Orthop Res., Vol. 8, pp. 651–661, 1990.

D.R. Carter, W.C. Hayes, The compressive behaviour of bone as a two phase porous structure, J. Bone Joint Surg. [Am], Vol. 59, Issue 7, pp. 954–962, 1977.

D.R. Carter, W.E. Caler, D.M. Spengler, V.H. Frankel, Uniaxial fatigue of human cortical bone. The influence of tissue physical characteristics, J Biomech, Vol. 14, Issue 7, pp. 461–470, 1981.

S.C. Cowin, D.H. Hegedus, Bone Remodeling I: Theory of Adaptive Elasticity, Journal of Elasticity, Vol. 6, pp. 313–326, 1976.

S.C. Cowin, W.C. Van Buskirk, Surface bone remodeling induced by a medullary pin, J Biomech., Vol. 12, pp. 269–276, 1979.

S.C. Cowin, Continuum Models of the adaptation of bone to stress, Mechanical properties of bone, ed. S.C. Cowin, American Society of Mechanical Engineers, New York, N.Y. (345 E. 47th St., New York 10017) pp. 193–210, 1981.

S.C. Cowin, R.T. Hart, J.R. Balser, D.H. Kohn, Functional adaptation in long bones: establishing *in vivo* values for surface remodeling rate coefficients, J Biomech., Vol. 18, pp. 665–684, 1985.

S.C. Cowin, Wolff's law of trabecular architecture at remodeling equilibrium, J. Biomech Eng., Vol. 108, pp. 83–88, 1986.

S.C. Cowin, The Mechanical Properties of Cortical Bone Tissue, Bone Mechanics, S. C. Cowin, Boca Raton, CRC Press, Inc., pp. 97–128, 1989.

S.C. Cowin, A.M. Sadegh, G.M. Luo, An evolutionary Wolff's law for trabecular architecture, J. Biomech Eng., Vol. 114, pp. 129–136, 1992.

J.D. Currey, The Validation of Algorithms Used To Explain Adaptive Remodelling in Bone, in Bone Structure and Remodelling (Edited by A. Odgaard and H. Weinans), World Scientific, Singapore, pp. 9–13, 1995.

D.T. Davy, R.T. Hart, A Theoretical Model for Mechanically Induced Bone Remodeling, American Society of Biomechanics, Rochester, MN, 1983.

C.M. Ford, T.M. Keaveny, The dependence of shear failure properties of trabecular bone on apparent density and trabecular orientation, J. Biomech., Vol. 29, pp. 1309–1317, 1996.

C.C. Gluer, C.Y. Wu, H.K. Genant, Broadband ultrasound attenuation signals depend on trabecular orientation: an *in vitro* study, Osteoporosis Int., Vol. 3, pp. 185–191, 1993.

R.T. Hart, D.T. Davy, K.G. Heiple, A Computational Method for Stress Analysis of Adaptive Elastic Materials with a View Toward Applications in Strain-Induced Bone Remodeling, Journal of Biomechanical Engineering, Vol. 106, pp. 342–350, 1984a.

R.T. Hart, D.T. Davy, K.G. Heiple, Mathematical modeling and numerical solutions for functionally dependent bone remodeling, Calcif. Tissue Int., Vol. 36, pp. S104–109, 1984b.

R.T. Hart, A.M. Rust-Dawicki, Computational Simulation of Idealized Long Bone Re-Alignment, in Computer Simulations in Biomedicine (Edited by H. Power and R. T. Hart) Computational Mechanics Publications, pp. 341–350, 1995.

R.T. Hart, Bone Modeling and Remodeling: Theories and Computation. In Bone Mechanics Handbook (Edited by S. C. Cowin), CRC Press, Boca Raton, Cap. 31, pp. 1–42, 2001.

R. Huiskes, H. Weinans, H.J. Grootenboer, M. Dalstra, B. Fudala, T.J. Slooff, Adaptive bone-remodeling theory applied to prosthetic-design analysis, J. Biomech., Vol. 20, pp. 1135–1150, 1987.

R. Huiskes, The Law of Adaptive Bone Remodelling: A Case for Crying Newton?, in Bone Structure and Remodelling (Edited by A. Odgaard and H. Weinans), World Scientific, Singapore, pp. 15–24, 1995.

W.S.S. Jee, Integrated Bone Tissue Physiology: Anatomy and Physiology, Bone Mechanics Handbook, (Edited by S.C. Cowin), 2nd edition, CRC Press LLC, Boca Raton, 2001.

J.L. Katz, Mechanics of Hard Tissue, The Biomedical Engineering Handbook, J. D. Bonzino, CRC Press, Inc., 1995.

J.L. Kuhn, J.L. nee Ku, S.A. Goldstein, K.W. Choi, M. Landon, M.A. Herzig, L.S. Matthews, The mechanical properties of single trabeculae, Trans. 33rd Annu. Meet. Orthop. Res. Soc., pp. 12–48, 1987.

C.M. Langton, C.F. Njeh, R. Hodgskinson, J.D. Currey, Prediction of mechanical properties of the human calcaneus by broadband attenuation, Bone, Vol. 18, pp. 495–503, 1996.

C. Mattheck, H. Huber-Betzer, CAO: Computer simulation of adaptive growth in bones and trees, in Computers in Biomedicine (Edited by K.D. Held, C.A. Brebbia and R.D. Ciskowski), Computational Mechanics Publications, Southampton, pp. 243–252, 1991.

B.P. McNamara, P.J. Prendergast, D. Taylor, Prediction of bone adaptation in the ulnar-osteotomized sheep's forelimb using an anatomical finite element model, J. Biomed Eng., Vol. 14, pp. 209–216, 1992.

A.N. Natali, E.A. Meroi, A review of the biomechanical properties of bone as a material, J. Biomed. Eng., Vol. 11, pp. 266–276, 1989.

P.H.F. Nicholson, M.J. Haddaway, M.W.J. Davie, The dependence of ultrasonic properties on orientation in human vertebral bone, Physics in Medicine and Biology, Vol. 39, pp. 1013–1024, 1994.

Z.M. Oden, R.T. Hart, M.R. Forwood, D.B. Burr, A Priori Prediction of functional adaptation in canine radii using a cell based mechanistic approach, Transactions of the 41st Orthopaedic Research Society, Orlando, FL, 296, 1995.

A. Odgaard, J. Kabel, B. van Rietbergen, M. Dalstra, R. Huiskes, Fabric and elastic principal directions of cancellous bone are closely related, J. Biomech., Vol. 30, Issue 5, pp. 487–495, 1997.

D.T. Reilly, A.H. Burstein, V.H. Fankel, The elastic modulus for bone, J. Biomech., Vol. 7, pp. 271–275, 1974.

J.C. Rice, S.C. Cowin, J.A. Bowman, On the dependence of the elasticity and strength of cancellous bone on apparent density, J. Biomech., Vol. 21, pp. 155–161, 1988.

A.M. Sadegh, G.M. Luo, S.C. Cowin, Bone ingrowth: an application of the boundary element method to bone remodeling at the implant interface, J. Biomech., Vol. 26, pp. 167–182, 1993.

H. Trebacz, A.N. Natali, The ultrasound velocity and attenuation in cancellous bone samples from lumbar vertebra and calcaneus, Osteoporosis Int, Vol. 9, Issue 2, pp. 99–105, 1999.

S.W. Tsai, E.M. Wu, A general theory of strength for anisotropic materials, J. of Composite Materials, Vol. 5, pp. 58–60, 1971.

C.H. Turner, The relationship between cancellous bone architecture and mechanical properties at the continuum level, Forma, Vol. 12, pp. 225–233, 1997.

W.J. Whitehouse, The quantitative morphology of anisotropic trabecular bone, Journal of Microscopy, Vol. 101, pp. 153–168, 1974.

E.M. Wu, Optimal experimental measurements of anisotropic failure tensors, J. Composite Materials, Vol. 6, pp. 472–489, 1972.

2 Mechanics of periodontal ligament

M Nishihira, K Yamamoto, Y Sato, H Ishikawa, AN Natali

2.1 INTRODUCTION

A tooth is secured to the alveolar bone by fibrous connective tissue that is called the periodontal ligament (PDL). The PDL not only strongly binds the tooth root to the supporting alveolar bone but also absorbs occlusal loads and distributes the resulting stress over the alveolar bone. The mechanical properties of the PDL are, therefore, essential parameters for understanding the mechanical behaviour of a tooth root and that of surrounding tissues. The PDL also plays an important role in the mechanical adaptation of the dentition, based on alveolar bone remodelling induced by a change in mechanical stress or strain around a tooth root. This adaptability is important for the maintenance of optimal occlusion at a proper vertical dimension and is also utilised for orthodontic treatment in which an optimal orthodontic force is applied so as to induce maximum cellular activities, resulting in the most efficient tooth movement.

It is of fundamental importance in the field of dental biomechanics to know how a force is transferred to a tooth root and the surrounding tissues. Because of the difficulty in measuring physical parameters in this region, stress–strain distributions have usually been estimated by finite element analysis. In this analysis, material constants of a tooth and the surrounding tissues, including the PDL, are indispensable parameters. Although there is an abundance of information on the mechanical properties of teeth and alveolar bone, little is known about those of the PDL, due to difficulties in examining this thin tissue, which is only about 0.2 mm in thickness.

In this chapter, theoretical and experimental approaches to investigating the mechanical properties of the PDL are discussed, and then measurements of the elastic properties of this thin tissue using a newly developed miniature testing machine are presented.

2.2 CONSTITUTIVE MODELS FOR THE PERIODONTAL LIGAMENT

Numerical techniques in the field of biomechanics allow for a prediction and a direct interpretation of the biomechanical response of biological tissues and also represent a useful tool for the comprehension of some physiological aspects. The method is based on the definition of mathematical models represented by relations between physical parameters, such as stress or strain, that can represent the mechanical responses of biological tissues.

With specific regard to the PDL, the biomechanical analysis is often based on strong simplifications about constitutive models. This is due to the relevant difficulties in obtaining data from experimental analysis, as well as in the formulation of the numerical problem. The assumption of simplified schemes for the material, for example, isotropic and linear elastic, can be justified by a specific analysis performed or by the conditions considered, as magnitude of loading, maximum strain attained, etc.. However, these assumptions cause a limitation since the biomechanical response of the periodontal ligament is characterised by a non-linear relation between stress and strain and by time-dependent behaviour.

Recently, particular attention has been paid to constructing more realistic constitutive models in order to describe PDL responses under a wide range of conditions, leading to reliable results. Efforts have also been made to investigate the response of the PDL under the application of long-lasting loads, such as typical conditions for orthodontic treatment. In spite of difficulties in providing experimental tests to get exhaustive information and in properly defining the models, these attempts represent a reliable and promising approach to the biomechanics of the PDL.

2.2.1 Hyperelastic constitutive models

For some rates of loading, for example, in the case of masticatory activity, the response of the PDL can be described in terms of elastic non-linear laws, i.e. as a relation between stress and strain. This behaviour can depend on the structure of the PDL, which, in a first approximation, can be considered to consist of a ground matrix reinforced by groups of collagen fibres. Due to the complex spatial organisation of the fibres, the PDL also shows an anisotropic response, which must be considered in addition to the non-linearity of the stress–strain relation.

Hyperelastic constitutive models prove to be adequate for describing the mechanical properties of the PDL under these conditions. In fact, they can effectively represent the above-mentioned characteristics even in the field of large strains. In addition, these models are particularly suitable for describing the possible almost-incompressible response of the material due to the liquid content present in the PDL.

Assuming that the PDL consists of an isotropic matrix reinforced by one family of fibres, the constitutive model is usually defined by the stored energy function, depending on the elastic deformation of the material:

$$W = W(I_1, I_2, I_3, I_4) \tag{1}$$

where I_1, I_2, I_3 are the principal invariants of the Cauchy-Green tensor **C**. The additional, with respect to an isotropic material, invariant I_4 is related to the family of fibres and is given by:

$$I_4 = \mathbf{a} \cdot \mathbf{C} \cdot \mathbf{a} \tag{2}$$

where **a** is the unit tensor representing the orientation of the undeformed fibres. The fourth invariant represents the square of a fibre stretch and is introduced to include the contribution of collagen fibres to the strain energy of the material. In order to describe the interaction between the fibres and the ground matrix, a further invariant should be introduced. However, only four invariants are used because of the limits in carrying out suitable experimental tests.

The stress response of the model can be represented in terms of the second Piola-Kirchhoff stress tensor as follows:

$$\mathbf{S} = 2\sum_{i=1}^{3} \frac{\partial W}{\partial I_i} \frac{\partial I_i}{\partial \mathbf{C}} \tag{3}$$

A particular form of the stored energy function is given by:

$$W = \tilde{W}_m + U_m + W_f \tag{4}$$

where the two terms related to the isotropic ground matrix are:

$$\tilde{W}_m = C_1(\tilde{I}_1 - 3) + C_2(\tilde{I}_2 - 3) \tag{5}$$

$$U_m = \frac{1}{D}(J - 1)^2 \tag{6}$$

The fibre stiffness in compression is neglected, while the contribution of the fibres in the tensile states is given as a function of the fourth invariant:

$$W_f = \frac{k_1}{k_2} \left\{ \exp\left[k_2(I_4 - 1)^2 - 1 \right] \right\} \tag{7}$$

The invariants $\tilde{I}_1$ and $\tilde{I}_2$ are functions of the iso-volumetric strain only, and the constants C_1 and C_2 can be related to the shear modulus in the undeformed state. The constant D is the inverse of the bulk modulus and J is the Jacobian, the measure of the volume change of the material.

The additive decomposition in the two parts (5) and (6) is typical of materials with incompressible or almost-incompressible behaviour and is related to the numerical analysis procedure. Term (7) makes it possible to include the effect of the spatial orientation of the fibres through unit tensor **a**.

The tensile stress-strain behaviour of the fibres is governed by the relation:

$$\mathbf{S}_f = 2k_1(I_4 - 1)\exp\left[k_2(I_4 - 1)^2 \right] \mathbf{a} \otimes \mathbf{a} \tag{8}$$

through the definition of the values for the two constants k_1 and k_2. The stress-strain relation (8) presents a small stiffness, toe region, near the undeformed configuration. This makes it possible to describe the mechanical response of the groups of collagen fibres, related to their typical initial configuration, known as crimp.

Several forms of the stored energy function have been proposed according to the requirement of fitting the numerical model to the experimental data. The choice of a particular constitutive model and the identification of its parameters are difficult tasks.

2.2.2   Visco-elastic constitutive models

The time-dependent response of the PDL can be ascribed to the movement of liquid phases and to the creep of the solid constituents of the PDL. The resulting effects are different degrees of stiffness depending on the rate of deformation, greater stiffness at a higher rate of deformation, and an increase in strain over time when a constant load is applied. A viscoelastic model can theoretically only properly describe the phenomena related to solid skeleton, but it can actually also be used to macroscopically simulate the effects of the liquid phase on the global behaviour of the PDL.

A viscoelastic model, accounting for large strains as well, can be defined by extending the rheological model depicted in Figure 2.1 to the three-dimensional case. The stress response is given by:

$$\mathbf{S} = \mathbf{S}_{x} + \sum_{i=1}^{M} \mathbf{Q}_i \tag{9}$$

where $\mathbf{Q}_i$ is the non-equilibrated stress of the viscous branches. The variation of this stress over time can be assumed to obey the following differential equations:

$$\dot{\mathbf{Q}}_i + \frac{1}{\alpha_i}\mathbf{Q}_i = \frac{d}{dt}\left[2\frac{\partial W_i(\mathbf{C})}{\partial \mathbf{C}}\right], \mathbf{Q}_i(0) = \mathbf{Q}_i^0 \quad (i = 1, M) \tag{10}$$

The integration of the above equation leads to the so-called convolution integral, giving the global stress response as a function of time:

$$\mathbf{S}(t) = 2\frac{\partial W_x}{\partial \mathbf{C}} + \sum_{i=1}^{M}\mathbf{Q}_i^0 \exp\left(-t/\alpha_i\right) +$$

$$+ \sum_{i=1}^{M} \int_{\tau=0}^{t} \left\{2\frac{\partial W_i}{\partial \mathbf{C}}\frac{d}{d\tau}\exp\left[(\tau - t)/\alpha_i\right]\right\}d\tau \tag{11}$$

Constants α_i affect the rate of viscous deformation, while terms W_i and W_∞ represent the stored energy functions of the elastic elements. A high value of a α_i constant corresponds to a rapid viscous deformation. For $t \to 0$ and $t \to \infty$, an elastic behaviour is recovered, with a low stiffness if time tends towards infinity.

The viscoelastic model presented here can also be modified in order to take into account the anisotropic response of the PDL by using stored energy functions like those described in the previous section.

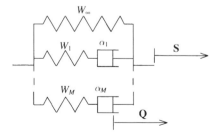

Figure 2.1 Rheological model.

2.2.3   Multi-phase constitutive models

The approach described in the previous sub-section interprets the overall response of the PDL and uses viscosity as a macro-modelling procedure for the complex behaviour related to the presence and movement of the liquid content in the PDL. A numerical model with more micro-mechanical coherence and a direct evaluation of the different components of the tissue can be represented by a multi-phase media approach. In this way, a more realistic description of the tissue is possible, considering the actual presence of different phases as interacting continuous media. The phases correspond to the solid network and fluid content. The effects on the global behaviour given by the coupling of the different phases are taken into account.

Assuming the PDL is an elastic solid, fully saturated by permeating liquids, the total stress $\mathbf{S}$ is given by the sum of the effective stress $\mathbf{S}'$ and the hydrostatic pressure p (positive if compressive):

$$\mathbf{S}' = \mathbf{S} + p\mathbf{C}^{-1} \tag{12}$$

The above equation is known as the principle of effective stress. It is assumed that Darcy's law governs the flux of different fluids:

$$\mathbf{v} = \mathbf{K}[-\text{grad}\,(p) + \rho_f \mathbf{g}] \tag{13}$$

where $\mathbf{v}$ is the relative velocity of the fluid with respect to the solid phase, ρ_f the density of the liquid, $\mathbf{g}$ the gravity acceleration and $\mathbf{K}$ the dynamic permeability matrix.

The constitutive equation of the solid matrix can be defined according to the previous approaches, taking into account viscoelastic and/or anisotropic schemes as well. These constitutive laws are defined by considering effective stress $\mathbf{S}'$ acting on the skeleton. The flux of the liquid phases in the PDL affects the response of the tissue over time. The variation in liquid pressure p, more rapid if the tissue shows high permeability, modifies the effective stress of the solid phase and its strain state.

It is therefore clear that the numerical formulation of this approach is rather complicated and also that there are difficulties in defining the parameters adopted by means of experimental testing.

However, this approach is certainly more accurate and useful for evaluating in detail the response of the PDL, as it keeps a valid connection to real tissue configuration.

2.3   REVIEW OF THE MECHANICAL PROPERTIES OF THE PDL

2.3.1   Experimental studies on the viscoelasticity of the PDL

Several approaches have been used to study the elastic properties of the PDL. The viscoelasticity and mechanical impedance of the PDL have been estimated based on tooth mobility when a force is applied to a tooth under quasi-static and dynamic conditions (Noyes and Solt, 1973). This method has the advantage of being applicable to *in vivo* measurements and has been used for evaluating the performance of the periodontium. However, it is difficult to directly obtain data on the mechanical properties of the PDL because tooth mobility greatly depends on the size and shape of the tooth root. Nonetheless, the viscoelasticity of the PDL can be estimated by making some geometrical simplifications.

The mechanical properties of the PDL are reflected in the force required to extract a tooth but also depend on the overall geometric configuration of the periodontium. Therefore, the ultimate tensile strength (UTS) of the PDL has been measured immediately before breaking using relatively small excised and trimmed samples (Atkinson and Ralph, 1977). When Atkinson and Ralph measured the UTS by stretching postmortem human PDL samples along fibre bundles, they obtained an average value of about 3.7 MPa by dividing the force by the cross-sectional area of each sample. However, as noted by the authors, even if the samples used are relatively small compared to root size, the influence of the curved nature of the ligament attachment may nonetheless be unavoidable. To eliminate this effect, Ralph (Ralph, 1982) improved the method so that the load is distributed over all of the fibre bundles by using transverse sections consisting of the root, ligament and alveolar bone. The thickness of each section was 1 mm, and the load was axially applied to the tooth root while supporting the alveolar bone. Ralph measured the UTS in terms of shear stress by dividing the load by the circumferential area of the ligament attachment and obtained an average value of 2.4 MPa. The deformation speed used was 0.25 mm/min.

Mandel et al. (Mandel et al., 1986) measured the whole stress–strain curves, instead of just maximum stress before breaking, on human mandibular premolars and determined the elastic stiffness of the PDL from the gradient of shear stress–strain curve. Mandel et al., used 1 mm thick transverse sections, as were used in the study by Ralph, for measurements at a deformation speed of 0.2 mm/min. They measured several stress–strain parameters at different root levels and found that elastic stiffness did not vary significantly (from 2.6 to 3.2 MPa), whereas other parameters, such as maximum shear stress and shear strain before breaking and the relative failure energy in shear, significantly varied along the root.

Chiba and Komatsu (Chiba and Komatsu, 1993) found that stress–strain curves of the PDL strongly depend on the strain rate in a study using a wide range of deformation speeds. They obtained the stress-strain curves of transverse sections of rat mandibular incisors at various speeds of 1 to 10^4 mm/24 h. They found that the curves were approximately sigmoid and that the linear part of the curve became steeper when the velocity was increased. The shear tangent modulus increased from 0.77 to 1115 kPa when the strain rate was increased from 1 to 10^4 mm/24 h, or from 0.012 μm/s to 0.12 mm/s.

2.3.2 Experimental studies on the elastic constants of the PDL

The experimental method using the transverse sections proposed by Ralph (Ralph, 1982) is a useful technique for determining the mechanical properties of the PDL because the sample preparation is relatively simple and the geometry-dependent error is greatly reduced. However, a modulus of elasticity, such as Young's modulus, which is used for finite element analysis, is not directly obtained using this technique.

To our knowledge, to date there are not many studies on the direct experimental determination of Young's modulus of the PDL. Dyment and Synge, (Dyment and Synge, 1935), determined it in four samples that had been scraped from the central teeth of calves and lambs. A travelling microscope was used to measure the changes in length with the change in load under quasi-static conditions. The Young's modulus was found to be about 1.5 MPa, but it was obtained by measuring the direction perpendicular to the fibre bundles. Ast et al. (Ast et al., 1966) obtained the force–deformation curves of the PDL using a tensile testing machine at an extension speed of 0.05–50 mm/min and estimated the tangent modulus to be 2–3 MPa. In their study, rectangular-shaped samples of a bone-ligament-bone complex were taken from the human mandible so that the tensile direction was along the fibre direction. The cross-sectional area of the samples was relatively large, about 13 mm^2. Zhu et al. (Zhu et al., 1995) estimated the tensile and compressive moduli of elasticity to be 3–5 MPa and 0.5 MPa, respectively, from measurements along the fibre direction in bone–ligament–bone samples collected from six adults. However, details of the measurement method were not given in their report.

A wide range of values for the elastic modulus of the PDL has been adopted in stress–strain analysis using the finite element method. Ree and Jacobson (Ree and Jacobson, 1997) surveyed and collected the elastic moduli of the PDL ranging from 0.1 to 1000 MPa, as reported in Table 2.1. Even in the most recent studies (Katona et al., 1995; Holmes et al., 1996; Cobo et al., 1996; Vollmer et al., 1999), the values are spread over a range of two orders in magnitude.

Finite element models were also used to estimate the elasticity of the PDL as an inverse problem. Tanne (Tanne, 1983) estimated the Young's modulus of the PDL to be 0.67 MPa, a value often referred to by many researchers, from the results of the finite element analysis of tooth displacement when applying a force to a tooth. Much lower values, i.e. 0.07 MPa (Andersen et al., 1991) and 0.05 MPa (Vollmer et al., 1999), determined from the analysis of excised specimens using a similar technique, have also been reported.

2.4 MEASUREMENTS OF THE ELASTIC MODULUS OF THE PDL

As mentioned in the previous section, there are very few experimentally determined values of longitudinal elasticity of the PDL. In this section, we will focus on the experimental determination of the elastic modulus of the PDL using a miniature tensile and compression testing machine developed by the authors.

Table 2.1 Material constants used in finite element analyses (Ree and Jacobsen, 1997; Vollmer, 1999)

Authors	Elastic modulus (MPa)	Poisson's ratio
Vollmer	0.05	0.3
	0.22	0.3
Andersen	0.07	0.49
	0.8–68.9	0.3–0.45
	13.8	0.49
Yettram	0.18	0.49
Tanne	0.67	0.49
Williams	1.5	0–0.45
	100	0–0.45
Korioth	2.5–3.2	0.45
Farah	6.9	0.45
Takahashi	9.8	0.45
Wright	49	0.45
Wilson	50	0.45
Ree	50	0.49
Cook	68.9	0.49
Ko	68.9	0.45
Atmaram	171.6	0.45
Thresher	1379	0.45
Goel	1750	0.49

2.4.1   Materials

Fourteen specimens consisting of tooth, PDL and alveolar bone were obtained from a maxillary canine of an adult cat, as shown in Figure 2.2, and used for mechanical tests. A saw with a 0.3 mm thick diamond blade was used to cut out small samples in conditions made wet with physiological saline. 0.7 mm thick slices were first obtained, and then four specimens, each 2 mm in length and 0.7 mm in width, were cut from each section. These small specimens were used for the mechanical tests so as to eliminate the effects of the curved nature of the tooth root. The specimens were frozen until they were to be used in the mechanical tests.

After the mechanical tests, the specimens were stained with eosin in order to distinguish the PDL from other tissues. Photographs of side views of each specimen were taken using a stereoscopic microscope, and the thickness and cross-sectional areas of the PDL were calculated from the photographs. The mean ($\pm$ S.D.) thickness and cross-sectional area of the PDLs were 0.19 ± 0.05 mm and 0.41 ± 0.06 mm^2, respectively.

2.4.2   Mechanical testing machine

A miniature testing machine that could be manipulated under a stereoscopic microscope was developed to carry out tensile and compression tests on the PDL. A schematic diagram of the testing machine is shown in Figure 2.3. The rotation of a stepping motor that was controlled by a personal computer was transmitted to a precise translation stage. The rate of translation was 500 μm per revolution, and the ratio of revolution to number of pulses fed to the motor was controlled in the range of 1/500 to 1/125,000. A force to deform the specimen by the stage was applied via a load cell. Signals from the load cell were stored in the personal computer after passing through a strain amplifier and an A/D converter. The deformation of the specimen was measured by a laser displacement meter that detected the distance from a reflector fixed to a sample holder with a resolution of 0.2 μm. The deformation signals were also stored in the computer. Photographs of the testing machine are shown in Figure 2.4.

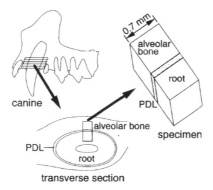

Figure 2.2 Sampling sites for specimens. Transverse sections, each about thick 0.7 mm, were cut out from the maxillary canines of a cat, including the surrounding periodontal ligament and alveolar bone. Four specimens, each about 0.7 mm in width and 2 mm in length, were obtained from each slice.

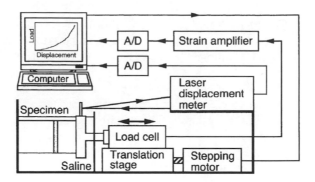

Figure 2.3 A schematic diagram of a mechanical testing machine. Samples were deformed by a translation stage actuated by a stepping motor. A load cell was placed between the stage and a sample holder. Deformation of the specimen was detected by a laser displacement meter. The output signals for loading and displacement were stored in a computer via A/D converters.

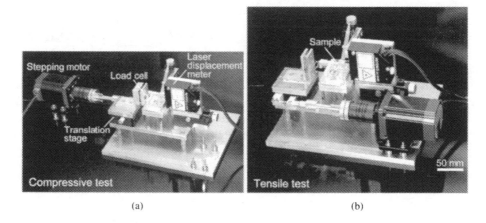

Figure 2.4 Set-up of the testing machine. Compression (a) and tensile (b) tests were separately performed after assembling a load cell-equipped part specially designed for each test. A sample was placed in the chamber and fixed with clamps as shown in Figure 2.5.

The strain rate was controlled by turning the pulse rate and the revolution ratio into a pulse. Since the deformation of the load cell during loading was not negligible compared to the deformation of the PDL, the load-deformation relationship of the load cell was measured and incorporated into the control of the strain rate for correction. The testing machine had a maximum sampling rate of 700 Hz, maximum load of 150 gf, maximum displacement of 500 μm, and minimum resolutions of 0.1 gf and 0.2 μm in load and displacement, respectively.

For the measurements, samples were mounted using clamps specially made for small samples, as shown in Figure 2.5. In tensile tests, both the edges of the tooth root and alveolar bone portions were fixed at the top and bottom with 0.5 mm thick movable knife

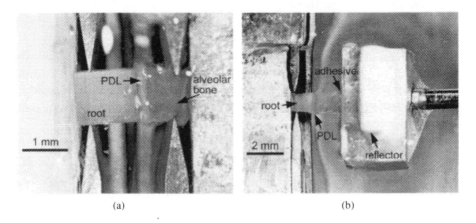

(a)   (b)

Figure 2.5 Clamping of samples in tensile (a) and compression (b) tests. Samples were clamped, using knife edges, at the top and bottom. In compression tests, a instant jellied adhesive was also used for fixing a portion of the alveolar bone.

edges. In compression tests, the end of the alveolar bone of a sample was fixed to the end of the moving portion of the holder with a instant jellied adhesive so as to be applicable to cracked bones.

We first evaluated the performance of the testing machine. The linearity of the machine was examined by conducting tensile and compression tests on a coil spring for a sample at various strain rates. The results obtained at a deformation rate of 6 μm/s are shown in Figure 2.6 (a). The machine had good linearity, and the slope, i.e. a spring constant, was not significantly different in the two tests. The slopes obtained at different deformation rates are also plotted in Figure 2.6 (b).

Although the slope slightly increased in the region of higher strain rates, the variation was ±2 per cent or less in both tests. It was confirmed that the machine operates with sufficient accuracy at deformation rates ranging from 0.01 to 1000 μm/s.

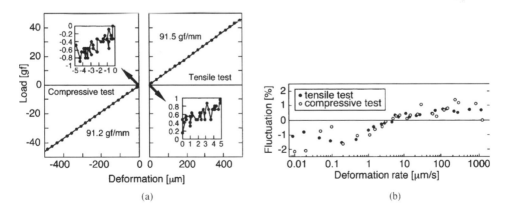

(a)   (b)

Figure 2.6 Results of a performance test on a coil spring for a sample. Slopes of load-deformation curves obtained at a deformation speed of 6 μm/s in tensile and compression tests (a) Variations in a spring constant obtained from the slopes of load-deformation curves obtained at various deformation rates (b).

2.4.3 Mechanical tests on the PDL

Each specimen was placed in the sample chamber and fixed with clamps under stereoscopic microscope observation. The sample chamber was then filled with physiological saline. Microscopic observation was used to check that the specimen was firmly clamped during testing.

Fourteen samples were divided into two groups and subjected to tensile or compression tests at six different speeds of deformation (0.014, 0.14, 1.4, 14, 140, 700 μm/s). Before each test, five preconditioning cycles were carried out at a deformation speed of 14 μm/s with a maximum load of 50 gf. The load-deformation curves obtained were converted into stress-strain curves using data on the thickness and cross-sectional area of each PDL sample, which were measured in the photographs described in the previous section. All the experiments were performed at a room temperature of 23 ± 2 °C.

2.4.4 Results

The stress–strain curves of a specimen obtained at various strain rates are shown in Figure 2.7. The strain rates are indicated by numbers inside the graph. In both tensile and compression tests, the curves showed remarkable nonlinearity unique to soft tissues. There was a great difference between the stress-strain curves obtained in tensile and compression tests. In the compression tests, the curves were strongly dependent on strain rate. The PDL greatly deformed without a significant increase in stress when the strain rate was low, whereas the curves obtained at a high strain rate shifted greatly toward the high-stress region, depending on the strain rate. On the other hand, the curves obtained in the tensile tests showed much less dependency on the strain rate than did those obtained in the compression tests.

The tangent modulus of each sample was obtained from the slope of each curve in two stress regions, 0–25 and 800–1000 kPa. The tangent moduli obtained are shown in Figure 2.8. In the tensile tests, the tangent modulus was not significantly dependent on the strain rate, although it tended to increase in the low-stress region of 0–25 kPa. In the

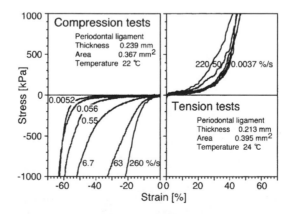

Figure 2.7 Typical stress-strain curves of the periodontal ligament obtained at various strain rates in tensile and compression tests. The values in the graphs denote strain rates.

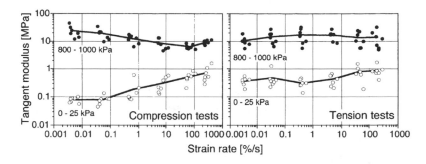

Figure 2.8 Tangent modulus of elasticity of the PDL obtained from gradients of stress–strain curves. Open and closed circles indicate moduli obtained in low- and high-stress regions, respectively.

compression tests, the tangent modulus in the low-stress region significantly increased as the strain rate increased: the elasticity increased ten fold with an increase of three–four orders in strain rate.

In the region of extremely low strain rate (less than 0.1 per cent/s), the curves were no longer dependent on the strain rate and quasi-static deformation was attained.

Under quasi-static (0.005 per cent/s) and low-stress (0–25 kPa) conditions, the tangent moduli of the PDL in tensile and compressive states were 0.37 ± 0.11 and 0.079 ± 0.017 MPa (mean ± S.D.), respectively. It should be noted that the tangent modulus in a tensile state was about five-times higher than in a compressive state (p < 0.001). In the region of 800–1000 kPa, the tangent moduli in the quasi-static tensile and compressive states were 11 ± 4 and 24 ± 12 MPa, respectively, thus indicating significantly lower elasticity in the tensile state than in the compressive state (p < 0.01).

2.4.5   Discussion

Research has shown that the elastic properties of soft tissues in a tensile state have little dependency on strain rate; the stress–strain relationships obtained in dog lung parenchyma (Vawter et al., 1978) and rabbit ligaments (Woo et al., 1990) were found to be almost insensitive to strain rate ranging over three orders in magnitude. The results obtained in the present study for the PDL also showed that stress-strain curves obtained in tensile tests had almost no dependency on strain rate even when it was varied over five orders in magnitude.

In contrast, stress–strain curves obtained in the compression tests showed strong dependency on strain rate. There have been few studies on the compressive viscoelastic behaviour of soft tissues other than articular cartilage, whereas there have been more on hard tissues because soft tissues, such as muscle, ligament, tendon and blood vessels, mainly fulfil their function in a tensile state. In this sense, the PDL is rather different from other soft tissues because the PDL also works in a compressive state. As for the compressive mechanical properties of articular cartilage, many biomechanical studies have been performed by Mow (Mow et al., 1984).

Articular cartilage is a connective tissue that covers the bony articulating ends inside a joint. It is a multi-phasic, non-linearly permeable, viscoelastic material consisting of two principal phases: a solid matrix and a movable interstitial fluid. It is widely accepted that the time-dependent response of cartilage can be represented by a multi-phase constitutive model such as the one described in section 1.3. The tensile stiffness of cartilage is derived primarily from its collagen fibre properties, which are flow-independent. However, when the interstitial fluid flow becomes significant, it causes flow-dependent viscoelastic effects. This is the main mechanism responsible for the compressive viscoelastic behaviour of cartilage (Mow et al., 1993).

As in cartilage, it is thought that the dependence of the compressive elasticity of the PDL on strain rate is due to the movement of water within and out of the PDL. This is also suggested from the stress-strain curves in the low-stress region shown in Figure 2.6. In the quasi-static compressive state, the tangent modulus abruptly increased at a strain of about 50 per cent in the specimen referred to in Figure 2.6 and 40 per cent on average in seven other specimens, presumably due to the compression of a solid phase after water excretion. As described in equations (12) and (13), under the condition of a high strain rate, the external force is also supported by the moving fluid and partially by the collagen fibres, resulting in viscoelastic behaviour that depends on the strain rate and permeability of the fluid. In our experiments, since small 0.7 mm × 0.7 mm samples were used, the water flow out of the tissue might have been unlike that in an *in vivo* state, where tissue fluid flows out of the ligament through the walls of capillary vessels and alveolar bone.

As described in section 2.1, Chiba et al. (Chiba et al., 1993) found that the shear tangent modulus greatly increased with an increase in the deformation speed. The tangent modulus, at the highest strain rate, increased by 1450 times that of the lowest one over the range of a four-order increase in strain rate. In transverse sections, the collagen fibres are straightened in the direction of load, so the loading condition might be similar to that in tensile tests. However, the mechanical behaviour of the PDL in a tensile state observed in the present study was almost independent of the strain rate and very different from that of the PDL in a shear state. Even when compared with the results of the compression tests, there is still a significant difference in the dependencies on strain rate. The reason for this is that the discrepancy between the two tests, longitudinal deformation and lateral deformation, is not known. The strong sensitivity to strain rate in the shear tests might simply result from the viscoelastic properties unique to shear deformation. It might also be due to the movement of water within tissue. In a shear test, when a part of the PDL sample is extended by loading, the remaining part, normal to the extended one, is compressed. To clarify and quantify the notable differences between time-dependent and time-independent responses of the PDL in different states, numerical analyses based on constitutive models are also needed while at the same time keeping a valid connection with the real configuration of the PDL.

The strain rate dependency and nonlinear elasticity of the PDL demonstrated in this study and discussed here suggest that these factors should be taken into account in the stress/strain analysis of a tooth. Under a high strain rate, the value of the tensile modulus is almost the same as that of the compressive modulus, as is shown in Figure 2.8. Therefore, the same value can be used in the analysis of, for example, dynamic tooth mobility measured at a relatively high frequency. In a high-stress region, a tangent modulus of about 10 MPa can also be used in both tensile and compressive regions. On the other hand, when analysing the stress–strain distribution in a quasi-static state, such as during orthodontic treatment, the five-fold difference between elasticities in tensile and compressive states should be taken into account: 0.08 MPa for a compressive region and 0.4 MPa for a tensile region. If these values are used in the analysis of the stress distribution in the PDL when applying an orthodontic force to a tooth, lower stress in a compressed region and higher stress in a tensile region will be obtained. Thus, it is important that adequate values of elasticity for an analysis must be chosen.

2.5 CONCLUSIONS

Despite the fundamental importance of material constants of the PDL in dental biomecahnics, there is little information on the mechanical properties of the PDL, compared to those of tooth or alveolar bone, mainly due to difficulties in obtaining data from experimental analysis. In this chapter, the experimental determination of the viscoelastic properties of the PDL was discussed. There is a significant difference between the stress–strain curves obtained in compression tests and those obtained in tensile tests. There is almost no dependency on strain rate in a tensile state but there is notable dependency on strain rate in a compressive state. This can be interpreted using a multi-phase constitutive model, also overviewed in this chapter, that can be introduced to describe flow-dependent viscoelastic effects. The PDL shows non-linear elastic properties as do other soft tissues. Under quasi-static and low-stress conditions, the tangent modulus of the PDL in a compressive state is significantly lower than in a tensile state, whereas the tangent modulus in a high-stress region is almost the same in both states. Although significant advances have been made in understanding the mechanical properties of biological tissues, much experimental work remains to be done in the field of studies on the PDL. The theoretical approach will also play an important role in understanding the mechanical properties of the PDL.

REFERENCES

K.L. Andersen, H.T. Mortensen and B. Melsen, Material parameters and stress profiles within the periodontal ligament, Am. J. Orthod. Dentofac. Orthop., Vol. 99, pp. 427–440, 1991.

D. Ast, R. Diemer and M. Hofmann, Untersuchungen über das elastische Verhalten der Wurzelhaut, des alveolären Knochens und der Wurzelhartsubstanzen (in German), Das Deutsche Zahnärzteblatt, Vol. 20, pp. 639–647, 1966.

H.F. Atkinson and W.J. Ralph, *In vitro* strength of the human periodontal ligament, J. Dent. Res., Vol. 56, pp. 48–52, 1977.

M. Chiba and K. Komatsu, Mechanical responses of the periodontal ligament in the transverse section of the rat mandibular incisor at various velocities of loading *in vitro*, J. Biomech., Vol. 26, pp. 561–570, 1993.

J. Cobo, J. Argüelles, M. Puente and M. Vijande, Dentoalveolar stress from bodily tooth movement at different levels of bone loss, Am. J. Orthod. Dentofac. Orthop., Vol. 110, pp. 256–262, 1996.

M.L. Dyment and J.L. Synge, The elasticity of the periodontal membrane, Oral Health, Vol. 25, pp. 105–109, 1935.

D.C. Holmes, A.M. Diaz-Arnold and J.M. Leary, Influence of post dimension on stress distribution in dentin, J. Prosthetic. Dent., Vol. 75, pp. 140–147, 1996.

T.R. Katona, N.H. Paydar, H.U. Akay and W.E. Roberts, Stress analysis of bone modeling response to rat molar orthodontics, J. Biomech., Vol. 28, pp. 27–38, 1995.

U. Mandel, P. Dalgaard and A. Viidik, A biomechanical study of the human periodontal ligament, J. Biomech., Vol. 19, pp. 637–645, 1986.

V.C. Mow, M.H. Holmes and W.M. Lai, Fluid transport and mechanical properties of articular cartilage: A review, J. Biomech., Vol. 17, pp. 377–394, 1984.

V.C. Mow, G.A. Ateshian and R.L. Spilker, Biomechanics of diarthrodial joints: A review of twenty years of progress, ASME J. Biomech. Engng., Vol. 115, pp. 460–467, 1993.

D.H. Noyes and C.W. Solt, Measurement of mechanical mobility of human incisors with sinusoidal forces, J. Biomech., Vol. 6, pp. 439–442, 1973.

J.S. Ree and P.H. Jacobson, Elastic modulus of the periodontal ligament, Biomaterials, Vol. 18, pp. 995–999, 1997.

W.J. Ralph, Tensile behaviour of the periodontal ligament, J. Periodont. Res., Vol. 17, pp. 423–426, 1982.

K. Tanne, Stress induced in the periodontal tissue at the initial phase of the application of various types of orthodontic force: three-dimensional analysis by means of the finite element method (in Japanese), J. Osaka Univ. Dent. Soc., Vol. 28, pp. 209–261, 1983.

D.L. Vawter, Y.C. Fung and J.B. West, Elasticity of excised dog lung parenchyma, J. Appl. Physiol., Vol. 45, pp. 261–269, 1978.

D. Vollmer, C. Bourauel, K. Majer and A. Jäger, Determination of the centre of resistance in an upper human canine and idealized tooth model, Europ. J. Orthod., Vol. 21, pp. 633–648, 1999.

S.L.-Y. Woo, R.H. Peterson, K.J. Ohland, T.J. Site and M.I. Danto, The effects of strain rate on the properties of the medial collateral ligament in skeletally immature and mature rabbits: a biomechanical and histological study, J. Orthop. Res., Vol. 8, pp. 712–721, 1990.

Z. Zhu, C. Du, M. Chen, Z. Wei and Y. Chao, Determination of modulus of elasticity of human periodontal membrane (in Chinese), J. West China Univ. Med. Sci., Vol. 26, pp. 160–162, 1995.

3 Computer tomography for virtual models in dental imaging

AN Natali, MM Viola

3.1 INTRODUCTION

This chapter presents an overview of the basic concepts of computer tomography and image processing in the development of virtual models. The tomographic image processing techniques addressed in this chapter are those used to develop software tools for surgical planning and to define numerical models for the prediction of biomechanical responses.

A description of the basic principles of tomographic relief is given, from the physical, technological and computational points of view, recalling the fundamental works that represent the basic knowledge in this field. Then the development of a virtual model is described, from geometry reconstruction to material behaviour estimation, using image processing techniques.

The most important limitations of the traditional projective radiological technique are low contrast resolution, which is the low capability to differentiate anatomical structures showing little difference in density, and the loss of in-depth information along the radiological projection. The former depends on the fact that measured X-ray attenuation is the sum of the X-ray attenuation coefficients of each tissue, weighted by the thickness of each tissue crossed by the beam. The latter depends on the methodology itself, which projects three-dimensional structures on a bi-dimensional detector. This makes it difficult to recover information regarding the position of the structures of interest in the direction of the X-ray propagation. In other words, the overlapping of structures makes it difficult to have a complete visualisation of them.

In order to overcome these limitations, many corrective methodologies have been introduced, such as the use of high contrast films or specific tomographic techniques. An important contribution came from the development of computer tomography. This methodology made it possible to obtain sectional views of the region of interest, with high contrast resolution, and acquire quantitative information of the tissue density. The CT technique, first proposed in the seventies, has been subjected to continuous technological evolutions and recently scan-machines have made it possible to quickly reconstruct large volumes with great accuracy.

The development of many post-processing software tools, which give detailed representations of the scanned volume, has offered advantages in diagnosing the dento-maxillo-facial district. Moreover, the growth in the tomographic survey has lead to the development of advanced computer models through a precise reconstruction of geometry and a reliable definition of properties. These models are of primary interest for the development of applications for surgical planning and numerical analysis.

3.2 FOUNDATIONS OF X-RAY COMPUTED TOMOGRAPHY

3.2.1 Physical principles of x-ray absorption

The attenuation of a narrow beam of mono-energetic photons with energy E and intensity I_o passing through a homogeneous medium of thickness x is described by equation (1) (Agati, 1976):

$$I = I_0 \cdot \exp\left(-\mu\left(\rho, Z, E\right) \cdot x\right) \tag{1}$$

where μ is the linear attenuation coefficient, which depends on absorbing medium density ρ, atomic number Z and beam energy E.

For inhomogeneous materials, such as biological tissues, the linear attenuation coefficient μ is no longer a constant, so it must be considered as the summation of all the attenuation coefficients along the X-ray path.

In the energy range used for diagnostic purposes (30–120 KeV), one of the following two interaction processes between photon radiation and the electrons of the material, occurs:

- the photoelectric effect, in which a photon collides with an atom and ejects a bound electron from external (K, L, M, or N) atomic shells, transferring all the energy to it;
- compton scattering, in which a photon is scattered by an electron of the medium; portion of the energy of the photon is transferred to the electron as kinetic energy.

The linear attenuation coefficient (Figure 3.1), a measurable quantity from an object in a X-ray tomography, is the sum of the photoelectric effect, μ_p, and of the Compton effect, μ_c, described by the following the equations:

$$\mu_p = K_1 \cdot \frac{\rho \cdot n_0 \cdot \tilde{Z}^{\,m-1}}{E^{3.1}} \tag{2a}$$

$$\mu_c = K_2 \cdot \rho \cdot n_0 \cdot f(E) \tag{2b}$$

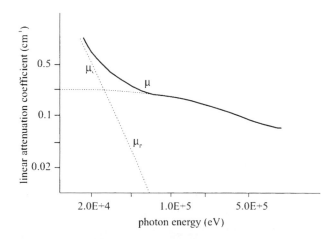

Figure 3.1 Linear attenuation coefficient of water and the contribution of each interaction to the total attenuation of X-rays as a function of energy. The photoelectric effect (μ_p) is dominant at lower energy, while the Compton effect (μ_c) is dominant at higher energy.

where K_1 and K_2 are constants, ρ is the density, n_0 the electron density per gram, $\tilde{Z}$ the effective atomic number, E the energy of the incident photon, m an empirical constant assumed to be 4.4 for biological materials at energy below 150 KeV and f(E) the Klein-Nishina function, which depends on energy E. The effective atomic number, $\tilde{Z}$, for a compound material such as water or human tissue, is a weighted average of the atomic numbers of each element (Johns and Cunningham, 1983). The contrast in an image depends on the differences in the attenuation coefficients of the different materials, and depends mainly on two factors: the effective atomic number $\tilde{Z}$ of the material in the low-energy region (see μ_p in equation (2a)) and the electron density at high energy, where the Compton interactions are the most important.

3.2.2 Data acquisition

Computed tomography reconstructs the image of an object by dividing it into contiguous parallel slices. The data, which represent the physical properties of a material strip, are acquired by a set of linear sampling at different projection angles (Figure 3.2).

The width of this strip is mainly determined by the spatial resolution of the detectors. The spatial resolution basically depends on the detector's dimension. The projection data can be measured by illuminating the object with an X-ray beam and moving the detector at different angles.

The idea behind computed tomography can easily be understood by the following example. Consider the distribution of the linear attenuation coefficient μ on a slice of the object shown in Figure 3.3.

It is assumed that the slice can be divided into four square components whose sides are d: each component is called a pixel and it is characterised by its own attenuation coefficient. Four equations along directions x and y can be written from equation (1) and easily solved with respect to variables μ_{11}, μ_{12}, μ_{21}, μ_{22}. It is thus possible to have a description of the properties of every pixel simply on the basis of the following measures:

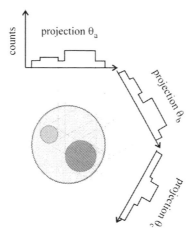

Figure 3.2 Linear samplings at different projection angles.

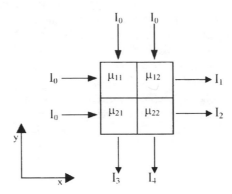

Figure 3.3 Division of the object into four pixels.

$$\begin{cases} I_1 = I_0 \cdot \exp\left(-(\mu_{11} + \mu_{12}) \cdot d\right) \\ I_2 = I_0 \cdot \exp\left(-(\mu_{21} + \mu_{22}) \cdot d\right) \\ I_3 = I_0 \cdot \exp\left(-(\mu_{11} + \mu_{21}) \cdot d\right) \\ I_4 = I_0 \cdot \exp\left(-(\mu_{12} + \mu_{22}) \cdot d\right) \end{cases} \qquad (3)$$

There are many algorithms that restore the images from scan projection profiles according to this approach; some notes regarding this are reported in the following paragraph.

3.2.3 Reconstruction algorithms

3.2.3.1 Iterative Method

Different methods can be used to obtain the properties of each pixel. One of the easiest to use is the iterative method describe here.

Initially, a preliminary distribution of values pertaining to μ is set. The values of μ then change until the calculated projection, generated using the estimated distribution of μ, reaches the measured projections. Many different iterative algorithms can be used to determine the value of μ, one of which is described below.

The following procedure first considers elements having a constant value, assumed, for example, as the average value. For each iteration the difference between the measured projection g_j and the projection estimated from the calculated elements $\left(\Sigma_{i=1}^{N} f_{ij}, \text{ where } f_{ij} \text{ represents a pixel belonging to the i-th line of projection}\right)$ is obtained.
This difference is divided by the number N of elements that contribute to the projection.

The iterative algorithm is analytically defined as:

$$f_{ij}^{q+1} = f_{ij}^q + \frac{\left(g_j - \Sigma_{i=1}^{N} f_{ij}^q\right)}{N} \qquad (4)$$

where q is the number of iterations (Figure 3.4). The process is stopped when the difference between the measured projection and the calculated projection is small enough, according to an assumed accuracy limit. Iterative methods present some problems, such as computational efficiency and convergence difficulties due to noise.

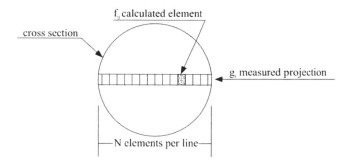

Figure 3.4 Iterative method scheme.

3.2.3.2 Filtered Back Projection

This method has a good computational efficiency and consists in back-projecting the measured value in each point along the projection, recalling the first description of the problem by Brooks and Di Chiro, 1975.

The back projection of scan profiles of distribution, defined by a bi-dimensional mapping using function f(x,y), gives a blurred image. It is possible to demonstrate (Phelps, 1986) that this distortion, for a punctiform object, is proportional to the inverse of the distance r, so that each point of a wide object will be blurred by this astigmatism.

In order to reconstruct the true image from the back projected image, the 1/r blurring factor must be eliminated from each point of the image (Figure 3.5). This can be done by applying a suitable correction filter, which is a ramp filter in the spatial domain, to the scan profiles before the back projection is carried out. This procedure is illustrated in Figure 3.6. Scan profiles at different angles are thus acquired (Figure 3.6 (a)). In the reconstruction of the object by simple back projection, the distortion around the object can be noticed (Figure 3.6 (b)); this blurring is eliminated by applying an appropriate filter to the scan profiles (Figure 3.6 (c)). As the number of scan profiles increases, the artifacts disappear and the original object distribution is restored. The object correctly reconstructed with an adequate number of angles is shown in (Figure 3.6 (d)).

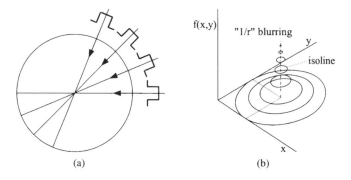

(a)   (b)

Figure 3.5 Back projection of profiles from a punctiform object (a) Point distortion, obtained by back projecting the scan profiles of the object (b).

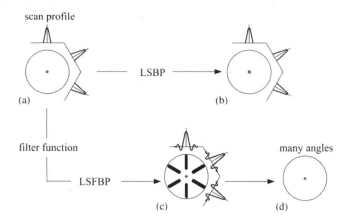

Figure 3.6 Illustration of the linear superposition of back projection (LSBP) and filtered back projection (LSFBP).

3.2.4 X-ray production

A CT system is essentially composed of a radiation source, some radiation detectors and a processing unit, which reconstructs the image from the measures. Radiation generation is provided by an X-ray tube. High energy electrons colliding with a medium can lose their energy by ionisation, excitation of medium atoms and irradiating X-rays. An X-ray generator is a tube in which there is a high vacuum with a cathode that emits electrons and an anode as a target. The emission of X-rays is due to two distinct effects:

- radiation emission caused by the significant deceleration (due to collision) of electrons when they pass through the field of anode nuclei (bremsstrahlung radiation), which in turn causes a continuous X-ray spectrum;
- radiation emission from the anode atoms ionised by incident electrons (characteristic radiation), which causes a line spectrum with a group of characteristic anode lines.

X-ray intensity depends on the electrons in the tube and can be changed either by varying the current intensity in the cathode filament or by adjusting the voltage. In Figure 3.7 it can be seen that X-rays emitted from a tube are polychromatic. This fact causes visible artifacts in the reconstructed image. X-rays generators for diagnostic purposes use voltage between about 30 and 120 kV while the current of the electrons is about 100 mA. When electrons hit the target a very small portion of the energy is converted into X-rays, while the rest is converted into heat. For this reason the target is made up of a high fusion point material such as tungsten.

3.2.5 X-ray detectors

Two types of X-ray detectors are commonly used: solid state and gas ionisation detectors. Xenon ionisation detectors are schematised in Figure 3.8. Each detector consists of a central collecting electrode with a high voltage strip on each side (Kak, 1979). X-ray photons entering a detector chamber cause ionisation with a certain probability. This probability depends on photon energy, detector length, type of gas and pressure. Electrons and ions are

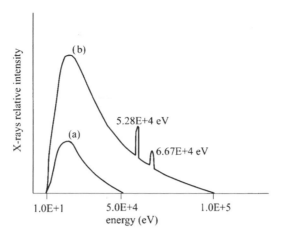

Figure 3.7 Energy spectra for a tungsten anode for the same anode current and for a voltage of 50 (a) and 100 KVp (b).

drawn towards positive and negative electrodes respectively, producing electric signals that can be registered. Usually the voltage applied between the electrodes is 170 V and the gas pressure is 10 atm. The resulting current through the electrodes is a measure of the incident X-ray intensity. The primary advantage of xenon gas detectors is that they can be packed closely. The entrance width defines the spatial resolution, so the image quality can be defined in accordance. For high X-ray beam intensity, the detector can saturate, producing wrong X-ray intensity measures.

The solid state detectors are usually scintillation detectors such as sodium iodide (NaI(Tl)), bismuth germanate (BGO) coupled to a photomultiplier tube (PMT) or cesium iodide crystals coupled to photo-diodes. Scintillation crystals produce flashes of light as they absorb X-ray photons. The light is then converted to electrical signals by a PMT or photodiodes. The performance offered by a PMT still remains limited by its low efficiency, the quantum efficiency, in converting scintillation light into electrons, that is about 25 per cent at 410 nm and lower than 15 per cent at 565 nm, which are the emission peaks of NaI(Tl) and CsI(Tl) crystals respectively. Moreover, the need for high voltages, the sensitivity to magnetic fields and the difficulty of closely packing small scintillator-PMT units in array, represent a practical limitation. Semiconductor photo-detectors represent a new promising solution for scintillation detection. These detectors

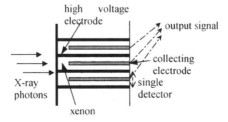

Figure 3.8 Xenon ionisation detectors.

are, in fact, characterised by a higher quantum efficiency with respect to scintillation light, up to 90 per cent at 565 nm. Moreover, they are more compact, immune to magnetic fields and can easily be integrated into monolithic arrays of single units available in a large range of active areas, from few mm^2 up to some cm^2.

3.2.6 Volume reconstruction in computed tomography

In order to get a volume reconstruction, different procedures can be followed:

* step and shoot fan-beam CT;
* single slice helical, or spiral, fan-beam CT;
* multi-slice helical, or spiral, small-cone-beam CT;
* cone-beam CT (CBCT).

The first method consists in two steps: the acquisition of the profiles of a patient slice in a defined position. This step lasts about 1 sec. After the patient is shifted, scan profiles of the contiguous slice are acquired. During the shifting there is no acquisition so as to avoid artifacts due to the patient motion.

The second method, single slice helical, or spiral, fan-beam, is more recent and consists in a continuous rotation of the system tube-detectors with continuous sampling of data during the patient motion in the gantry. The efficiency in the volume coverage is better than that of the previous method and the duty-cycle is about 100 per cent. The pitch is defined as the ratio between the distance path of the patient-carrying table during a 360° rotation of the system's tube-detectors and the slice thickness determined by the beam narrowness. In comparison to the previous method, acquisition time is faster but with a decrease in transverse sampling. In order to have a good image quality it is necessary to work with a pitch value of 1:1. Recently, in order to acquire several slices in a single rotation, multiple-row detectors and a small-cone-beam, in place of a fan-beam, have been adopted.

Finally, the cone-beam mode (CBCT) uses X-ray area detectors and allows for a simultaneous sampling of an entire volume without the patient having to move. Among the volume reconstruction algorithms, the most widespread is the one proposed by Feldkamp (Feldkamp et al., 1984) and consists in an extension of the traditional Filtered Back Projection algorithm.

3.2.7 CT-relief accuracy

An image obtained by computed tomography is characterised by factors such as spatial resolution, uniformity, artifacts, signal to noise ratio (SNR) and contrast, which define the diagnostic image quality. Spatial resolution is the ability of the scanner to distinguish two points under ideal conditions without noise. It depends on many factors such as the entrance width of the detectors, width of the anode focal spot, motion of the patient, and linear and angular sampling. Spatial resolution is an important feature in dental-maxillo-facial imaging, above all in implant planning, because it must correspond to reality. Recent scanners have about 1/10 mm resolution. This parameter is usually obtained by measuring the Modulation Transfer Function (MTF) of the scanner. Suitable phantoms with groups of small cylinders parallel to scanner axes are used to calibrate the scanner. To do this, the cylinders are placed closer and closer to one another, increasing the number of cylinders in a specific space, thus increasing the spatial frequency. The spatial resolution of the scanner is defined as the frequency value where the MTF has its initial value at 50 per cent.

Noise mainly comes from the fluctuations of detected photons number, as quantum noise. If a detector measures N photons, then the error of this measure is $\sqrt{N}$ and the relative error is $\sqrt{N}/N$. The relative error becomes smaller with a higher number of photons and, therefore, with a higher dose for the patient. The quantum noise limits the image contrast and, when the difference between two tissues is comparable to it, they cannot be distinguished.

The image quality is also affected by the different artifacts, which can be caused by the following terms.

- Non-uniform slice thickness can occur when there is a small beam divergence between the source and the detectors. Even if the beam is collimated, it will not be exactly parallel, so some voxels (three-dimensional pixels) intercept different X-ray quantities, according to their position. The central voxels will be thinner than external voxels, causing small distortions in image linearity and resolution.
- Rings can be caused by system calibration problems, imperfect homogeneity of the detectors or low component stability.
- Streaks can be caused by insufficient projection data sampling or beam hardening due to the beam polychromaticity, as low energies are attenuated more than high energies. This effect produces artifacts such as streaks and flares in the vicinity of thick bones and between bones, as observed by Joseph and Spital, 1978, Duerinckx and Macovski, 1978. The beam hardening artifacts can be reduced by using the dual-energy technique, as proposed by Alvarez and Macowski, 1976.
- Streaks can also be caused by scattering radiation (Glover, 1982; Joseph, 1982).
- A cause of defect is the patient motion: this defect can be reduced by improving the velocity of the acquisition procedure.

Some of these artifacts can be limited by the use of adequate filters in acquisition, which reduce the radiation spectrum and the dynamic range of the beam itself. Moreover, there are some error estimation algorithms that can be used once the image has been acquired to reduce the effects of artifacts.

3.3 CT SOFTWARE FOR DENTO-MAXILLO-FACIAL IMAGING

CT-scan-machine software has been significantly improved, not only in relation to new machine parameter control modalities, but mostly for the possibility it offers of producing new types of images. Some of the particular characteristics are represented by 3D visualisation techniques (Figure 3.9). These methodologies reconstruct, from the primary sequence of axial views, a pseudo-three-dimensional representation of a certain region by means of volume rendering techniques.

Moreover, other software tools can be adopted for specific applications in order to exploit the potential of the CT technique in consideration of particular diagnostic needs.

With regard to the dental-maxillo-facial district, in addition to traditional view modes, as axial, coronal and sagittal, two new typology of images are available: panoramic views (PV) and cross-sectional views (CSV). Both these views are obtained by tracing the arc of a parabola, following the route of dental arches, on an axial slice. Panoramic views can then be obtained by interpolating axial views in correspondence with the curve surface orthogonal to the axial plane, identified by the traced arc of the parabola. The result is

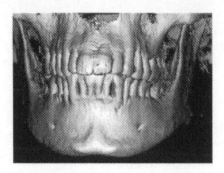

Figure 3.9 Three dimensional rendering of maxillo-facial region

similar to traditional panoramic images, but without the overlapping of structures which is present on film. CSV images are arranged on normal planes with reference to the PVs. They are used to view sections of mandibular or maxillar bone. The characteristics of both types of view modes can be modified in terms of number and distance of images, thickness of interpolation, etc..

Different software packages allow for the simulation of implant positioning in order to verify their dimension and orientation and to evaluate their compatibility with the anatomical site. There has been an increasing interest in CAOS techniques (Computer Aided Oral Surgery), which use CT data to control machines which manufacture masks and guides for the *in vivo* positioning of implants.

3.4 NOTES ON NMR APPLICATIONS IN MAXILLO-FACIAL AREA

Nuclear Magnetic Resonance imaging has not been used very much in maxillo-facial area modelling with regard to applications related to bone tissue. NMR offers a significant contrast resolution for soft tissue, but, at the same time, NMR resolution is less refined than CT resolution. NMR applications for numerical modelling could potentially help in characterising soft tissues, such as the periodontal ligament, the gum and the temporomandibular articulation, if and when resolution capabilities are improved. Moreover, the importance of the application is also more evident for surgical planning in the case of aesthetic or reconstructive surgery.

Integration of information between CT and NMR images will make it possible to develop more complex models, discriminating between hard and soft tissues.

3.5 VIRTUAL MODEL GENERATION

Acquired tomographic images can be used to develop a virtual model of the anatomical region of interest. A virtual model is defined mostly by using the geometrical characteristics; however, the properties related to constitutive materials can also be taken into account. A valid virtual model can be the basis for surgical planning and numerical modelling. A good anatomical representation is the first step in developing a numerical simulation for interpreting the response of the biological tissues belonging to a specific anatomical site.

3.5.1 Geometric model

3.5.1.1 Segmentation techniques

Within the analysis of an image it is essential to first distinguish the specific region of interest from the background. The techniques used to do this are called segmentation techniques. There are several segmentation techniques which represent an important and interesting research topic (Duncan and Ayache, 2000). Depending on the characteristic of the problem treated, one or more techniques can be used together. Each technique is more reliable with regard to specific aspects and it is not possible to define a unique, perfect technique able to cover the general demands of all the technical problems that can be encountered.

3.5.1.1.1 Thresholding technique

This technique is based on the evaluation of a parameter T, called the threshold of brightness, applied to an image to distinguish the region of interest, foreground pixels, from the rest, background pixels. Image values greater than T are object pixels; the others are background pixels.

The main problem is the definition of the limit value to be assumed. There is no unique procedure for this purpose, but rather there are many alternatives. One alternative is the fixed threshold procedure, in which the threshold is chosen independently from the image. If the image is a high contrast image, where the difference between the object of interest and the background is relevant, a constant threshold in the middle of the value range could be precise enough. Another alternative is the histogram-derived threshold. In many cases the threshold is chosen from the brightness histogram of the region of interest, as adaptive thresholding; the brightness histogram reports the number of pixels for each brightness value. The algorithms used benefit from a smoothing of the raw data, to remove small local fluctuations without moving the peak position. Some of the algorithms are described here below.

- The isodata algorithm (Ridler and Calvard, 1978) is an iterative technique. The histogram is first segmented into two parts with an initial threshold value of half of the maximum dynamic range. The sample mean value of brightness in the foreground and background pixels is calculated. The new threshold value is the average of the calculated values. This process is repeated iteratively until the threshold values reach a significant convergence.
- For the gaussian-peak algorithm, it is assumed that there is a single dominant peak and the distribution around the peak is gaussian. Once the maximum is detected, the threshold is evaluated from the standard deviation (σ) of the distribution around the peak itself: $T = \max \pm 2 \bullet \sigma$. The sign depends on the direction of the displacement.
- For the triangle algorithm (Zack et al., 1977), a line between the maximum and the minimum is traced. The distance between this line and the histogram is calculated and the maximum distance (d) is the threshold (Figure 3.10). This methodology is especially effective if modest peaks are present.

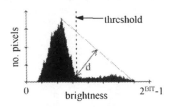

Figure 3.10 Triangle algorithm: d is the maximum distance which determines the threshold.

3.5.1.1.2 *Edge finding techniques*

These techniques are used to try to identify pixels that belong to the edge of the object of interest, according to the following procedures.

- The gradient-based procedure. The main aim of edge finding techniques is to find close borders around the region of interest. In objects with a particularly high signal to noise ratio (SNR), this can be obtained by calculating the gradient, for example with the Sobel gradient operator, and then applying a suitable threshold.
- Zero-crossing based procedure (Canny, 1986). In noisy images, zero-crossings of laplacian images are considered. The principle is based on a model of an ideal step edge (Figure 3.11). The location of the border is where the laplacian crosses zero. Since the laplacian operator involves second derivatives, this leads to a noise increase in images with high spatial frequencies. In order to limit this phenomenon, a smoothing correction is necessary. The most appropriate filter for this smoothing should be as narrow as possible both in frequency domain, to eliminate high frequency noise, and in spatial domain, for a more precise edge localisation. A gaussian filter can be used to obtain minimum bandwidth and spatial width. This means that the image has to be smoothed using an appropriate gaussian procedure, followed by the application of a laplacian filter: laplacian-of-gaussian filter (Marr and Hildreth, 1980).

The performance of each procedure depends on the characteristic of the image under consideration, and often the combined use of different techniques is necessary to have an adequate result.

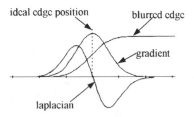

Figure 3.11 Edge position and shape of the first derivative, the gradient, and of the second derivative, the laplacian (not in scale).

3.5.1.2 Border definition

Once the object of interest has been identified, it is necessary to develop its geometrical representation, i.e. a virtual model. The main problem is the geometrical representation of an object using its borders, which in the case of bi-dimensional objects are curves and in three-dimensional objects surfaces.

It is possible to trace a closed linear piecewise curve around the point obtained by the segmentation. Unfortunately, this curve is often irregular, fragmented and practically useless for any application. Therefore, an approximation system is needed to convert a number of points acquired from the segmentation into a mathematical expression, which can represent the object's geometry. The underlying mathematical representation is called a Non-Uniform Rational B-Splines (NURBS) representation (Piegl, 1991). NURBS curves are piecewise polynomial curves which approximate free-form boundaries (Figure 3.12).

NURBS curves offer many advantages. They make it possible to represent arbitrary shapes keeping mathematical precision. Moreover, they make it possible to carry out and maintain a valid control of the curve's shape through its knots and control points, which can be directly manipulated. In this way, complex shapes can be represented with little data. Control points can be thought of as little magnets that attract the curve. The more control points used, the better the fit will be. Some caution in increasing the number of control points is advised because, if the number of points is too high, the fit becomes can actually be worse because, in the case of too many control points, the curve tends to create waving forms.

The definition of a NURBS curve is:

$$C(u) = \frac{\sum_{i=0}^{n} w_i \cdot P_i \cdot N_{i,p}(u)}{\sum_{i=0}^{n} w_i \cdot N_{i,p}(u)} \tag{5}$$

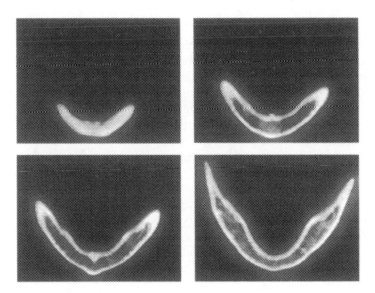

Figure 3.12 Segmented tomographic images, with border lines.

A NURBS curve is, therefore, a vector-valued piecewise rational polynomial where the $w_i \in \mathbb{R}$ are the weights, the $P_i \in \mathbb{R}^3$ are the control points and $N_{i,p}(u)$ are the B-spline basis functions of order p (degree p-1). The B-spline basis functions is defined as:

$$N_{i,0}(u) = \begin{cases} 1 & \text{if } u_i \leq u \leq u_{i+1} \\ 0 & \text{otherwise} \end{cases} \qquad (6)$$

$$N_{i,p}(u) = \frac{u - u_i}{u_{i+p} - u_i} \cdot N_{i,p-1}(u) + \frac{u_{i+p+1} - u}{u_{i+p+1} - u_{i+1}} \cdot N_{i+1,p-1}(u) \qquad (7)$$

where u_i are the knots which form the knots vector $U = \{u_0, u_1, \ldots, u_r\}$. The equation $r = n + p + 1$ defines the relationship between the number of knots, the number of control points and the order of the curve. It can be noticed that an important property of this mathematical representation is the dependence of the curve, in a specific point, on a finite number of control points just before or just after the point. In fact, the movement of a control point affects the curve only in the range $[u_i, u_{i+p+1}]$.

NURBS curve properties make them particularly suitable for modelling, above all because of their invariance to affine transformations. This means that an affine transformation of the entire curve can be obtained easily by applying the transformation to the control points. In addition, every NURBS curve is contained within the convex hull of all the control points. Finally, the curves are differentiable on the interior of the knot spans, and p-k times differentiable at a knot of multiplicity k.

For these reasons, NURBS curves are used to create a series of level curves of the object of interest (Figure 3.13). These cross-section curves are then skinned to develop a three-dimensional surface model (Dimas and Briassoulis, 1999). As an alternative to skinning, to make a three-dimensional model, it is possible to interpolate or approximate a cloud of points obtained from segmentation. This representation implies a careful definition of curve parameters. The configuration of the curves themselves causes computational problems in the application of some algorithms, like those for intersections calculation. A disadvantage of the NURBS mathematical representation regards the increased storage requirements for shapes such as circles and spheres.

It is important to recall that, in order to obtain numerical models such as finite element models from virtual models, the virtual models must be exported in an adequate format to share the geometry with CAD systems. For example, this can be done by using the IGES format (Initial Graphics Exchange Specification).

It is interesting to keep in mind a fundamental consideration: the development of the geometry of a model is not a separate procedure but rather is strictly correlated to the final aim of the model itself. For this reason there is not a standard procedure, nor are there standard parameters, but the model is defined through many compromises that lead to an acceptable level of approximation.

3.5.2 Material characteristics estimation

A model is identified not only by its geometric characteristics, but also on the basis of the properties and behaviour of its materials. Material identification offers great possibilities for development since it is possible to evaluate material properties from a tomographic analysis.

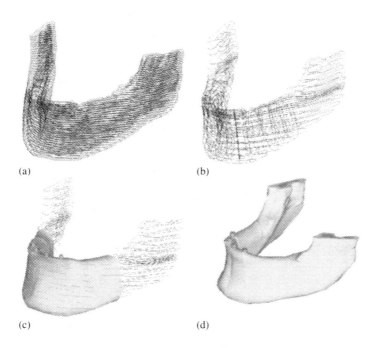

Figure 3.13 Virtual model development: cross-section curves (a) transversal approximation curves (b) surfaces development with the insertion of four implants for surgical planning (c) model with both of cortical and cancellous bone (d).

Even if these techniques have not yet achieved high reliability, they represent a step forward from using the mean values found in literature, in order to obtain a more accurate model for numerical simulation. Custom-made modelling can be obtained completely from medical images, both for site characterisation and for mechanical properties assignment.

3.5.2.1 Densitometry

The tomographic survey gives a map of linear attenuation coefficient μ. In living tissues, the relationship between tomographic measure and density is monotonic and the linear attenuation coefficient is strictly correlated to density. However, there are many other influencing factors, such as atomic number and energy: $\mu = \mu(\rho, Z, E)$.

Methodologies for the quantitative determination of bone density through CT (QCT) (Bacarini et al., 1992) are based on calibration techniques. A calibration phantom is positioned near the object of interest as a reference term. However, the simple comparison with the phantom sometimes leads to an over-estimation of the mineral component because the phantom reproduces the mineral and water components in a limited way, but it excludes the fat component, which is always present. In order to avoid this error, dual energy techniques are used.

New methodologies coming from other fields of application (Van Geet et al., 2000) are very promising for future development, in order to obtain better reliability.

3.5.2.2 *Mechanical properties*

Many efforts have been made to find empirical relationships between the mechanical properties and physical properties of bones. Generally, bone mechanical properties, both cancellous and cortical, seem to be significantly correlated to tissue density. Empirical relationships between mechanical properties of the material and CT-numbers have been developed and are easily available in literature.

3.6 CONCLUSIONS

Computer tomography represents a fundamental task in the approach to dental biomechanics for development of virtual models, rapid prototyping processes, numerical modelling, etc.. Clearly, the evaluation of the accuracy of a virtual model is quite a difficult task because it involves different aspects within a complicated procedure. First of all, it is necessary to consider the quality of the tomographic survey, which depends both on the quality of the instrumentation, as hardware and reconstruction software, and on the nature of the subject. A good survey is the first pre-requisite for a good model, but it isn't always enough. It is also necessary to evaluate the accuracy of the geometry, which is strongly dependent on the segmentation techniques used, which also depend from the characteristics of the subject. Moreover, it must be considered that making an approximation using NURBS curves introduces a new error that clearly depends on the degree and parameters of the curve. Acceptable approximation changes significantly from application to application. For example, in the planning of a virtual model for certain rapid-prototypes, a very detailed mathematical description is not needed because the model is the final product of the application, and, in this case, a good tessellation is enough. On the other hand, in the case of a finite element model for numerical analysis a significant precision is often required, mostly in certain regions. The virtual model is just a step in the analysis that precedes the meshing process that, in and of itself, should entail further approximation. In the end, the assignment of appropriate mechanical properties to materials must be considered. In order to weigh the influence of the approximations assumed on the final reliability of a procedure, a sensitivity analysis can be carried out with regard to different terms affecting the results.

REFERENCES

G. Agati, Elementi di fisica delle radiazioni, Edizioni Libreria Cortina, Torino, 1976.

R.E. Alvarez, A. Macovski, Energy-selective reconstruction in x-ray computerized tomography, Phys. Med. Biol., Vol. 21, pp. 733–744, 1976.

L. Bacarini, R. Giacomich, C. Saccavini, Misura della componente minerale dell'osso: riflessioni sulle apparecchiature – Bone mineral content measurement: reflections on the equipment, Radiol. Med., Vol. 84, pp. 716–724, 1992.

R.A. Brooks, G. Di Chiro, Theory of image reconstruction in computed tomography, Radiology, Vol. 117, pp. 561–572, 1975.

J. Canny, A Computational Approach to Edge Detection, IEEE Transactions on Pattern Analysis and Machine Intelligence, PAMI-8(6), pp. 679–698, 1986.

E. Dimas, D. Briassoulis, 3D geometric modelling based on NURBS: a review, Advances in Engineering Software, Vol. 30, pp. 741–751, 1999.

A.J. Duerinckx, A. Macovski, Polychromatic streak artifacts in computed tomography images, J. Computed Assist. Tomog., Vol. 2, pp. 481–487, 1978.

J.S. Duncan, N. Ayache, Medical image analysis: progress over two decades and the challenges ahead, IEEE Transactions on Pattern Analysis and Machine Intelligence, Vol. 22, Issue 1, pp. 85–106, January 2000.

L.A. Feldkamp, L.C. Davis, J.W. Kress, Practical Cone-Beam Algorithm, J. of Optical Society of America, Vol. A6, pp. 612–619, 1984.

G.H. Glover, Compton scatter effects in CT reconstruction, Med. Phys., Vol. 9, pp. 860–867, 1982.

H.E. Johns, J.R. Cunningham, Physics of radiology, C.C. Thomas, Springfield (Illinois), 1983.

P.M. Joseph, R. Spital, A method for correcting bone induced artifacts in computed tomgraphy scanner, J. Computed Assist. Tomog., Vol. 2, pp. 100–108, 1978.

P.M. Joseph, The effects of scatter in x-ray computed tomography, Med. Phys., Vol. 9, pp. 464–472, 1982.

A.C. Kak, Computerized tomography with x-rays emission and ultrasound sources, Proc. IEEE, Vol. 67, pp. 1245–1727, 1979.

D. Marr, E.C. Hildreth, Theory of edge detection, Proc. R. Soc. London Ser. B., Vol. 207, pp. 187–217, 1980.

M.E. Phelps, Positron Emission Tomography and Autoradiography, Raven Press, New York, 1986.

L. Piegl, On NURBS: a survey, IEEE Computer Graphics and Applications, Vol. 11, Issue 1, pp. 55–71, 1991.

T.W. Ridler, S. Calvard, Picture thresholding using an iterative selection method, IEEE Trans. on Systems, Man, and Cybernetics, SMC-8(8), pp. 630–632, 1978.

M. Van Geet, R. Swennen, M. Wevers, Quantitative analysis of reservoir rocks by microfocus X-ray computerised tomography, Sedimentary Geology, Vol. 132, pp. 25–36, 2000.

G.W. Zack, W.E. Rogers, S.A. Latt, Automatic Measurement of Sister Chromatid Exchange Frequency, Vol. 25, Issue 7, pp. 741–753, 1977.

4 Computer-aided, pre-surgical analysis for oral rehabilitation

*H Van Oosterwyck, J Vander Sloten, J Duyck,
J Van Cleynenbreugel, B Puers, I Naert*

4.1 INTRODUCTION

When the oral function of a person is restored by means of implant-supported oral prostheses different factors must be taken into account for an optimal placement of the oral implants. During pre-surgical planning the restorative dentist and/or the surgeon will determine the position and number of implants that have to be installed, based on the following factors:

- quality and quantity of the host bone;
- anatomical constraints, as mandibular canal or sinuses;
- aesthetics;
- biomechanical factors.

As to the latter, prosthesis design and implant placement may strongly affect implant loading and the mechanical stresses and strains to which the periimplant bone tissues will be subjected. A number of animal experiments, in which adverse loading conditions were applied to oral implants, have shown that excessively high implant loading can lead to pathological overload of the bone tissue, resulting in increased marginal bone loss or even complete loss of osseointegration (Hoshaw et al., 1994; Isidor, 1996; Isidor, 1997; Duyck et al., 2001). In the clinic it has been hypothesised that marginal bone loss can be correlated with unfavourable prosthesis design and parafunctional habits, as clenching or bruxism, both possibly leading to overload. Lindquist et al., 1988 and Ahlqvist et al., 1990, detected increased marginal bone loss around fixtures with long cantilevers, giving raise to high bending moments at the position of the most distal implants, i.e. the implants that are closest to the cantilever. They found a significant difference in bone loss between medially located fixtures and the two distal ones. Quirynen et al., 1992, found that excessive marginal bone loss, more than 1 mm, after the first year of loading and/or fixture loss correlated well with prosthetic and loading conditions that may enhance the risk of overload. These conditions were identified as a lack of anterior contact, the presence of parafunctional habits and full fixed prostheses in both jaws. The risk of excessive marginal bone loading due to high bending moments has been recognised by many authors. Rangert et al., 1989, 1995, have identified a number of hazardous prosthetic conditions and have presented some biomechanical guidelines for treatment planning in order to reduce bending moments:

- inclination of implant axis with respect to direction of vertical occlusal force: avoid large inclinations, since they give raise to large transverse forces and bending moments;

- alignment of the implants along the mandibular or maxillary arch: the straighter the alignment, the larger the bending moment;
- restorative height: increase of bending moments when restorative height (e.g. abutment length) is increased;
- prosthesis with cantilevers extensions: long extensions cause large bending moments;
- cuspal inclination: flatten inclination in order to eliminate large transverse force components;
- bucco-lingual width of the prosthesis: avoid discrepancy between dimensions of occlusal surface and implant diameter;
- centring the occlusal contact: avoid eccentric occlusal forces.

The risk of pathological bone overload not only depends on the *in vivo* encountered occlusal loading, but also must be seen in relation to quality and quantity of the jawbone. If overload should be of major concern, then one should expect a higher failure rate in case of lower bone quality and quantity. This is confirmed by a study of Jaffin and Berman, 1991, who reported high failure rates for Brånemark implants placed in type IV bone. In case of the Brånemark implant the failure rate is two to three times higher in the maxilla than in the mandible, the former having thinner cortical bone and less dense trabecular bone. Esposito et al., 1997, mentioned that the failure rate for Brånemark implants in partially edentulous patients are only half of that in fully edentulous patients. Again, this coincides with the fact that partially edentulous patients normally have less resorbed jaws. The jaw bone quality and quantity will not only have an effect on the risk of overload during function, but also on the initial implant stability, therefore influencing the healing process and early failure rate.

Although biomechanical factors already play a role during pre-surgical planning of oral restoration in the form of certain guidelines, e.g. to reduce the magnitude of bending moments, quantitative information on periimplant bone tissue stresses and strains is completely lacking. It would be of interest to the restorative dentist or the surgeon to quantify pre-operatively the biomechanical effect of varying certain oral restoration parameters, like the number, inclination or position of the oral implants. By applying the finite element method a pre-surgical analysis could be performed to optimise oral restoration parameters from a biomechanical point of view. Since jaw anatomy, bone quality and quantity can strongly vary from patient to patient, it is clear that a patient-dependent approach is necessary for the construction of such finite element models. In this chapter the methodology to develop patient-dependent image-based finite element models of the mandible will be described. Afterwards, results will be shown that illustrate the application of these models in the study of periimplant bone stresses and strains and their dependence on oral restoration parameters. Finally, some aspects of the integration of a biomechanical analysis in a pre-surgical planning environment and the transfer of such a planning to the clinical practice will be shown.

4.2 METHODOLOGY

For the creation of patient-dependent finite element models of skeletal parts like the mandible, both the geometry and the bone tissue distribution, as cortical bone thickness or trabecular bone density, must be implemented patient-dependently. When a patient has to be treated with oral implants it has become a regular clinical procedure to take a preoperative CT scan in order to assess the bone quality and quantity. The CT slices are a representation of the spatial distribution of the linear attenuation coefficient within an object or patient. The absolute image grey-values (CT numbers) are normally given in Hounsfield units (HU) that are defined as $[(\mu - \mu_{H_2O})/\mu_{H_2O}] \bullet 1000$, in which μ is the attenuation coefficient of a material and μ_{H_2O} is the attenuation coefficient of water. The digital preoperative CT data can be used to implement the patient-dependent anatomy of the mandible and the bone heterogeneity. The implementation of both aspects will be further described in the next paragraphs.

4.2.1 CT-based anatomical modelling

Different approaches in the development of CT-based finite element models have been applied in orthopaedics, such as the geometry-based and the voxel-based approach. With the first method a geometrical model, consisting of either curves or surfaces is constructed before meshing (Marom and Linden, 1990; Merz et al., 1996; Lengsfeld et al., 1998). This method results in smooth bone surfaces and implant-bone interfaces, but can be time-consuming and less robust. In case of the voxel-based method groups of voxels in the CT data are converted into hexahedral elements. The method gives rise to stair-like surfaces and interfaces with implants, but is fast and robust, therefore easy to automate. Examples of the voxel-based approach in the field of orthopaedics are the work of Keyak et al., 1990, 1998, Guldberg et al., 1998 and Lengsfeld et al., 1998. Since we are interested in the stress transfer at the implant-bone interface, the voxel-based method is less suitable for our applications, because the description of the actual stress field within the periimplant bone tissue can result very coarse. Therefore, the geometry-based approach was preferred. The modelling procedure will be illustrated here for an oral restoration, consisting of a fixed partial prosthesis in the right side of the mandible.

CAD model of the jaw bone

In a first step the bone tissue must be segmented in the CT images, which was done by specifying a threshold CT value, that separates bone from soft tissue. In some regions of the mandible it is very difficult to distinguish between cortical bone and dense trabecular bone, suggesting that a thresholding operation is insufficient to segment cortical from trabecular bone. Therefore, no attempt was made to segment cortical from trabecular bone or to build separate models for cortical and trabecular bone. The discrimination between cortical and trabecular bone was accomplished in a later stage of the modelling procedure, when the CT-based elastic properties were implemented. In order to convert the segmented bone tissue into a geometrical model of the jaw, contours, mathematically represented as polylines, that define the outer periosteal surface of the jaw are determined in each CT slice. Bone segmentation and contour determination were performed within a medical image processing software package. The set of contours was transferred by means of a neutral file format (IGES) to a computer-aided design (CAD) software package, where a solid model of the jaw was created by fitting a surface to the contours. However, difficulties arise when a certain contour branches into two or more contours in an adjacent image slice, as depicted in Figure 4.1 (a). For such situations it is not possible to create one continuous surface through the set of curves automatically. One could create separate surfaces for the original set of contours and the branching set of contours, and then join them together by adding small surfaces that bridge the gaps between the different surfaces. In this way, surface discontinuities and very small surface entities would originate, that lead to substantial difficulties in finite element mesh definition.

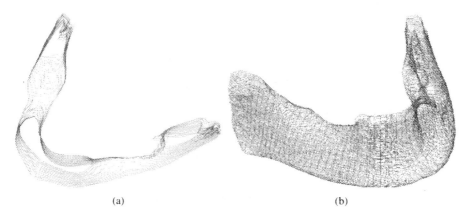

(a)   (b)

Figure 4.1 Contours of the outer surface of a patient's mandible: one contour branches into three
groups of contours (a), original set of contours, lying in parallel planes and re-sliced
set of contours (b).

A more elegant solution is to define a new set of contours by intersecting the old set with
a fan of planes lying perpendicular to the mandibular arch. This new set does not contain any
branching contours, so that it is now easy to construct a surface. The result of the re-slicing
operation is depicted in Figure 4.1 (b), together with the original set of contours. In a final step
a NURBS (Non-Uniform Relational B-Spline) surface was fitted to the re-sliced contours.

CAD model of implants

Many of the commercially available oral implants have a screw-shaped geometry. In order to
limit the total number of elements in the finite element model the implant geometry was simplified to a cylinder with a conical apex. Both fixture and abutment were modelled. Most screw-
type implants, like e.g. the Brånemark implant, have a smooth collar or neck that precedes the
threaded part of the implant. In order to discern both fixture parts in the solid model the fixture
model consisted of two different cylinders. In this way different implant-bone interface conditions could be implemented for the different fixture parts, as will be discussed below.

The way the position of the implants is incorporated in the CAD model depends on the
type of application. If the patient-dependent finite element analysis is performed preoperatively, as part of a biomechanical optimisation of the implant position, the implant position
in the CAD model must correspond to the planning of the restorative dentist. This planning
can be performed in a CT image-based preoperative planning environment, and can be easily transferred, by means of a neutral file format, like IGES, to the CAD environment, if the
same coordinate system is used in both environments.

If the analysis is performed post-operatively the real implant positions must be incorporated correctly. This can be done based on a postoperative CT of the same patient, after the
postoperative CT data has been transformed and matched to the preoperative CT data
(Maes et al., 1997). In this way identity of the coordinate system in preoperative and
postoperative CT is ensured. This approach was followed for the patient model shown in
this chapter. Implant position was derived from the postoperative CT, matched to the
preoperative CT, by segmenting the implants.

Finite element model

Tetrahedral meshes were generated for every part of the CAD model by making use of automatic mesh generators by pre and post processors. Before the mesh was constructed for the mandible, the CAD model of the mandible was split into different parts. In this way, different mesh densities can be applied to different mandibular regions. Since we are merely interested in the stress and strain distribution around the implants, a fine mesh must be created here. On the other hand, much coarser meshes are acceptable in more distal regions, so that the total number of elements can be limited. The final mesh is shown in Figure 4.2 and consists of 153,934 4-noded tetrahedral elements and 30,190 nodes.

Different implant-bone interface conditions were implemented for the smooth and the threaded part of the fixture. For the smooth neck a finite interfacial strength was implemented, allowing relative motion, both in the tangential and the normal direction, at the interface when interfacial stresses exceed the interfacial strength. An infinite interfacial strength was utilised for the threaded part, impeding all relative motion.

4.2.2 CT-based bone properties

Many researchers have studied the relation between CT values and apparent Young's modulus of trabecular bone for excised bone samples from various anatomical locations, giving raise to different equations and different correlation coefficients, varying between 0.43 and 0.9 (Hvid et al., 1989; Ciarelli et al., 1991; Rho et al., 1995). Others have investigated a possible relation between cortical bone mechanical properties and CT values, but generally found only a weak correlation (Snyder and Schneider, 1991; Rho et al., 1995). One must be aware of certain limitations of these relations.

The CT values of bone tissue, or any other material, are dependent on the CT scan protocol that is clinically applied: when different settings are applied, different CT values would be obtained for the same material. Therefore, the absolute CT values, and thus the relation between CT value and Young's modulus, are only useful when the CT scanner is calibrated with a phantom, containing known material densities. A relationship between CT

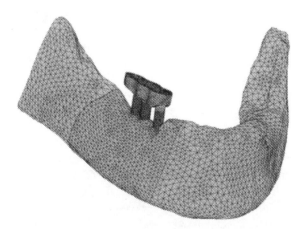

Figure 4.2 Finite element model for a patient wearing a fixed partial prosthesis in the mandible. A finer mesh has been constructed for the part of the mandible around the implants.

value and Young's modulus reported in literature can be applied by other researchers, provided that the relation between CT value and phantom density is given.

The relation between CT values and Young's modulus has been established for excised bones or bone samples without soft tissues surrounding the bone. Although efforts can be made to simulate the soft tissues, e.g. by embedding the bone in a plastic cylinder filled with water, the experimental situation cannot entirely mimic the clinical situation. Moreover the relations are site-dependent: different relations are found for e.g. the femur and the vertebra. As a result, it seems logical that these relations will only allow for a qualitative rather than a quantitative assessment of bone elastic properties. Nevertheless, by applying CT-based properties, the heterogeneity of trabecular bone can be implemented in the finite element model, which is already much closer to reality than assuming a homogeneous bone tissue distribution.

For each tetrahedral element of the bone mesh the Young's modulus was calculated individually, based on the CT number in the patient's preoperative CT data. Per element nine entry points were selected: the four vertices of the tetrahedron; the centroid of the tetrahedron, which is the element integration point; for a tetrahedron with given vector coordinate $v_i(x_i, y_i, z_i)$ of the i-th vertex, the vector coordinate of the centroid $v_c(x_c, y_c, z_c)$ was calculated as quarter portion of the summation of v_i terms; the centroids of four subtetrahedrons: in order to have additional entry points the centroids of four subtetrahedrons were calculated for each element; each subtetrahedron was constructed by replacing one of the four tetrahedral nodes by the tetrahedral centroid.

For each entry point the CT number in the corresponding point in the preoperative CT data was determined. The corresponding Young's modulus was then calculated by applying either a linear or a quadratic relation between CT number and Young's modulus. One relation was used over the entire range of CT numbers, pertaining to bone, i.e. for CT numbers larger than a predefined threshold value that separates bone from soft tissue. The relations that were implemented are shown graphically in Figure 4.3.

The maximum CT number for cortical bone, encountered in the CT data for the specific patient was attributed a Young's modulus of 15500 MPa (Dechow et al., 1993). For CT numbers lower than the threshold value between bone and soft tissue a very low Young's modulus was attributed, typically 0.01–1 MPa. As can be noticed in Figure 4.3, the choice of the threshold value also influences the relation between CT number and Young's modulus.

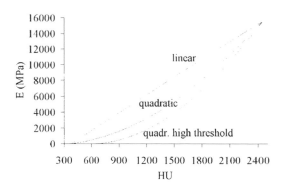

Figure 4.3 Relations between CT number expressed in HU and Young's modulus, used for the calculation of CT-based elastic bone properties: one linear relation and two quadratic relations (with different thresholds between soft tissue and bone) were evaluated.

Once the Young's modulus was calculated in all entry points, the Young's modulus in each element was determined by averaging the values. For the elements at the surface of the mandible, a different approach was followed.

The CT numbers at the bone perimeter are unreliable and are an underestimation of the real values. If the element Young's modulus would be calculated here as the average of all entry points, the Young's modulus would be underestimated as well. To compensate for this error, the Young's modulus for the elements at the bone perimeter were calculated, based on the maximum CT number of its entry points.

In order to reduce the number of different Young's moduli in the finite element model, fixed values were defined between the minimum and maximum Young's modulus and each element modulus is rounded to the nearest fixed value. Suppose δ is a small value, then the fixed values were taken as E_{min}, $E_{min}(1 + \delta)$, $E_{min}(1 + \delta)^2, \ldots$, E_{max}. In this way, the maximum relative error that was introduced is smaller than $\delta/2$. The value of δ was taken here as 0.1, so that the maximum relative error is smaller than 5 per cent.

The Young's modulus distribution in the finite element model was compared with the patient's CT data. Qualitatively, linear and quadratic relations between CT number and Young's modulus produce similar distributions, but quantitatively the calculated Young's moduli are dependent on the choice of the relation. The example in Figure 4.4, taken for a quadratic relation between HU and Young's modulus, illustrates the good resemblance between the Young's modulus distribution in the finite element model and the bone tissue distribution in CT. Especially in the implant region, the correspondence is very good, since smaller finite elements were used here. As a result, even tiny dense trabecular bone islands can be captured in the finite element model.

The cortical bone at the alveolar bone ridge is in general much thinner than the basal bone. This also appeared in the patient's CT data. Besides, the CT values of the alveolar bone ridge were generally much lower than the CT values of cortical bone at other locations.

Low Young's moduli were calculated for the alveolar process and implemented in the finite element model, as can be seen in Figure 4.5. Especially in case of a quadratic relation, low values, lower than 4000 MPa, appeared in the molar region at both sides of the mandible.

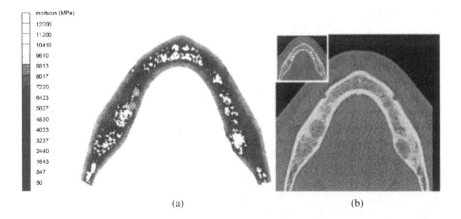

(a)   (b)

Figure 4.4 Comparison between the Young's modulus distribution in the finite element model (a) and the tissue distribution in the preoperative CT (b) for an xy plane. The Young's modulus was calculated for a quadratic relation. Tissue with a modulus smaller than 50 MPa is omitted from the modulus distribution. The postoperative CT image is shown in the inset.

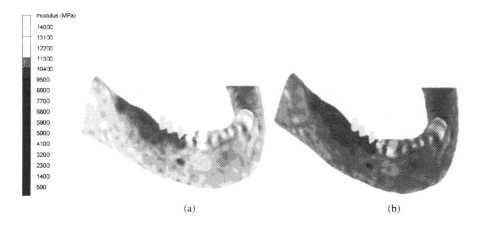

Figure 4.5 Young's modulus distribution at the periosteal surface for a linear (a) and a quadratic (b) relationship.

4.3 ANALYSIS DEVELOPED

4.3.1 Influence of oral restoration parameters on bone loading

The influence of the following parameters was investigated:

- prosthesis material properties: metal alloy, E = 88000 MPa, acrylic resin, E = 2260 MPa;
- number of supporting implants: three versus two supporting implants; in case of two implants the abutment of the middle implant was omitted in the model, so that the middle fixture was not connected to the prosthesis;
- implant inclination: the effect of implant inclination on bone loading was examined here by varying the inclination of the distal implant; with respect to the original situation the inclination was increased of 10° towards the oral-lingual side of the mandible, as shown in Figure 4.6.

Instead of using the finite element model of the entire mandible (Figure 4.2), a model that only takes into account the right and frontal region of the mandible, was applied in order to

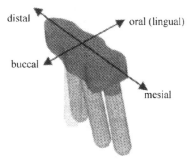

Figure 4.6 The inclination of the distal implant is varied of 10° towards the oral-lingual side of the mandible.

reduce the total number of elements. This does not compromise the validity of the results, since we were merely interested in the relative effect of the investigated parameters. For this study homogeneous instead of heterogeneous elastic properties were assigned to cortical, E = 15500 MPa, v = 0.31, and trabecular bone, E = 300 MPa, v = 0.3. In this way, the different stress and strain results only reflect the influence of the considered parameters and are more generally applicable. If bone heterogeneity were incorporated in the model, then this heterogeneity could interfere with the general tendencies in the results. In particular, when implant inclination is changed, the implant could be placed in bone tissue with elastic properties that strongly differ from the original situation. Therefore, a patient-dependent pre-surgical biomechanical analysis of the influence of oral restoration parameters will require that not only the anatomy, but also the bone heterogeneity be CT-based.

Influence of prosthesis material and number of implants

The use of a resin prosthesis resulted in higher stresses and strains in the marginal bone region around all implants than in case of a metal prosthesis. The effect of prosthesis stiffness was studied for three different loading conditions with either three or two supporting implants. A 50 N bite force was applied perpendicular to the occlusal surface of the prosthesis at three different locations: above the mesial implant, above the middle implant and between middle and distal implant. The bite forces were applied as distributed forces on a number of selected element faces. The effect of prosthesis stiffness on the average Von Mises stress at the marginal bone edge is presented in Figure 4.7. One average value was calculated by evaluating the Von Mises stress along a path that runs along the marginal bone edge of the three implants. In general the stress increase due to the use of a resin prosthesis is higher when the prosthesis is supported by only 2 implants, especially if the bite force is applied in the middle of the prosthesis.

Based on these results one can conclude that a resin prosthesis may produce less favourable stress distributions in the marginal bone, with respect to the risk of marginal bone overload, when a static biting force is applied.

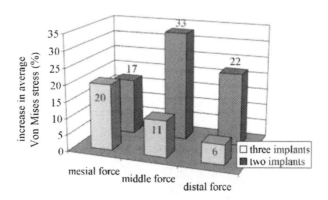

Figure 4.7 Influence of prosthesis material on the average Von Mises stress at the marginal bone level. The increase (in per cent) of the average Von Mises stress in case of a resin prosthesis, relative to the value in case of a metal prosthesis, is calculated for three different loading conditions: a 50 N bite force is applied at respectively the mesial, middle and distal occlusal point. Results are presented for 3 and 2 supporting implants, respectively.

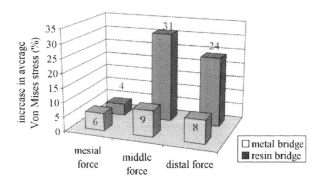

Figure 4.8 Influence of number of supporting implants on the average Von Mises stress at the marginal bone level. The increase (in per cent) of the average Von Mises stress in case of two implants, relative to the value in case of 3 implants, is calculated for three different loading conditions: a 50 N bite force is applied at respectively the mesial, middle and distal occlusal point. Results are presented for respectively a metal and a resin prosthesis.

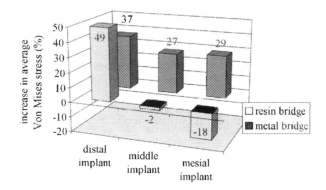

Figure 4.9 Increase (in per cent) of the average Von Mises stress, with respect to the original situation, due to an increased inclination of the distal implant in case of a 100 N vertical force. Average values are calculated at the marginal bone level around each individual implant.

Functional loads during chewing are however dynamic, so that the viscous properties of the acrylic resin might dampen the impact loads. Anyway, the evaluation of this aspect requires the use of more refined finite element analyses.

The use of two instead of three supporting implants leads to higher peak and average stresses for all loading conditions. This is illustrated in Figure 4.8 for the average Von Mises stress in the marginal bone. The effect is much more pronounced in case of a resin prosthesis. Since the stress increase for a metal prosthesis is only very moderate, one can argue that from a biomechanical point of view two instead of three supporting implants are acceptable with respect to bone loading in case of a metal prosthesis.

Influence of implant inclination

The effect of implant inclination was studied for a 100 N vertical force, perpendicular to the occlusal surface, applied between the middle and the distal implant. Results strongly depend on the prosthesis material, as shown in Figure 4.9. Average Von Mises stresses were calculated at the marginal bone level around each individual implant, in contrast to the diagrams in Figures 4.7 and 4.8, where overall average values were calculated. A larger inclination of the distal implant results in higher average Von Mises stresses around all implants when a metal prosthesis is used. A different situation originates when a resin prosthesis is used: for the same loading condition substantially higher stresses exist around the distal implant, but for the unchanged mesial and middle implant, stresses are reduced.

As to the distal implant results seem logical. Indeed, if the implant inclination is increased the misalignment between implant axis and force vector is raised as well, so that the transverse force component, perpendicular to the implant axis, becomes more important. Other researchers have also reported a considerable marginal bone stress increase in case of horizontal (transverse) force application (Clift et al., 1992; Holmes et al., 1992; Clift et al., 1993; Meyer et al., 1993; Meyer et al., 1996). The influence on the stresses in the marginal bone around the other implants, which orientation was not changed, is less obvious. In case of the stiffer metal prosthesis the misalignment of one implant has a negative influence on the stress distribution around all implants, while a different condition is accounted for the resin prosthesis.

4.3.2 *In vivo* bone loading patterns

The results in the previous paragraph illustrate the use of patient-dependent modelling as a tool to compare different oral restorations from a biomechanical point of view. In this way patient-dependent finite element models can contribute to a pre-surgical planning of the oral restoration for an individual patient. These results do however not provide an answer to the following questions:

- is there a direct connection between clinically observed marginal bone loss and peri-implant bone loading?
- which loading levels are tolerable for the bone, i.e. does not impede osseointegration or even enhances osseointegration?
- can we identify clinical situations where the encountered bone loading conditions lead to excessive marginal bone loss or even complete loss of osseointegration?

Again, a patient-dependent approach is needed to try to answer to these questions. In this case not only the jaw anatomy and bone heterogeneity, but also the implant position and implant loading must be incorporated patient-dependently. The implant position can be implemented correctly based on a postoperative CT, as was previously described.

The *in vivo* implant loads were measured by means of strain-gauged abutments. Three strain gauges were mounted on the outer surface of the abutment cylinder wall, each 120° apart, at the same height. All strain gauges were aligned parallel to the abutment axis and measure the local axial normal strain of the abutment cylinder. These measurements allow to calculate the magnitude of the axial force and the magnitude and direction of the bending moment for each abutment (Duyck et al., 2000a, 2000b).

By applying the *in vivo* measured implant loads to the CT-based finite element model, the corresponding bone stresses and strains can be calculated. The CT-based model, described in the previous paragraphs can serve here as an example. The *in vivo* load measurements, performed for this patient, involved functional tasks, like chewing, maximal biting and clenching. From a clinical point of view, it is most interesting to calculate the bone loading patterns for a loading regime that produces the highest implant loads, in order to verify whether bone overload could be a clinical risk for the patient. For this reason, results for maximal clenching are presented here. The applied *in vivo* measured implant loads are summarised in Table 4.1.

As mentioned in paragraph 2.2 either a linear or quadratic relation between CT number and Young's modulus was implemented, which resulted in different values of Young's modulus. Besides, the choice of the threshold value between bone and soft tissue influenced these values as well. The effect of the choice of relation (linear versus quadratic) and of the threshold value on the calculated bone stresses and strains was assessed for the maximal clenching task. Similar stress and strain distributions at the periosteal bone surface were calculated for the implemented relations, as can be appreciated from Figure 4.10. Quantitative results did not strongly differ as to their absolute values: the maximum Von Mises stress in the marginal bone region, which occurred around the middle implant, amounted to 5.3 and 4.7 MPa for the linear and quadratic relation respectively. Choosing a higher threshold value between soft tissue and bone (300 HU higher than in the first series of analyses) resulted, for a quadratic relation, in a maximum Von Mises stress of 5.7 MPa, which presents an increase of 21 per cent, compared to the results for a quadratic relation with a lower threshold.

Table 4.1 Implant loads, corresponding to maximal clenching for a selected patient, wearing a fixed partial prosthesis: axial force (Ax), x and y component of bending moment (My, Mz). Positive axial forces are compressive forces. The components of the bending moment are given within a local coordinate system, fixed to the abutment

	Mesial implant	*Middle implant*	*Distal implant*
Ax (N)	− 0.30	169.02	− 5.97
My (Ncm)	0.45	− 0.52	− 1.59
Mz (Ncm)	− 5.33	− 5.76	− 1.78

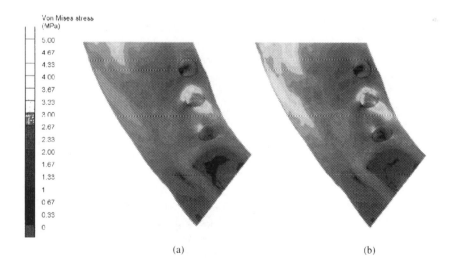

(a) (b)

Figure 4.10 Von Mises stress distribution in cortical bone around the implants in case of maximal clenching (cf. table 4.1) Only the mandibular part around the implants is shown. Heterogeneous bone properties were implemented by means of a linear (a) and a quadratic (b) relation between CT number and Young's modulus.

4.4 PRE-SURGICAL ANALYSIS

Results were shown that illustrate the influence of a number of oral restoration parameters on bone stresses for a patient wearing a fixed partial prosthesis in the mandible. These results clearly demonstrate the added value of a presurgical patient-dependent finite element analysis to a presurgical planning. Such an analysis can quantify the biomechanical effect, in terms of bone stresses or strains, of a change of oral restoration parameters for this patient, like the number of supporting implants and implant position. Furthermore, the results demonstrate that in many cases these biomechanical effects should be carefully evaluated. Again, this proves the validity of a pre-surgical analysis to gain insight in the biomechanical effect of an oral restoration planning. As to the influence of prosthesis material, one could have expected that a stiffer prosthesis would impede more the free deformation of the mandible and that for this reason the metal prosthesis would lead to higher stress concentrations around the implants. Another hypothesis could have been that when a bite force is applied above a certain implant that is connected via a resin prosthesis, the load is less evenly distributed over the connected implants than in case of a metal prosthesis. As a result, one could have expected that the stresses around the directly loaded implant would be higher for a resin prosthesis, while the stresses around the distal implants would be lower. In fact, these hypotheses are not confirmed by the results. A resin prosthesis may produce higher stress concentrations at the marginal bone level around every implant in case of a static bite force. As to the influence of implant inclination, less obvious results were found as well.

The integration of a pre-surgical finite element analysis in a pre-surgical planning environment could be an additional tool to discriminate between different alternative oral restorations. Suppose a restorative dentist and/or surgeon determine the position and number of implants for a patient's oral treatment, based on anatomical and esthetical grounds, and a number of valid alternatives would be retained. An additional biomechanical analysis of these alternatives by means of patient-dependent finite element modelling could help the restorative dentist or surgeon to decide for the most optimal oral restoration. This implies that biomechanical criteria exist to select the biomechanically most optimal treatment. Since animal experimental and clinical research suggest that overload could be a cause of marginal bone loss or even loss of integration, a possible criterion could be to minimise the overall maximum stress or strain.

A difficulty lies in the selection of relevant loading conditions to be analysed presurgically. Indeed, a standardised oral implant loading condition probably does not exist due to large inter-patient variability. Even within the same patient, a large variability can be expected during different (para)functional tasks. One way to deal with this problem is to select a number of arbitrary loading conditions and to study the influence of oral rehabilitation parameters for these loading conditions.

In order to be fully effective in a pre-surgical planning environment not only accuracy and validity, but also robustness, speed and flexibility are important aspects for patient-dependent modelling. The creation of a patient-dependent, CT-based finite element model with the currently developed procedures is still a matter of days, which is unacceptable for an efficient integration in a planning environment. A geometry-based (CAD-based) approach was followed here to create anatomical finite element models. The creation of a CAD surface to describe the jaw anatomy is the most time-consuming and less robust step in the procedure. Therefore, it will be interesting to investigate alternative methods that interface directly between CT and modelling, without the necessity of an intermediate CAD step, and still produce smooth model boundaries. Furthermore, when oral restoration parameters, like implant position, length or inclination are varied, the finite element mesh for the jaw must be adaptable in an efficient way, without the need of creating a completely new mesh. To a certain extent, this was already implemented in the current procedure: the model of the mandible was divided in different parts and only the mesh for the part around the implants was reconstructed when implant inclination was varied. Another important aspect can be computation time.

The validity of a pre-surgical biomechanical analysis will only increase if the knowledge of the role of mechanical load in periimplant bone response is increased. Although clinical studies suggest the role of mechanical (over)load, much more quantitative data is needed in the study of the relation between *in vivo* bone loading and *in vivo* bone response.

4.5 FROM PLANNING TO CLINICAL PRACTICE: A TECHNOLOGICAL CHALLENGE

From the previous paragraphs and from literature it is clear that bone stresses and strains are sensitive to the exact placement of the implant in cases of dental rehabilitation with oral implants. During the presurgical planning phase the implants are positioned, taking into account aesthetic, anatomical and biomechanical constraints (Verstreken et al., 1996; 1998, 2000). It is certainly not obvious that the surgeon can, during surgery, reproduce this planning with the required accuracy. Technology may here contribute to achieve a sufficient amount of accuracy when placing the implants in the oral cavity.

Medical images are the basis for the presurgical planning, and may be used to guide the surgeon when introducing the implants in the bone. Indeed, more and more medical images are becoming the central database for patient treatment: they play a key role in the planning of surgery, but also in the surgery itself and in the post-operative follow-up. Among the technological tools that have been developed to assist the surgeon, we mention navigation systems, robotics and personalized mechanical guides. In navigation systems, a camera system monitors the position of markers attached to the bone and of markers attached to the surgical instruments. Hence it is possible to track the relative position of the instruments with respect to the bone, and compare this with the data of a presurgical planning (Hassfeld and Muhling, 2001). Robotic surgical devices have also been developed. The data of a presurgical planning are translated into robot commands, and here too planned trajectories are realised with very high accuracy (Davies, 2000). In all computer assisted surgery systems, registration is a very important phase. It refers to the establishment of the transformation matrix between the anatomic volumes, as they are visualised and available in the presurgical planning system, and the anatomic volumes that are available during surgery itself. Registration is most often based upon digitising a number of anatomic reference points or markers during surgery, and comparing these with the medical image information of the same anatomic object. It is often a long and tedious procedure, which may be repeated a couple of times to achieve a sufficient amount of accuracy. Medical image based, personalized mechanical guides to assist the surgeon in implant placement provide an attractive alternative (Van Brussel et al., 1999). They incorporate an interface to the bone, assuring a stable, unique and correct fit of the guide upon the bone. Also, mechanical guiding elements are integrated (e.g. metal cylinders) to assure a correct position and orientation of the drill with respect to the jawbone. The mechanical drill guide that has been developed (Figure 4.11) covers a rather large area and metal

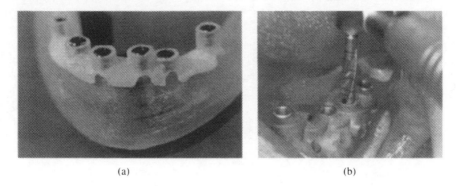

(a)   (b)

Figure. 4.11 Example of a medical image to assist the surgeon in the placement of dental implants (a). Example of a clinical application (b).

cylinders, incorporated in the guide, have an interface with the drill. Cost-effective production is assured by applying rapid prototyping techniques to manufacture the drill guides, such as stereolithography or selective laser sintering.

The implants are planned by the surgeon using a dedicated software, and this planning is the basis for the semi-automatic generation of the mechanical drill guide geometry. During the clinical trial phase, over 50 guides were designed, produced and successfully used. Besides of a design for conventional oral implant placement in the mandible or the maxilla, also a special design for the placement of zygomatic implants was developed and evaluated (Vrielinck, 2001). Compared with navigation and robotic systems, the application of a mechanical drill guide does not require an additional step of registration, since the positioning of the drill guide upon the bone itself assures a proper registration because of the uniqueness of the fit upon the bone. To the best of our knowledge, neither navigation systems nor robotic solutions are available in clinical practice for oral implant placement.

4.6 CONCLUSIONS

A procedure was developed to create patient-dependent finite element models of a jaw, restored with oral implants. CT data was used to implement the patient-dependent jaw anatomy and bone heterogeneity. Patient-dependent models were applied to study the influence of oral restoration parameters on the periimplant bone stress distribution and to study *in vivo* bone loading patterns for a selected patient. Results illustrate the value of patient-dependent modelling, both as a pre-surgical tool to optimise oral treatment from a biomechanical viewpoint and as a tool to investigate the relation between *in vivo* bone loading and *in vivo* bone response for an individual patient. Finally, it should be noted that even the best and most reliable pre-surgical planning system loses its value when the planning cannot be transferred to the surgery. We have described in this chapter a medical image based, personalized drill guide to assist the surgeon to transfer a pre-surgical plan exactly to the surgical theatre.

REFERENCES

J. Ahlqvist, K. Borg, J. Gunne, H. Nilson, M. Olsson, P. Åstrand, Osseointegrated implants in edentulous jaws: a 2-year longitudinal study, International Journal of Oral and Maxillofacial Implants, Vol. 5, pp. 155–163, 1990.

M.J. Ciarelli, S.A. Goldstein, J.L. Kuhn, D.D. Cody, M.B. Brown, Evaluation of orthogonal mechanical properties and density of human trabecular bone from the major metaphyseal regions with materials testing and computed tomography, Journal of Orthopaedic Research, Vol. 9, pp. 674–682, 1991.

S.E. Clift, J. Fisher, C.J. Watson, Finite element stress and strain analysis of the bone surrounding a dental implant: effect of variations in bone modulus, Proceedings of the Institution of Mechanical Engineers, Part H: Journal of Engineering in Medicine, Vol. 206, pp. 233–241, 1992.

S.E. Clift, J. Fisher, C.J. Watson, Stress and strain distribution in the bone surrounding a new design of dental implant: a comparison with a threaded Brånemark type implant, Proceedings of the Institution of Mechanical Engineers, Part H: Journal of Engineering in Medicine, Vol. 207, pp. 133–138, 1993.

B. Davies, A review of robotics in surgery, Proceedings of the Institution of Mechanical Engineers, Part H: Journal of Engineering in Medicine, Vol. 214, pp. 129–140, 2000.

P.C. Dechow, G.A. Nail, C.L. Schwarts-Dabney, R.B. Ashman, Elastic properties of human supra-orbital and mandibular bone, American Journal of Physical Anthropology, Vol. 90, pp. 291–306, 1993.

J. Duyck, S. Lievens, H. Van Oosterwyck, M. De Cooman, J. Vander Sloten, R. Puers, I. Naert, Three-dimensional force measurements on oral implants: a methodological study, Journal of Oral Rehabilitation, Vol. 27, pp. 744–753, 2000a.

J. Duyck, H. Van Oosterwyck, M. De Cooman, J. Vander Sloten, R. Puers, I. Naert, Magnitude and distribution of occlusal forces on oral implants supporting fixed prostheses: an *in vivo* study, Clinical Oral Implants Research, Vol. 11, pp. 465–475, 2000b.

J. Duyck, H.J. Rønold, H. Van Oosterwyck, I. Naert, J. Vander Sloten, J.E. Ellingsen, The influence of static and dynamic loading on the marginal bone behaviour around implants: an animal experimental study, Clinical Oral Implants Research, Vol. 12, pp. 207–218, 2001.

M. Esposito, J.M. Hirsch, U. Lekholm, P. Thomsen, Epidemiology of biological failures of osseointegrated oral implants, 13th European Conference on Biomaterials, Göteborg, Sweden, 1997, pp. 38.

R.E. Guldberg, S.J. Hollister, G.T. Charras, The accuracy of digital image-based finite element models, Transactions of the ASME: Journal of Biomechanical Engineering, Vol. 120, pp. 289–295, 1998.

S. Hassfeld, J. Muhling, Computer assisted oral and maxillofacial surgery – a review and an assessment of technology, International Journal of Oral and Maxillofacial Surgery, Vol. 30, pp. 2–13, 2001.

D.C. Holmes, W.R. Grigsby, V.K. Goel, J.C. Keller, Comparison of stress transmission in the IMZ implant system with polyoxymethylene or titanium intramobile element: a finite element stress analysis, International Journal of Oral and Maxillofacial Implants, Vol. 4, pp. 450–458, 1992.

S.J. Hoshaw, J.B. Brunski, G.V.B. Cochran, Mechanical loading of Brånemark implants affects interfacial bone modelling and remodelling, International Journal of Oral and Maxillofacial Implants, Vol. 9, pp. 345–360, 1994.

I. Hvid, S.M. Bentzen, F. Linde, L. Mosekilde, B. Pongsoipetch, X-ray quantitative computed tomography: the relations to physical properties of proximal tibial trabecular bone specimens, Journal of Biomechanics, Vol. 22, pp. 837–844, 1989.

F. Isidor, Loss of osseointegration caused by occlusal load of oral implants. A clinical and radiographic study in monkeys, Clinical Oral Implants Research, Vol. 7, pp. 143–152, 1996.F. Isidor, Histological evaluation of periimplant bone at implants subjected to occlusal overload or plaque accumulation, Clinical Oral Implants Research, Vol. 8, pp. 1–9, 1997.

R.A. Jaffin, C.L. Berman, The excessive loss of Brånemark fixtures in type IV bone: a 5-year analysis, Journal of Periodontology, Vol. 62, pp. 2–4, 1991.

J.H. Keyak, J.M. Meagher, H.B. Skinner, C.D. Mote, Automated three-dimensional finite element modelling of bone, Journal of Biomechanics, Vol. 12, pp. 389–397, 1990.

J.H. Keyak, S.A. Rossi, K.A. Jones, H.B. Skinner, Prediction of femoral fracture load using automated finite element modelling, Journal of Biomechanics, 1998, Vol. 31, pp. 125–133, 1998.

M. Lengsfeld, J. Schmitt, P. Alter P, J. Kaminsky, R. Leppek, Comparison of geometry-based and CT voxel-based finite element modelling and experimental validation, Medical Engineering and Physics, Vol. 20, pp. 515–522, 1998.

L. Lindquist, B. Rockler, G.E. Carlsson, Bone resorption around fixtures in edentulous patients treated with mandibular fixed tissue-integrated prosthesis, Journal of Prosthetic Dentistry, Vol. 59, pp. 59–63, 1988.

F. Maes, A. Collignon, D. Vandermeulen, G. Marchal, P. Suetens, Multimodality image registration by maximisation of mutual information, IEEE Transactions on Medical Imaging, Vol. 16, pp. 187–198, 1997.

S.A. Marom, M.J. Linden, Computer aided stress analysis of long bones utilising computed tomography, Journal of Biomechanics, Vol. 23, pp. 399–404, 1990.

H.J.A. Meijer, F.J.M. Starmans, W.H.A. Steen, F. Bosman, A three-dimensional, finite element analysis of bone around dental implants in an edentulous human mandible, Archives of Oral Biology, Vol. 38, 491–496, 1993.

H.J.A. Meijer, F.J.M. Starmans, W.H.A. Steen, F. Bosman, Loading conditions of endosseous implants in an edentulous mandible: a three-dimensional, finite element study, Journal of Oral Rehabilitation, Vol. 23, pp. 757–763, 1996.

B. Merz, P. Niederer, R. Müller, P. Rüegsegger, Automated finite element analysis of excised human femora based on precision-QCT, Transactions of the ASME: Journal of Biomechanical Engineering, Vol. 118, pp. 387–390, 1996.

M. Quirynen, I. Naert, D. van Steenberghe, Fixture design and overload influence marginal bone loss and fixture success in the Brånemark system, Clinical Oral Implants Research, Vol. 3, pp. 104–111, 1992.

B. Rangert, J. Gunne, P.O. Glantz, A. Svensson, Vertical load distribution on a three-unit prosthesis supported by a natural tooth and a single Brånemark implant. An *in vivo* study, Clinical Oral Implants Research, Vol. 6, pp. 40–46, 1995.

B. Rangert, T. Jemt, L. Jörneus, Forces and moments on Brånemark implants, International Journal of Oral and Maxillofacial Implants, Vol. 4, pp. 241–247, 1989.

J.Y. Rho, M.C. Hobatho, R.B. Ashman, Relations of mechanical properties to density and CT numbers in human bone, Medical Engineering and Physics, Vol. 17, pp. 347–355, 1995.

S.M. Snyder, E. Schneider, Estimation of mechanical properties of cortical bone by computed tomography, Journal of Orthopaedic Research, Vol. 9, pp. 422–431, 1991.

K. Van Brussel, Ph. Lauweryns, J. Vander Sloten, R. Van Audekercke, G. Fabry, W. Vancraen, Medical image based drill guides can achieve a sub-millimeter accuracy in pedicle screw placement : a clinical study, Proc. Fifth Conference of the European Society for Engineering and Medicine, Barcelona, Spain, May 30-June 2, pp. 49–51, 1999.

K. Verstreken, J. Van Cleynenbreugel, G. Marchal, I. Naert, P. Suetens, D. van Steenberghe, Computer-assisted planning of oral implant surgery: a three-dimensional approach, International Journal of Oral and Maxillofacial Implants, Vol. 11, pp. 806–810, 1996.

K. Verstreken, J. Van Cleynenbreugel, K. Martens, G. Marchal, D. van Steenberghe, P. Suetens, An image-guided planning system for endosseous oral implants, IEEE Transactions on Medical Imaging, Vol. 17, pp. 842–852, 1998.

K. Verstreken, J. Van Cleynenbreugel, D. van Steenberghe, G. Marchal, P. Suetens, An image-guided planning system for endosseous oral implants, In: Computer technology in biomaterials science and engineering (J. Vander Sloten, ed), John Wiley & Sons, Chichester, pp. 192–240, 2000.

R. Vrielinck, La retention des prothèses maxillaries supérieures au moyen d'implants zygomatiques et/ou pérygoïdiens, Le point, mensuel d'information dentaire, Vol. 17, Issue 154, pp. 23–26, 2001.

5 Materials in dental implantology

*E Fernández, FJ Gil, C Aparicio, M Nilsson, S Sarda,
D Rodriguez, MP Ginebra, JM Manero, M Navarro,
J Casals, JA Planell*

5.1 INTRODUCTION

The number of families of biomaterials that can withstand the aggressive environment of the oral cavity is limited. However, implants and medical devices keep growing both in number and in complexity, and there must therefore be a sustained effort in research and development to understand the local and systemic effects of the interaction between the material and the oral cavity. For this reason, the biological, mechanical, physical and chemical properties of dental materials should be considered as forming part of a problem that affects quality, safety and the long-term performance of the medical device.

The purpose of this chapter is to point out some of the ideas and developments that have been carried out recently, to define the key properties of dental implants, in order to improve the reliability of medical devices for dental applications.

Dental implants are usually manufactured in pure commercial titanium because of its biocompatibility and suitable mechanical and corrosion properties (Albrektsson et al., 1981; Mish, 1994; Proubasta et al., 1997). Nowadays, there are two different tendencies in designing implant surfaces. Some techniques have been developed to further increase the roughness of the surface of the implant (Wennerberg, 1996). In the long run, these techniques improve fixation by creating better interaction between the implant and the surrounding tissue. Another approach concerns the techniques that create a coating on the implant (Brånemark et al., 1977; Posner et al., 1980; Carlsson et al., 1986; Brånemark et al., 1987; De Groot et al., 1990; Ducheyne et al., 1990; Lausmaa, 1991; Bruijn et al., 1992; Oshida et al., 1993; Hero et al., 1994; Mann et al., 1994; Metals handbook, 1995; Cook et al., 1998; Park et al., 1998; Cleries, 1999; Loh, 1999). The coating should be able to chemically link with the bone tissue and should not provoke a foreign-body reaction after implantation. The biomaterials that chemically link to the bone are called bioactive and the one most often used is hydroxyapatite, which has been mainly coated using plasma-spray techniques (Cook et al., 1998; Cleries, 1999).

In this context, new ideas keep pushing the development of further innovative technologies to be applied to a new generation of dental implants with better performance in service. These ideas mostly consist in optimising the shot-blasting technique, widely used to increase the surface roughness of dental implants. The objective is to improve not only the bone-implant fixation but also the mechanical and corrosion resistance properties of the implant. Research has also been carried out to develop a two-step treatment. This process combines an increase in surface roughness by the shot-blasting technique with chemical treatments to make the implant surface bioactive. Not only would it take advantage of its surface roughness for the bone-implant fixation, but it would also take advantage of the possibility of inserting an apatite coating, which is chemically linked to the new bone tissue. This method should overcome the problems associated with the degradation of the bioactive coating obtained by traditional methods.

Before going into detail on the aspects highlighted, the next section first presents an overview of relevant information concerning the types and properties of the metallic materials used to manufacture medical devices.

Metals are used in many engineering applications as external and/or internal structural components. Their mechanical properties provide stiffness to the structure and their ability to withstand plastic deformation make it possible to carry out many manufacturing methods (Brunski, 1996).

Metals and alloys for structural applications are characterised by both their high elastic modulus and yield stress. When they come into contact with human tissue, properties such as biocompatibility, corrosion resistance, high static and fatigue strength and fracture toughness are also required.

The main degradation processes, which may lead to the eventual failure of the medical device, are due to fatigue, corrosion, wear and any interaction among them. Though few metallic alloys can be used as biomaterials in dental use, some families of metals and alloys exhibit good properties of fatigue, corrosion and wear. Such properties may even be improved by means of surface modification.

The development of new alloys has significantly contributed to an evolution of surgical procedures in medicine in general, and in hard tissue substitution in particular. Materials which have traditionally been used, such as gold, stainless steel or chromium-cobalt-nickel alloys have been substituted by a new generation of alloys with excellent characteristics of toughness and strain recovery as well as suitable properties of mechanical strength, fatigue and corrosion. These new metal alloys are based on titanium and, jointly with its pure commercial grade, offer great advantages for their use in several biomedical fields such as oral implantology, traumatology, orthopaedics, maxillofacial surgery, etc.. It is important to highlight that, at present, pure grade titanium is the best material used to manufacture dental implants. The following paragraphs will briefly describe conventional alloys and give detailed information on commercial pure grade titanium.

5.2 METALS AND ALLOYS FOR DENTAL IMPLANT DEVICES

The conventional alloys used for medical devices belong to three main metallic systems: austenitic stainless steels, cobalt alloys and titanium alloys (Table 5.1) (Proubasta et al., 1997). These systems exhibit an excellent combination of high strength, relative workability and good resistance to corrosion. The improvements made mainly consist in variations in the chemical

Table 5.1 Conventional alloys used for medical devices

Alloy	Chemical composition	Type
Stainless steel	18 Cr, 12 Ni, 2.5 Mo, < 0.03 C, Fe-balance	AISI – 316L
Cobalt	28 Cr, 6 Mo, 2 Ni, Co-balance	ASTM F75 – CoCr
	20 Cr, 35 Ni, 20, 10 Mo, Co-balance	ASTM F5758 – CoNiCr
Titanium	6 Al, 4 V, Ti-balance	ASTM F136
Pure titanium	100 Ti	ASTM F67

composition, heat treatments and processing technologies in order to improve aspects such as fatigue behaviour, wear, corrosion, ion release and stress transmission to the surrounding tissues.

5.3 TITANIUM AND ITS ALLOYS FOR MEDICAL DEVICES

Commercially pure titanium (CP-Ti) has been used since 1950 in applications requiring mechanical resistance, high corrosion resistance, good shape-ability and good welding capacity (Brunski, 1996). CP-Ti is available in different grades, with different amounts of impurities such as carbon, hydrogen, iron, nitrogen and oxygen. Some CP-Ti alloys can incorporate small amounts of palladium (Ti-0.2Pd) and nickel-molybdenum (Ti-0.3Mo-0.8Ni). These elements report improvements to the corrosion resistance and/or mechanical resistance. Generally speaking, CP-Ti's main impurities consist in more than 1000 ppm of oxygen, iron, nitrogen, carbon and silicon.

Considering that small amounts of interstitial impurities considerably affect the mechanical properties of CP-Ti, looking at the chemical composition of the alloy is not a proper method to differentiate titanium grades. That is why the American Standards for Testing and Materials (ASTM) recommends CP-Ti alloys be classified in four different groups according to their mechanical properties, as shown in Table 5.2. Some of the main characteristics for these different CP-Ti grades are explained in the following subsections.

The limitations related to monophasic-α alloys, such as CP-Ti grades, with low mechanical strength, low formability and fragility lead to the study and development of biphasic-α/β alloys, such as Ti-6Al-4V. Nowadays, the most used titanium alloy is Ti-6Al-4V, representing more than 50 per cent of all titanium tonnage in the world. Its use for medical prostheses is its second largest application.

Ti-6Al-4V is produced in a number of formulations. The oxygen content may vary from 0.08 to more than 0.2 per cent, the nitrogen content may be adjusted up to 0.05 per cent, the aluminum content may reach 6.75 per cent, and the vanadium content may reach 4.5 per cent. The higher the content of these elements, particularly oxygen and nitrogen, the higher is the strength and the lower the ductility and fracture toughness. The ELI grade (Extra Low Interstitial) for surgical applications is a special grade whose principal compositional characteristics are low oxygen and iron contents (5.5–6.5 per cent Al; 0.08 per cent C; 0.25 per cent Fe; 0.012 per cent H; 0.05 per cent N; 0.13 per cent O; 3.5–4.5 per cent V).

ELI Wrought Ti-6Al-4V is a useful material for surgical implants because of its low modulus, good tensile and fatigue properties (Table 5.3), and biological compatibility. It is used for bone screws and for partial and total hip, knee, elbow, jaw, finger, and shoulder replacement joints. It is not used as much as CP-Ti in dental applications because loads borne by the dental implants are not as high as in other surgical applications, and Ti-6Al-4V is not as corrosion resistant as CP-Ti.

Table 5.2 CP-Ti grades according to the ASTM classification

ASTM-grade	Tensile strength (MPa)	Yield strength (MPa)
Grade-1	240	170–310
Grade-2	345	275–450
Grade-3	440	380–550
Grade-4	550	480–655

Table 5.3 Young modulus and tensile strength of Ti-6Al-4V alloys compared to other metallic materials

Material	Young's modulus, E (GPa)	Tensile strength (MPa)
Ti-6Al-4V	105–116	895–1250
Titanium alloys	70–128	240–1500
Aluminum	66–81	70–700
Stainless steel	190–215	400–1500

5.3.1 Grade-1 CP-titanium

The ASTM Grade-1 CP-titanium is chemically the purest. As a consequence of its low content of interstitial elements, it has the lowest mechanical strength and the highest ductility, shape-ability and workability, at room temperature, of all four grades.

Grade-1 is used when maximum workability is required and the main concern is to increase corrosion resistance by reducing both the iron content and the interstitial elements. It has an excellent behaviour from high oxidising environments to medium reducing ones, including chlorides. Grade-1 can be used in continuous service up to 425°C and in discontinuous service up to more than 540°C. Moreover, it has good impact properties even at low temperatures.

The maximum limits by weight of its impurities are 0.18 for oxygen, 0.20 for iron, 0.03 for nitrogen and 0.10 for carbon. The equivalent compositions for specifications other than the ASTM ones should be accounted for by estimating the mechanical properties. As it has been explained, small amounts of interstitial elements can increase the yield strength and decrease the ductility below the specifications for this property. For example, it has been reported that amounts of hydrogen as low as 30–40 ppm can make CP-titanium very brittle.

Grade-1 CP-titanium can be used in all standard-manufacturing processes and has the best ability to be shaped of the four grades. It can be appropriately welded, mechanised, cold-worked, hot-worked and moulded. Its yield strength is comparable to the fully annealed stainless steel AISI-304.

5.3.2 Grade-2 CP-titanium

The ASTM Grade-2 CP-titanium is an ideal material for industrial applications because it has a guaranteed yield strength of a minimum value of 275 MPa. This strength is comparable to the annealed austenitic stainless steel and is used in applications where excellent ductility and shape-ability are needed. Grade-2 has low contents of interstitial elements and as a consequence the corrosion resistance is also improved. It also has good impact properties at low temperatures and an excellent wear and corrosion resistance to saline solutions. It can be used in continuous service up to 425°C and in discontinuous service above 540°C.

Grade-2 has the same maximum content in weight of nitrogen (0.03 per cent) and iron (0.30 per cent) as Grade-1. The maximum allowed concentration of oxygen for Grade-2 is 0.25wt per cent, which is approximately the average value of the interval allowed for Grade-3 (0.18wt per cent-0.40wt per cent). Compared to Grade-1, the concentrations of iron and oxygen in Grade-2 are greater. This results in an increase in tensile strength (240 MPa vs. 345 MPa) and yield strength (170 MPa vs. 275 MPa) but a decrease in ductility (20 per cent vs. 24 per cent) and corrosion resistance. The effect of hydrogen in Grade-2 is similar to that in Grade-1. In fact, hydrogen contents as low as 30–40 ppm make titanium very brittle.

Grade-2 CP-Ti is available in all forms of production. As with the other grades of titanium, it can be welded, mechanised, moulded and cold-worked. Moulded products in Grade-2 CP-Ti make up five per cent of all moulded titanium products. Grade-2 has an annealed *alpha* structure in all its forms of production and it cannot be heat-treated. Figures 5.1 and 5.2 show two magnifications of a single-phase *alpha* structure of Grade-2 CP-Ti; the first has been cold worked, while the second cold worked and then annealed. In general, depending on the amount of cold working done and the time and temperature of the annealing process, equiaxed *alpha* grains with different grain diameters and amount of twins inside the grains can be produced.

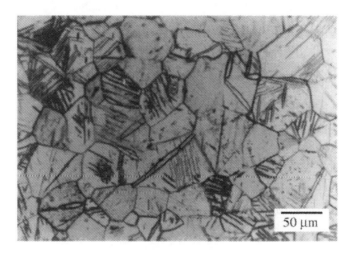

Figure 5.1 Microstructure of cold-worked Grade-2 CP-Ti used in an oral implant.

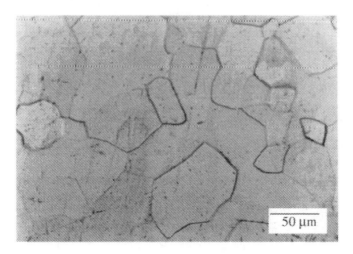

Figure 5.2 Microstructure of annealed Grade-2 CP-titanium used in an oral implant.

5.3.3 Grade-3 CP-titanium

The ASTM Grade-3 CP-titanium has excellent corrosion resistance in environments going from high oxidising to medium reducing, including chlorides. It has excellent specific strength and this is why Grade-3, as well as other titanium alloys, is halfway between high resistance steels and light aluminum alloys. It has good fracture toughness to impact at low temperatures. The maximum limits in weight of iron in Grade-3 is lower than in Grade-4 (0.3 per cent vs. 0.5 per cent) and Grade-3 has the second highest value of oxygen (0.35 per cent) of the four grades. Only Grade-4 has greater mechanical strength than Grade-3.

As has already been said, excessive levels of interstitial/substitutional impurities can increase yield strength and decrease ductility far below the minimum values allowed. Moreover, the corrosion resistance can also be affected by the presence of values of iron and interstitial impurities higher than those allowed. Hydrogen amounts as low as 30–40 ppm will affect Grade-3 in the same manner as the other grades, giving very brittle materials.

Grade-3 is available in all forms of production and can be welded, mechanised and cast. Most of the conformational processes are carried out at room temperature. However, hot production reduces elastic recovery and decreases the effectiveness of the operation. Grade-3 has an annealed *alpha* structure in all its forms of production.

5.3.4 Grade-4 CP-titanium

The ASTM Grade-4 CP-titanium has the highest values of mechanical strength of the four grades. It also has acceptable ductility and conformation. The benefits of high mechanical strength and low density of Grade-4 can be maintained up to moderate temperatures. Its specific mechanical strength is superior to that of stainless steel AISI-301 even at temperatures above 315°C.

Grade-4 has excellent corrosion-fatigue resistance in saline solutions. The stress required to attain fracture after a few million cycles is 50 per cent higher than the stress needed for stainless steel AISI-341.

Grade-4 has the highest content in weight of oxygen (0.40 per cent) and iron (0.50 per cent) of the four CP-Ti grades. A further increase in the iron content and interstitial elements decrease the corrosion resistance. The presence of 30–40 ppm of hydrogen has the same result as in the other grades, creating very brittle materials.

Grade-4 is available in all forms of production and can be mechanised, moulded, welded and cold-worked. All these processes can be performed at room temperature but hot production (between 150 and 425°C) is normally used to reduce the elastic recovery and energy required during production. This method is used to produce complex shapes during manufacturing. Grade-4 has an annealed equiaxed structure in all its forms of production.

5.4 MANUFACTURING PROCESSES OF TITANIUM ALLOYS

Generally speaking, there are two basic ways of generating required shapes following a metal-working process, recalling Dieter, 1976. The first one is the plastic deformation process in which the volume and mass of the metal are preserved. The second way is metal removal or machining processes in which the metal is removed in order to give it the required shape. This is the most commonly used method to manufacture dental implants. However, before describing this process in detail, an overview of the other manufacturing processes used for titanium alloys is presented to highlight the advantages of machining. A look inside on machining dental implants is performed, aiming at knowing how an inappropriate use of the process can alter significantly the properties of the surface and the implant performance itself. This point of view should later introduce the new treatments proposed to increase surface bioactivity of titanium dental implants.

5.4.1 Casting titanium alloys

There are many technological difficulties involved in casting titanium alloys because of the high affinity of melting titanium for the oxygen, nitrogen and hydrogen in the atmosphere as well as for the constituents of the crucibles and moulds. That is why melting should be performed in a vacuum and moulds should be made of compact graphite. The moulding pieces can have the normal defects associated with this process, such as the presence of interior pores due to solidification. Casting titanium alloys can also present a specific defect: the high tendency of interstitial elements to segregate. In this case, the corrosion resistance and mechanical strength of dental implants can be drastically reduced.

5.4.2 Welding titanium alloys

Titanium alloys can be welded by melting if the inert atmosphere or vacuum conditions are rigorously controlled. Welding is limited to titanium alloys with a hexagonal crystalline structure, or *alpha* phase, or to those titanium alloys with less than 20 per cent of cubic structure, or *beta* phase. During welding, oxyacetylene flames cannot be used due to gas contamination; instead, electric arc welding with consumable or not electrode, plasma, electron beam or laser welding techniques can be applied. The low specific heat and low thermal conductivity of titanium are the main factors to consider during welding processes.

Another process to weld titanium alloys is diffusion. This technique has the advantage of dissolving the oxide layer and the surface contaminants at the same time during a dissolving treatment performed at usual conditions, i.e. at 900°C, with a pressure of 1 MPa, for one hour. Since welded joints have about 90 per cent of the bulk strength, this technique is also applied in combination with superplasticity processes.

For certain applications, strong welding conditions can be produced at 1000°C in an inert atmosphere and the contribution of silver, copper and/or titanium-copper alloys.

5.4.3 Forging titanium alloys

Forging is the working of metal into a required shape by hammering or pressing. It is carried out at high temperatures, although certain metals may be cold-forged. There are two major classes of equipment for forging operations. The forging hammer delivers rapid impact blows to the surface of the metal, while the forging press subjects the metal to a slow-speed compressive force.

Titanium alloys can be deformed plastically to obtain different shapes. However, cold forging is difficult if the hexagonal crystalline phase of titanium (*alpha* phase) is the main phase present phase in the alloy. As it is known, hexagonal structures cannot be deformed plastically beyond a certain point. Furthermore, they are textured resulting in severe differences of behaviour in different directions. As far as hot forging is concerned, when the allotropic transformation temperature for titanium (882°C) is surpassed, the *beta* phase, which is cubic, is reached and thus plastic deformation can occur more easily. The hot forging process of titanium is equivalent to the stainless steel one and some alloys can present the superplasticity behaviour.

5.4.4 Powder metallurgy and titanium alloys

The use of the powder metallurgy technology for titanium alloys can reduce the cost of implant production by up to 50 per cent. A titanium powder, which is extremely pure and has a low content of interstitial elements, is needed for this procedure. The powder obtained from a previously prepared titanium sponge is pressed with stresses up to 400 MPa and densities of 90 per cent of the theoretical ones are attained. However, it is difficult to obtain the powder with the proper content of the necessary elements due to the high reactivity of liquid titanium with the gases and refractory materials of the mould. To minimise this problem, techniques such as atomisation by vacuum centrifugation have been developed.

The hot isostatic pressing (HIP) technique, used initially to eliminate defects in moulding pieces, is applied to obtain good pieces sintered to a high density. This technique is performed at a temperature where the cubic crystalline structure for titanium (*beta* phase) is obtained. Normal treatment is at 900°C for two hours in an argon atmosphere at 105 MPa of pressing. The advantage of this type of process is that it produces titanium alloys with greater homogeneity and no texture or anisotropy.

5.5 MACHINING TITANIUM ALLOYS

Machining processes make it possible to obtain the required shape by removing selected areas of the workpiece. Most machining is accomplished by straining a local region of the workpiece by relative motion of the tool and the workpiece. Although mechanical energy is the usual input to most machining processes, some of the newer metal-removal processes use chemical, electrical, or thermal energy. Machining is usually used to produce shapes with high dimensional tolerance, good surface finish, and having a complex geometry. However, machining is often adopted as a secondary processing operation since it is conducted on a workpiece that has already been produced by a primary process such as hot rolling, forging or casting.

Machining titanium alloys has difficulties similar to those for stainless steel. Moreover, the possible local heating caused by machining, which is due to the low thermal properties of titanium alloys, can be a problem. Titanium alloys also have the tendency to block the machine tool due to the high affinity of titanium for other chemical elements. Since machining is the most widely used method to manufacture dental implants, the following subsections give an overview of the typical defects encountered during the process. These defects can be overcome by carefully controlling the factors affecting the machining process. Figure 5.3 shows different details observed in a Scanning Electron Microscope of an endosseous dental implant, which was obtained by machining Grade-3 CP-titanium.

The information that can be gathered by Scanning Electron Microscopy makes it possible to know what the real state of the implant surface is after the machining and sterilisation processes. It can give information regarding the presence of impurities on the surface resulting from the use of lubricants during machining, or even from possible bacterial contamination. It also gives information regarding the effects of the cutting, polishing and finishing processes on the final aspect of the implant surface. As is known from fracture mechanics, any scratch on the surface can act as a stress concentration factor. As a consequence, it can be the origin of a propagating crack initiating at the surface under fatigue conditions. In this situation, when unstable crack propagation

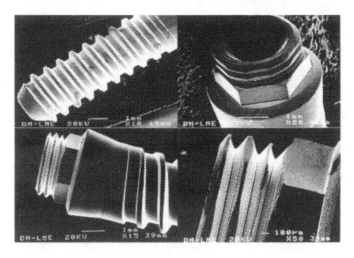

Figure 5.3 Details of an endosseous dental implant observed by electron microscopy.

conditions are attained, the implant will suddenly fail even under mechanical conditions, which are not particularly severe. For example, the image in the lower right-hand corner of Figure 5.3 shows that the upper part of the dental implant can be the weakest one, from a mechanical point of view, because any of the screw rings can be the origin of propagating cracks under fatigue conditions. For this reason, it is very important to polish and finish the surface as well as possible.

Figure 5.4 shows a detail of the body of the screw, as shown in the upper left-hand corner in Figure 5.3, of the dental implant after poor cleaning. Energy Dispersive Spectrometry shows that the chemical composition of the particles and residues caused by machining and/or brushing are made of iron, copper and/or aluminum. These particles on the surface of the dental implant can be dangerous because of their toxicity after implantation.

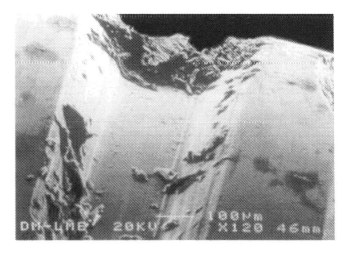

Figure 5.4 Metal particles on the surface of a dental implant after machining and brushing.

Figure 5.5 is another example of the incorrect machining and finishing of a dental implant. In this detail, a chip of metal during shaping, and even after brushing, has not been removed from the surface of the dental implant. The usual practice to avoid this problem is to include a chip-breaker on the rake face of the tool to deflect the chip and cause it to break into short pieces. The accumulation of chip material, as shown in Figure 5.5, is known as a *builtup edge*. It is also important to consider that the machining process is performed using a cutting fluid whose primary functions are to decrease friction and wear and reduce the temperature generated in the cutting area. Furthermore, it washes away the chips produced in the cutting area and protects the newly machined surface against corrosion. Though cutting fluids are usually liquids, they may also be gases.

The procedures here described offer increased tool life, improved surface finish, reduced cutting forces and power consumption, and reduced thermal distortion of the dental implant. Solid lubricants also play a role in improving machinability.

Other steps may also be necessary to avoid contamination of the surface of the implant by deleterious elements, which may have unwanted effects during implantation. These include the use of metallic brushes to remove the chips still attached to the implant (Figure 5.5) and detergents and surfactants to properly clean the entire surface from possible contaminants.

Figure 5.6 shows a dental implant after machining carried out using lubricant oil. Scanning Electron Microscopy shows that a significant amount of lubricant oil has accumulated on several areas of the implant.

Even after cleaning the implant with detergent, Energy Dispersive Spectrometry shows traces of sulphur and toxic elements from the lubricant as well as chlorides and calcium ions from the detergent, as shown in Figure 5.7.

It is important to mention that a metal surface is composed of different films having different thickness. Working outward from the metal substrate, first there is a work-hardened layer of nearly 10000 Å, produced by impact treatment. On the top of this, there is an oxide layer of 100 Å produced by the reaction of the metal to the oxygen in the air. This layer is common in all metals except noble ones, such as gold. Then, there is a three Å absorbed layer, generally of molecules of water vapour and oxygen, produced by the atmosphere. The outmost layer, there are usually greasy or oily films of nearly 30 Å which are a contaminant layer.

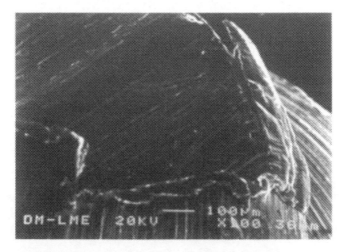

Figure 5.5 Detail of a builtup edge after machining a dental implant.

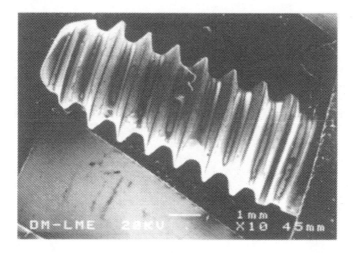

Figure 5.6 Dental implant showing accumulation of lubricant oil in several areas.

Though many believe that unwanted grease film can be removed from a metal surface using a good solvent such as acetone or carbon tetrachloride, this is not the case. The outer layers of the grease film dissolve easily in the solvent. However, the last layer, about 30 Å, is so strongly attached to the metal that it will not go be dissolved by the solution unless the solvent itself is completely free of all grease-type material. In fact, if a perfectly grease-free metal surface is washed in a good commercial purity grade solvent, the metal surface itself will pick up monolayer thickness contaminants from the solvent, because of the high affinity that greasy substances have for clean metal surfaces.

Two simple tests are often used to confirm the cleanliness of a metal surface. In one test a drop of water is placed on the metal surface; this will spread uniformly on a clean surface, but form a well-defined globule on a contaminated surface. The second test consists

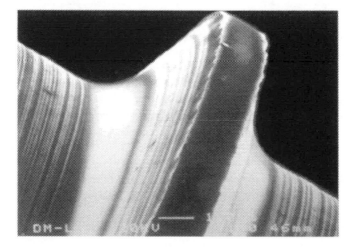

Figure 5.7 Convex area of dental implant with toxic elements, even after cleaning.

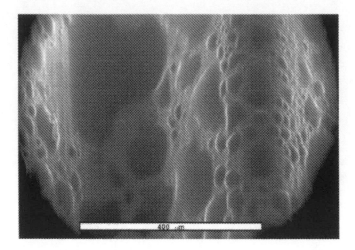

Figure 5.8 Detail of a dental implant showing contamination by accumulation of water drops.

of breathing gently on the surface, thus condensing moisture on it. If the moisture is formed as a mist, rather than as a uniform and invisible film, the surface is contaminated. Both of these tests depend on the fact that water does not wet a grease film but does wet a clean metal surface.

Figure 5.8 shows the results of the second test described above carried out on the surface of a dental implant after careful cleaning, observed in an Environmental Scanning Electron Microscope. As can be seen, the surface is still contaminated.

5.6 SURFACE TREATMENTS ON TITANIUM ALLOYS

5.6.1 Mechanical treatments

It is known that cells attach better to a rough surface than to a smooth one and that rough implants osseointegrate better than smooth ones after implantation. In order to improve long term fixation, the topography of an implant can be modified by increasing its surface roughness; this leads to better interlocking between the implant and bone at the micrometric level. It is generally recognized that the type of surface of the implant affects cell differentiation. Several processes, such as rectification, titanium plasma-spray, surface coatings and photolithography can be used to increase the surface roughness of implants. However, the shot-blasting treatment is the one used most in dental implants. It consists in the projection of small sized abrasive particles against the titanium surface at a high pressure. The energy of the impacting particles cause the plastic deformation of the surface, thus increasing its roughness. Figures 5.9 and 5.10 show a detail of a dental implant before and after the shot-blasting treatment.

It is evident from Figure 5.10 that an enormous increase in surface roughness has been produced by the treatment. This increase should improve the long term bone-implant fixation. It can also be observed that shot-blasting improves surface finishing and cleaning

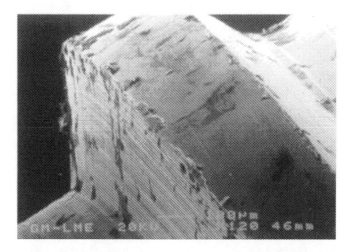

Figure 5.9 Detail of a dental implant before the shot-blasting treatment.

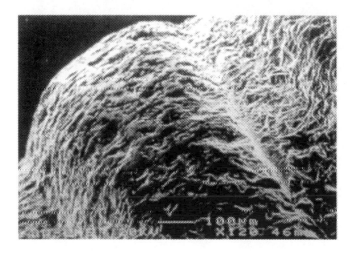

Figure 5.10 Detail of a dental implant after the shot-blasting treatment.

by eliminating the small cracks, bumps, chips and contaminants caused by machining shown in Figures 5.4 to 5.6. Moreover, from a mechanical point of view, shot blasting improves fatigue strength and stress-corrosion resistance of the implant because of the presence of a hardened layer created during hammering. By delaying crack nucleation, the formation of this layer helps improve the service life of the implant. It is also evident that many factors during the shot-blasting process, such as the chemical composition and morphology of the abrasive particles, their biocompatibility, the impact pressure and time of treatment, can modify the roughness of the implant and the possibility of osseointegration. It is necessary to optimise the process and therefore these factors should be carefully controlled.

5.6.2 Diffusion treatments

When acids are used to clean the surfaces of implants, even small amounts of the hydrogen left on the surface of the implant can create a brittle effect. For some applications, refractory metal coatings can be produced to avoid oxidation at high temperatures. In the same way, copper or platinum coatings produced by electrolysis are used to improve wear. For applications where wear and friction are important, surface hardening methods have been applied to titanium alloys. Among them, nitrogen hardening seems to be the most promising technique. Figure 5.11 shows, on the right-hand side, a detail of a hard layer created on titanium by nitrogen diffusion.

Another surface treatment of titanium is anodization, which gives different colour appearances to titanium surfaces as a consequence of the interference of light through the titanium oxide layer formed during the process. Figure 5.12 shows that a proper control of the voltage and intensity during the anodization treatment can modulate the thickness of the oxide layer, and hence the light interference, giving a full gradation of colour.

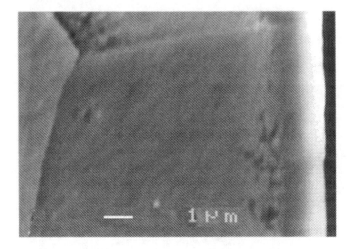

Figure 5.11 Detail of *alpha* titanium after nitrogen diffusion hardening treatment.

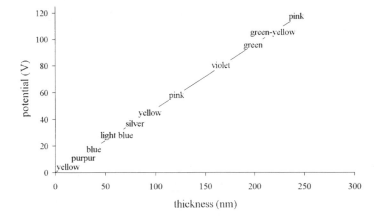

Figure 5.12 Titanium colouring by anodization treatment.

5.6.3 Chemical deposition

This section presents a summary of information on the deposition methods of bioactive coatings (Li and De Groot, 1993; Campbell et al., 1996; Kokubo et al., 1996; Ohtsuki et al., 1997; Wen et al., 1997; Li and Ducheyne, 1998; Peltola et al., 1998) that have been developed to overcome some of the drawbacks of the standard deposition of hydroxyapatite, when using the plasma spray technique (De Groot et al., 1990). The main disadvantage of this method is related to the high temperature used to plasma spray the hydroxyapatite mineral phase onto the implant surface. Due to the low thermal properties of titanium alloys, local heating of the surface is produced, thus changing the structure and mechanical properties of the metal surface.

Another main problem concerns the control of the chemical composition and crystallinity of the hydroxyapatite coating, as well as its physical and mechanical properties during and after deposition. Hydroxyapatite is thermally unstable during cooling, thus producing amorphous calcium phosphate phases. The presence of amorphous phases in the coating works against the long term stability of the coating after implantation. As it is known, amorphous calcium phosphates, and even phases such as tetracalcium and tricalcium phosphates, which are also formed during cooling, dissolve faster than hydroxyapatite, thus leading to the complete mechanical disintegration of the coating and loosening of the implant fixation.

It has also been reported that adhesion of the coating to the implant is very limited, leading to early decohesion of the coating even shortly after implantation (De Groot et al., 1990). This is related to the absence of any chemical link between the titanium surface and the hydroxyapatite coating. And this is precisely what the new methods attempt to do: improve adhesion by modifying the surface of the metal with different chemical agents, so that apatite crystals can be deposited chemically. For example, commercially pure titanium can be made bioactive by attacking its oxide layer so that a gel of sodium titanate is produced, which is able to induce the nucleation of apatite crystals.

Many researchers have developed methods to obtain bioactive metals. These methods have offered a real solution to the problem of the complete absence of any chemical link between titanium and bone tissue in normal conditions after implantation. Moreover, they overcome some of the problems associated with the standard chemical and physical apatite deposition methods. Some of these standard methods, besides the plasma spray method mentioned above, include electrophoretic deposition (Ducheyne et al., 1990), laser ablation (Cleries, 1999) and isostatic pressing (Hero et al., 1994).

The following subsections briefly explain the main characteristics of the new methods to chemically coat titanium metal substrates with bioactive apatite.

5.6.3.1 The Method of Ohtsuki

This method, developed by Ohtsuki (Ohtsuki et al., 1997), uses CP-titanium treated with hydrogen peroxide at 30 per cent in weight including 5mM of tin chloride solution, over the course of 24 hours at a temperature of 60°C. Titanium samples are then immersed in a Simulated Body Fluid (SBF). This fluid has a similar composition to that encountered in blood plasma (Kokubo et al., 1990), as is shown in Table 5.4. According to Ohtsuki, after three days apatite crystals were detected by X-Ray Dispersive Energy and then observed by Scanning Electron Microscopy.

Table 5.4 Ionic concentration (in mM) of SBF and of human plasma

Ion	SBF	Human plasma
Na^+	142.0	142.0
K^+	5.0	5.0
Mg^{2+}	1.5	1.5
Ca^{2+}	2.5	2.5
Cl^-	147.8	103.0
HCO_3^-	4.2	27.0
HPO_4^{2-}	1.0	1.0
SO_4^{2-}	0.5	0.5

5.6.3.2 The Method of Kokubo

The method proposed by Kokubo (Kokubo et al., 1996) also uses CP-titanium, which is chemically treated in a 5M sodium hydroxide solution over the course of 24 hours at a temperature of 60°C. Then, it is dried in an oven at 40°C for another 24 hours. After drying, the treated titanium is heated up to 600°C for one hour and cooled inside the oven. When this treatment is completed the titanium is immersed in SBF (see Table 5.4). According to Kokubo, titanium samples showed apatite crystal formation after three days of immersion. The apatite crystals were detected by Low-Angle X-Ray Diffraction and observed by Scanning Electron Microscopy.

5.6.3.3 The Method of Li

This method (Li and De Groot, 1993) uses a sol-gel solution prepared by adding water and acid chloride to a diluted ethanol solution containing $Ti(C_3H_7O)_4$ and $C_4H_{10}O_2$. The mixing is carried out at 0°C. Titanium samples are then immersed for one hour and thereafter dried for five minutes at room temperature. Then, a thermal treatment is performed at 500°C for ten minutes followed by cooling inside an oven. Once the surface of the titanium has been prepared using this method, the samples are immersed in SBF. According to Li, apatite crystals were detected by Low-Angle X-Ray Diffraction after three days. However, a drawback to this method is the low adhesion of the apatite crystals to the titanium oxide layer. This is a serious problem when the coating is quite thick.

5.6.3.4 The Method of Campbell

This method is also known as the Surface Induced Mineralization Method (Campbell et al., 1996). It was tested with Ti6Al4V titanium alloy. The idea is to deposit a self-assembled monolayer of calcium phosphates on the surface. Samples are treated for 30 seconds in 1 wt per cent solution of silane/cyclohexane, cleaned in two-propanol and immersed in chloroform for five minutes for further cleaning using ultrasound. The deposition of calcium phosphates is carried out with a supersaturated solution of calcium and phosphate ions prepared by the slow addition of KH_2PO_4 into a solution of calcium chloride. This method is very sensitive to the calcium and phosphate ion concentration in the solution and, depending on this, the rate of deposition can be controlled.

5.6.3.5 *The Method of Klas De Groot*

This is known as the Supersaturated Calcification Solution Method (Wen et al., 1997). The commercially pure titanium is chemically etched by a 1:1 molar solution of acid chloride (18 wt per cent) and sulphuric acid (48 wt per cent) for 30 minutes. Then, it is immersed in a sodium hydroxide solution (0.2 N) at 140°C and at a pressure of three bars for five hours. After this, there is a pre-calcification treatment in an Na_2HPO_4 solution (0.5 N) over the course of 12 hours and in calcium hydroxide saturated solution for five hours. The final deposition of the calcium phosphate is carried out in a Hank's balanced salt solution at 37°C. The rate of deposition was estimated at 0.4 μm/day.

5.6.3.6 *The Method of Ducheyne*

This method was carried out for CP-titanium (Li and Ducheyne, 1998). Both sides of the titanium samples were polished and one of them pre-coated with gold. Then, the samples were immersed in SBF. The presence of calcium, phosphorus, magnesium and chlorine on the surface was detected by chemical analysis. According to Ducheyne, the calcium phosphate coating had a width of 1 μm after four weeks of treatment.

5.7 IMPROVING THE RELIABILITY OF IMPLANT OSSEOINTEGRATION

As has already been said, there are two technological approaches to optimising the fixation of dental implants: one changes the topography of the implant surface and the other changes its chemical composition. The former approach increases the surface roughness in order to improve long-term fixation by assuring better implant-bone interlocking. As a consequence, the bone grows as near as possible to the titanium implant and no fibrous tissue is observed between the implant and the bone when using optical microscopy, as first given by Brånemark et al., 1977. In fact, this kind of interlocking should lead to a structural and functional direct connection between the bone tissue and the surface of an implant, i.e. osseointegration of the dental implant (Carlsson et al., 1986). This includes several processes, among which is the shot-blasting treatment. With this method a direct link between the material and the surrounding bone is not produced. Nonetheless, in this case a thin coating of fibrous tissue, which can only be observed by electron microscopy (Lausmaa, 1991), surrounds the implant.

As to the latter approach, the absence of a chemical link between titanium and bone tissue has lead to the development of several techniques to try to modify the chemical composition of the implant. Some of these processes include electrophoretic deposition (Ducheyne et al., 1990), plasma-spray (Loh, 1999), ion beam or radiofrequency attack (Cook et al., 1998), laser ablation (Cleries, 1999) and isostatic pressing (Hero et al., 1994). However, none of these has been able to produce coatings chemically linked to the substrate.

Nowadays, a common procedure used for clinical applications is the coating of hydroxyapatite by plasma-spray (De Groot et al., 1990). As mentioned before, since hydroxyapatite is a bioactive material (Bruijn et al., 1992), a hydroxyapatite-coated implant can stimulate bone cellular activity without any foreign-body reaction, offering the possibility of complete osseointegration of the implant. However, one drawback to this method is the high temperature needed during the plasma projection of the hydroxyapatite onto the titanium surface.

Others are related to the difficult control of the chemical composition, the crystallinity and the physical structure of the hydroxyapatite during deposition because of its thermal instability. As a result, the coating degrades over time. Moreover, the coating has only limited mechanical adhesion to the surface and this can lead to decohesion of the coating both during and after implantation (Mann et al., 1994; Park et al., 1998). Nonetheless, as previously reported, some new treatments have been developed to overcome the problems associated with the degradation of the plasma-spray coatings (Li and De Groot, 1993; Campbell, 1996; Kokubo, 1996; Ohtsuki, 1997; Wen, 1997; Li and Ducheyne, 1998; Peltola, 1998).

The osseointegration of a dental implant can be evaluated by *in vitro* and *in vivo* studies. *In vitro* studies are performed to evaluate the adhesion, proliferation and differentiation of bone cells either from human or animal bone tissue (Naji and Harmand, 1991; Puleo, 1991; Keller et al., 1994; Anselme et al., 1997) or some bone cancer cell lines such as osteosarcome (Martin et al., 1995; Kieswetter et al., 1996; Weiland et al., 1997; Batzer et al., 1998). These studies are carried out as preliminary tests because they are less expensive than *in vivo* tests and the results are produced in a shorter time. Moreover, *in vitro* studies give information on the influence of the state of the surface on cell behaviour. In fact, many studies have been performed comparing different materials with different topographies and thermal treatments. These studies have shown that an increase in surface roughness of the implant improves the cellular behaviour. However, there is still much work to be done to clarify how this surface roughness should be in order to obtain an optimum cellular response to the implant during the osseointegration process.

In vivo studies have been performed in order to establish the relationship between histomorphometry and mechanical fixation. Parameters such as the percentage of the implant in direct contact to new bone tissue at different healing times after implantation, and the maximum torque and push-out strength during implant extraction have been measured (Gross et al., 1990; Piattelli et al., 1990; Buser et al., 1991; Wong et al., 1995; Feighan et al., 1995; Wennerberg et al., 1995, 1996, 1997; Johansson et al., 1996, 1997; Dhert et al., 1998). However, the results reported for plasma-sprayed hydroxyapatite coated implants and for shot-blasted implants show unclear results about which treatment is the most suitable for dental implants. Hydroxyapatite coated implants show better short-term behaviour because more of the implant surface is in direct contact with bone and there is greater torque and push-out strength. However, the shot-blasted implants show better osseointegration than the plasma-spray hydroxyapatite implants four months after implantation as well as after one year, though these implants show unfilled bone tissue areas. This behaviour has been attributed to the surface roughness of the implant, in the order of micrometers, and probably to the morphology of the surface after the shot-blasting treatment. It is thought that, after the shot-blasting treatment, a mechanical fixation at the micrometer level is added to the normal fixation due to the macroscopic design of the implant (Brånemark et al., 1987). On the other hand, some references state that for dental implants coated with plasma-spray hydroxyapatite there is faster resorption of the surrounding maxillar bone. This phenomenon has been related to the release of hydroxyapatite particles to the surrounding bone as result of the degradation of the coating (Park et al., 1998). For this reason, clinical failures due to the loosening of coated dental implants has also been related to the degradation of the coating itself.

As far as the *in vivo* behaviour of commercially pure titanium is concerned, smooth implants coated with a precipitated bone-like apatite, following the method of Kokubo, improved their histomorphometry and the bone-implant fixation compared to the smooth implants without coating (Yan et al., 1997; Kim et al., 1997).

5.8 CONCLUSIONS

Many factors affect the osseointegration of dental implants, e.g. the quality of the receptor bone, the surgical technique during operation, the conditions of load, the geometric design of the implant, the type of material and the surface quality of the implant. The present chapter offered a short summary of the materials used in dental implantology, with main regard to titanium and its alloys, highlighting the manufacturing procedures, as casting, welding forging and machining, and reporting on their characteristics. Furthermore, special attention was given to the surface quality of implants, as it greatly influences the success of fixation. Notes on mechanical treatments, diffusion and, in particular, chemical treatments are reported. In fact, new research on surface modification to improve osseointegration is constantly being proposed. This confirms that this field must to be both constantly reviewed and properly considered for reliability evaluation of dental implant devices.

REFERENCES

T. Albrektsson, P. I. Brånemark, H.A. Hansson, J. Lindström, Osseointegrated titanium implants, Acta Orthop. Scand., Vol. 52, pp. 155–170, 1981.

K. Anselme, M. Bigerelle, B. Noel, M. Duquesne, D. Judas, A Iost, P. Hardouin, Qualitative and quantitative study of human osteoblast adhesion on Ta6V samples with different surface roughness, 13th European Conference on Biomaterials, p. 93, Göteborg, 1997.

R. Batzer, Y. Liu, D. Cohran, S. Moncler, D. Dean, B. Boyan, Z. Schwartz, Prosteoglandins mediate the effects of titanium surface roughness on MG63 osteoblast-like cells and alter cell responsiveness to $1\alpha,25$-(OH)2D3, J. Biomed. Mater. Res., Vol. 41, pp. 489–496, 1998.

P.I. Brånemark, B.O. Hansson, R. Adell, U. Breine, J. Lindström, A. Olsson, Osseointegrated implants in the treatment of edentulous jaw. Experience from a 10-year period, Scand. J. Plast. Reconstr. Surg., Vol. 11, 1977.

P.I. Brånemark, G.A. Zrab, T. Albrektsson, Prótesis tejido-integradas. La osteointegración en la odontología clínica, Quintessenz Verlag GmbH, Berlin, 1987.

J.D. Bruijn, J.E. Davies, C.P. Klein, K. De Groot, C.A. Van Blitterswijk, Biological responses to calcium phosphate ceramics, In: Bone-bonding. Ed. P. Ducheyne, T. Kokubo, C.A. Van Blitterswijk, pp. 57–72, 1992.

J.B. Brunski, Classes of materials used in medicine. Metals. In: Biomaterials Science, An Introduction to Materials in Medicine. Edited by: B. Rutner, A. Hoffman, F. Schoen, J. Lemons, Academic Press, San Diego, CA, 1996.

D. Buser, R.K. Schenk, S. Steinemann, J.P. Fiorellini, C.H. Fox, H. Stich, Influence of surface characteristics on bone integration of titanium implants. A histomorphometric study in miniature pigs, J. Biomed. Mater. Res., Vol. 25, pp. 889–902, 1991.

A.A. Campbell, G. Fryxell, J. Linehan, G. Graff, Surface-induced mineralization: anew method for producing calcium phosphate coatings, J. Biomed. Mater. Res., Vol. 32, pp. 111–118, 1996.

L. Carlsson, T. Röstlund, T. Albrektsson, P.I. Brånemark, Osseointegration of titanium implants, Acta Orthop. Scand., Vol. 57, pp. 285–289, 1986.

L. Cleries, In vitro studies of calcium phosphate coatings obtained by laser ablation, PhD Thesis, University of Barcelona, Spain, 1999.

S.D. Cook, K.A. Thomas, M. Jarcho, Hydroxyapatite-coated porous titanium for use as an orthopaedic biologic attachment system, Clin. Orthop., Vol. 230, pp. 303–312, 1998.

K. De Groot, C.P. Klein, J.G. Wolke, J.M. Blieck-Hogervorst, Plasma sprayed coatings of calcium phosphate, In: CRC Handbook of Bioactive Ceramics, Vol. II. Calcium phosphate and hydroxyapatite ceramics, Ed. T. Yamamuro, L. Hench, J. Wilson. CRC Press, Inc., pp. 133–142, 1990.

W. Dhert, P. Thomsen, A. Blomgren, M. Esposito, L. Ericson, A. Verbout, Integration of press-fit implants in cortical bone: A study on interface kinetics, J. Biomed. Mater. Res., Vol. 41, pp. 574–583, 1998.

G.E. Dieter, Mechanical Metallurgy, 2nd Edition, Mc Graw-Hill Ltd., 1976.

P. Ducheyne, S. Radin, M. Heughbaert, C. Heughbaert, Calcium phosphate ceramic coating on porous titanium: Effect of structure and composition on electrophoretic deposition, vacuum sintering and in vitro dissolution, Biomaterials, Vol. 11, pp. 244–254, 1990.

J. Feighan, V. Goldberg, D. Davy, J. Parr, S. Stevenson, The influence of surface blasting on the incorporation of titanium-alloy implants in a rabbit intramedullary model, J. Bone Joint Surg., Vol. 77ª, pp. 1380–1395, 1995.

U. Gross, Ch. Müller-Mai, Th. Fritz, Ch. Voigt, W. Knarse, H.G. Schmitz, Implant surface roughness and mode of load transmission influence periimplant bone structure, Clin. Implant Mater., Vol. 9, pp. 303–309, 1990.

H. Hero, H. Wie, R.B. Jorgensen, I.E. Ruyter, Hydroxyapatite coating on titanium produced by isostatic pressing, J. Biomed. Mater. Res., Vol. 28, pp. 344–348, 1994.

C.B. Johansson, A. Wennerberg, C.H. Han, T. Albrektsson, A quantitative comparison of titanium implants, Fifth World Biomaterials Congress, p. 478, Toronto, 1996.

C.B. Johansson, I. Cho, S.J. Heo, T. Sawai, A. Sawase, A. Wennerberg, N. Meredith, Techniques to quantify the incorporation of machined and blasted implants in bone, 13th European Conference on Biomaterials, p. 33, Göteborg, 1997.

J.C. Keller, C.M. Stanford, J.P. Wightman, R.A. Draughn, R. Zaharias, Characterization of titanium implant surfaces III, J. Biomed. Mater. Res., Vol. 28, pp. 939–946, 1994.

K. Kieswetter, R. Batzer, Y. Liu, Z. Schwartz, D. Cochran, D.D. Dean, S. Szmuckler, J. Simpson, B.D. Boyan, Surface roughness modulates the response of MG63 osteoblast-like cells to vitamin D3 stimulation, Fifth World Biomaterials Congress, p. 941, Toronto, 1996.

H. Kim, F. Miyaji, T. Kokubo, T. Nakamura, Bonding strength of bonelike apatite layer to Ti metal substrate, J. Appl. Biomater., Vol. 38, pp. 121–127, 1997.

T. Kokubo, H. Kushitani, S. Sakka, T. Kitsugi, T. Yamamuro, Solutions able to reproduce in vivo surface-structure changes in bioactive glass ceramic A-W, J. Biomed. Mater. Res., Vol. 24, pp. 721–734, 1990.

T. Kokubo, F. Miyaji, H. Kim, Spontaneous formation of bonelike apatite layer on chemically treated titanium metals, J. Am. Ceram. Soc., Vol. 79, pp. 1127–1129, 1996.

J. Lausmaa, Surface oxides on titanium: Preparation, characterisation, and biomaterial applications, PhD Thesis, Chalmers University of Technology, Göteborg, 1991.

P. Li, K. De Groot, Calcium phosphate formation within sol-gel prepared titania *in vitro* and *in vivo*, J. Biomed. Mater. Res., Vol. 27, pp. 1445–1500, 1993.

P. Li, P. Ducheyne, Quasi-biological film induced by titanium in a simulated body fluid, J. Biomed. Mater. Res., Vol. 41, pp. 341–348, 1998.

I.H. Loh, Plasma surface modification in biomedical applications, Medical Devices Technology, Issue Jan/Feb, pp. 24–30, 1999.

K.A. Mann, A.A. Edidin, R.K. Kinoshita, M.T. Manley, Mixed mode fracture characterisation of hydroxyapatite-titanium alloy interface, J. Appl. Biomater., Vol. 5, pp. 285–291, 1994.

J.Y. Martin, Z. Schwartz, T.W. Hummert, D.M. Schraub, J. Simpson, J.J. Lankford, D.D. Dean, D.L. Cochran, B.D. Boyan, Effect of titanium surface roughness on proliferation, differentiation, and protein synthesis of human osteoblast-like cells (MG63), J. Biomed. Mater. Res., Vol. 29, pp. 339–401, 1995.

Metals handbook. Volume 5: Surface Engineering, ASM, Toronto, 1995.

C.E. Mish. In: Implantología contemporánea, Mosby/Doyma Libros, Madrid, Spain, 1994.

A. Naji, M.F. Harmand, Cytocompatibility of two coating materials, amorphous alumina and silicon carbide, using human differentiated cell cultures, Biomaterials, Vol. 12, pp. 690–694, 1991.

C. Ohtsuki, H. Iida, S. Hayakawa, A. Osaka, Bioactivity of titanium treated with hydrogen peroxide solutions containing metal chlorides, J. Biomed. Mater. Res., Vol. 35, pp. 39–47, 1997.

Y. Oshida, R. Sachdeva, S. Miyazaki, J. Daly, Effects of shot-peening on surface contact angles of biomaterials, J. Mater. Science: Mater. Med., Vol. 4, pp. 443–447, 1993.

E. Park, S.R. Condrate, D.T. Hoelzer, G.S. Fischman, Interfacial characterisation of plasma-spray coated calcium phosphate on Ti6Al4V, J. Mater. Sci. Med., Vol. 9, pp. 643–649, 1998.

T. Peltola, M. Pätsi, H. Rahiala, I. Kangasniemi, A. Yli-Urpo, Calcium phosphate induction by sol-gel derived titania coatings on titianium substrates *in vitro*, J. Biomed. Mater. Res., Vol. 41, pp. 504–510, 1998.

A. Piattelli, L. Manzon, A. Scarano, M. Paolantonio, M. Piatelli, Histologic and histomorphometric analysis of the bone response to machined and sand-blasted titanium implants: An experimental study in rabbits, Int. J. Oral. Maxill. Impl., Vol. 13, pp. 805–810, 1990.

A.S. Posner, N.C. Blumenthal, F. Betts, In: Proceedings of the 2nd International Conference on Phosphorous Compounds, Ed. Eon, C. Imphos, Paris, p. 25, 1980.

I. Proubasta, F.J. Gil, J.A. Planell, In: Fundamentos de Biomecánica y Biomateriales, Ergon, Madrid, Spain, 1997.

D.A. Puleo, L.A. Holleran, R.H. Doremus, R. Bizios, Osteoblast response to orthopaedic implant materials in vitro, J. Biomed. Mater. Res., Vol. 25, pp. 711–723, 1991.

M. Weiland, C. Sittig, M. Textor, V. Schenk, S.W. Ha, B.A. Keller, E. Wintermantel, N.D. Spencer, Influence of the structure and chemical composition of titanium alloy surfaces on the adhesion of osteoblasts, 13th European Conference on Biomaterials, p. 100, Göteborg, 1997.

H.B. Wen, J.R. De Wijn, K. De Groot, F.Z. Cui, A simple method to prepare calcium phosphate coatings on Ti6Al4V, J. Mater. Sci. Mater. Med., Vol. 8, pp. 765–770, 1997.

A. Wennerberg, T. Albrektsson, B. Andersson, An animal study of CP titanium screws with different surface topographies, J. Mater. Science. Mater. Med., Vol. 6, pp. 302–309, 1995.

A. Wennerberg, On surface roughness and implant incorporation, PhD Thesis, Dpt. of Biomaterials, Göteborg University, Göteborg, 1996a.

A. Wennerberg, T. Albrektsson, C. Johansson, B. Andersson, Experimental study of turned and grit-shaped implants with special emphasis on effects of blasting material and surface topography, Biomaterials, Vol. 17, pp. 15–22, 1996b.

A. Wennerberg, T. Albrektsson, J. Lausmaa, Torque and histomorphometric evaluation of cp titanium screws blasted with 25 and 75 μm sized particles of Al2O3, J. Biomed. Mater. Res., Vol. 30, pp. 251–260, 1996c.

A. Wennerberg, C. Hallgren, C.B. Johansson, S. Danelli, A histomorphometrical evaluation of 40 implants prepared with two surface roughness each, 13th European Conference on Biomaterials, p. 21, Göteborg, 1997.

M. Wong, R. Eulenberger, R. Schenk, E. Hunziker, Effect of surface topology on the osseointegration of implant materials in trabecular bone, J. Biomed. Mater. Res., Vol. 29, pp. 1567–1575, 1995.

W. Yan, T. Nakamura, M. Kobayashi, H. Kim, F. Miyaji, T. Kokubo, Bonding of chemically treated titanium implants to bone, J. Biomed. Mater. Res., Vol. 37, pp. 267–275, 1997a.

W. Yan, T. Nakamura, K. Kawanabe, S. Nishigochi, M. Oka, T. Kokubo, Apatite layer-coated titanium for use as bone-bonding implants, Biomaterials, Vol. 18, pp. 1185–1190, 1997b.

6 Dental devices in titanium-based materials via casting route

F Bonollo, AN Natali, PG Pavan

6.1 INTRODUCTION

Casting processes are probably the most common method for producing titanium dental devices. These manufacturing techniques have to be tailored with reference to the peculiarities of titanium and its alloys. In fact, on the one hand, the high melting points of such materials make it necessary to use very efficient melting systems and suitable casting methods in order to compensate for the high viscosity of the melt. On the other hand, because of the high chemical reactivity between titanium and oxygen processes must be carried out in a vacuum or under inert gas.

A significant support in designing these casting processes and in evaluating the quality of the cast component is now offered by numerical simulation techniques. In fact, computational codes have recently been introduced which are able to calculate the mass, velocity, momentum and temperature fields established during all the stages of the casting process once the boundary and initial conditions have been correctly defined.

This chapter initially presents a review of the metallurgical features of titanium alloys and the casting technologies usually used for producing dental devices, followed by an explanation of the potential of process simulation applied to this field. Then, with reference to a titanium grade two cast framework, the fluid dynamics and thermal fields induced during manufacturing are presented to simulate the evolution of the process. Finally, the results of the thermal field calculation are shown. These results can be related to the microstructural evolution of the device and to its metallurgical quality. Since the microstructure is directly correlated to the mechanical properties, as is the case in all metallic materials, the output of process simulation can be used to carry out a biomechanical evaluation of the component.

6.2 MICROSTRUCTURE AND PROPERTIES OF TITANIUM AND ITS ALLOYS

The properties which make titanium and its alloys excellent materials for biomedical applications are related to their mechanical behaviour and corrosion resistance (Polmear, 1981; Collings, 1984; Black, 1992; Park and Lakes, 1992; Brunski, 1996). From a very general viewpoint, alloyed titanium presents tensile strength up to about 1000 MPa. On the other hand, though commercially pure titanium only reaches up to about 500 MPa, it has better corrosion resistance properties. Tables 6.1 and 6.2 show the mechanical properties of titanium and its alloys as well as a comparison of them with other metals and alloys (Polmear, 1981; Boyer and Hall, 1993; Okazaki et al., 1993; Lampman, 1994; Niinomi, 1998).

Titanium is a transition metal; its incomplete shell in electronic structures enables it to form solid solutions with most substitutional elements (size factor within 20 per cent). The melting point of pure titanium is quite high (1678°C).

From a structural point of view, titanium presents a hexagonal and closed packed crystal structure (hcp), called α, up to 882.5°C, whereas for higher temperatures, there is a body centered cubic (bcc) structure, called β.

The classification of titanium alloys is consequently related to their microstructure at room temperature (Polmear, 1981; Boyer and Hall, 1993; Niinomi, 1998):

- α alloys;
- near-α alloys;
- α–β alloys;
- metastable β alloys;
- stable β alloys.

The values of elastic modulus and fatigue strength for these different families of titanium alloys are schematically reported in Figures 6.1 and 6.2 (Polmear, 1981; Rundinger and Fisher, 1985; Boyer and Hall, 1993; Mishra et al., 1993; Okazaki et al., 1993; Wang et al., 1993a; Wang et al., 1993b; Lampman, 1994; Kobayashi et al., 1995; Long and Rack, 1998; Niinomi, 1998).

Table 6.1 Mechanical properties of titanium alloys

Alloy		UTS [MPa]	YS [MPa]	Elongation [%]	RA [%]	E [GPa]	Type of alloy
Pure Ti Gr.1		240	170	24	30	102.7	α
Pure Ti Gr.2		345	275	20	30	102.7	α
Pure Ti Gr.3		450	380	18	30	103.4	α
Pure Ti Gr.4		550	485	15	25	104.1	α
Ti-6Al–4V	(*annealed*)	895–930	825–869	6–10	20–25	110–114	$\alpha + \beta$
Ti-6Al–7Nb		900–1050	880–950	8–15	25–45	114	$\alpha + \beta$
Ti-5Al–2.5Fe		1020	895	15	35	112	$\alpha + \beta$
Ti-5Al–1.5B		925–1080	820–930	15–17	36–45	110	$\alpha + \beta$
Ti-15Zr–4Nb–4Ta–0.2Pd							
	(*annealed*)	715	693	28	67	99	$\alpha + \beta$
	(*aged*)	919	806	18	72	94	$\alpha + \beta$
Ti-13Nb-13Zr (*aged*)		973–1037	836–908	10–16	27–53	79–84	β
Ti-12Mo-6Zr-2Fe							
	(*annealed*)	1060–1100	1000–1060	18–22	64–73	74–85	β
Ti-15Mo	(*annealed*)	874	544	21	82	78	β
Ti-15Mo-5Zr-3Al	(*ST*)	852	838	25	48	80	β
	(*aged*)	1060–1100	1000–1060	18–22	64–73	74–85	β
Ti-15Mo-2.8Nb-0.2Si							
	(*annealed*)	979–999	945–987	16–18	60	83	β
Ti-35.3Nb-5.1Ta-7.1Zr		597	547	19	68	55	β
Ti-29Nb-13Ta-4.6Zr (*aged*)		911	864	13.2		80	β

Table 6.2 Comparison of the properties of various engineering materials

Material	Yield strength [MPa]	Density [g/cm³]	Yield strength to density ratio	% ratio relative to Ti-Grade 2	% ratio relative to Ti-Grade 5
Ti-Grade 2	275	4.51	61	100	32
Ti-Grade 5	830	4.42	188	308	100
AISI 316	230	7.94	29	48	15
254 SMO	300	8.00	38	62	20
2205 duplex	450	7.80	58	95	31
Monel 400	175	8.83	20	32	11
Inconel 625	415	8.44	49	80	26
Hastalloy C-276	355	8.89	40	66	21
70/30 Cu-Ni	120	8.90	13	21	7

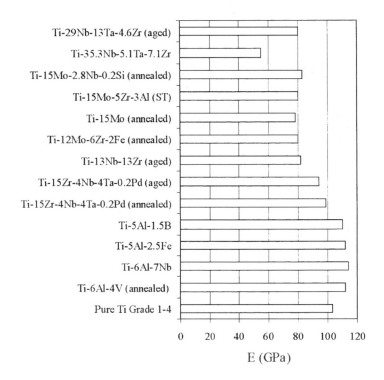

Figure 6.1 Values of the modulus of elasticity for different titanium-based materials.

Alloying elements for titanium can be grouped into three categories:

- α-stabilisers, such as Al, O, N, C;
- β-stabilisers, such as Mo, V, Nb, Ta, (isomorphous), Fe, W, Cr, Si, Ni, Co, Mn, H (eutectoid);
- neutral, such as Zr.

according to their capability of promoting α or β structures, as schematically shown in Figure 6.3. α and near-α titanium alloys exhibit superior corrosion resistance with relatively

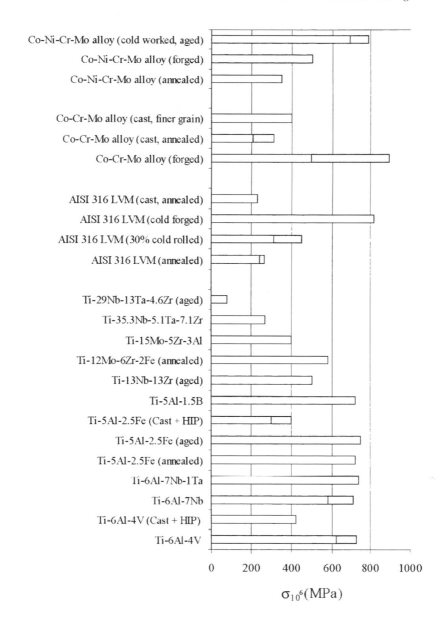

Figure 6.2 Values of the fatigue strength for different alloys.

low strength with respect to α–β alloys (Polmear, 1981; Steinemann, 1985; Boyer and Hall, 1993; Kovacs and Davidson, 1993; Schutz, 1993).

Their properties depend on composition, the relative proportions of the α/β phases, and the thermal treatment and thermo-mechanical processing conditions (Polmear, 1981; Boyer and Hall, 1993; Vassel, 1993). β alloys (metastable or stable) are titanium alloys which have high strength and hardness and good formability. β alloys also present low elastic modulus and superior corrosion resistance. Figure 6.4 compares yield strength and elongation for the titanium alloys most commonly used for biomedical applications.

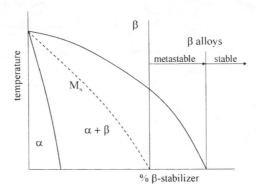

Figure 6.3 Definition of α, α + β and β titanium alloys as a function of temperature.

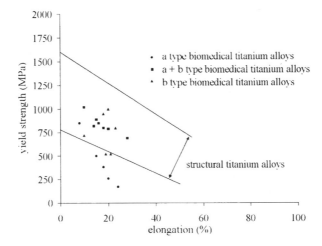

Figure 6.4 Relation between yield strength and elongation for different titanium biomedical alloys.

The manufacturing and treatment processes must be controlled in order to obtain the best possible alloy microstructure for the application requirements and thus optimise the titanium alloy properties, i.e. ductility, strength, fatigue resistance or fracture toughness. The characteristics of various microstructures are then correlated with the engineering properties. The most common microstructural features studied in metastable β alloys are β grain size and the size and distribution of aged α grains.

6.3 SHAPING OF TITANIUM COMPONENTS BY CASTING PROCESSES

There are several techniques available for shaping titanium and its alloys, including casting, hot forming and forging, extrusion and rolling, welding, and powder metallurgy. The manufacturing cycle used depends on design requirements, economical evaluation, and feasibility. Among those mentioned, casting processes are potentially very good since they offer near net shape, good dimensional control, repeatability, possibility of carrying out mechanical adaptation and surface treatments, controlling adhesion and consequently the mechanical behaviour of titanium devices (Williams and Wood, 1971; Hernandez de Gatica et al., 1993).

It is worth mentioning, however, that the corrosion resistance of titanium, which is one of the best properties of this material, is due to its high chemical affinity with oxygen creating a very stable and resistant oxide film on its surface (Table 6.3) (Polmear, 1981; Steinemann, 1985; Manusli et al., 1988). The characteristics of this oxide film play a fundamental role in giving titanium excellent biocompatibility (Manusli et al., 1988; Morton and Bell, 1989; Hernandez de Gatica et al., 1993; Raikar et al., 1995). On the other hand, this affinity is also the main reason of the difficulty in shaping titanium components by means of casting processes. In fact, the rapid interaction between molten titanium and oxygen, leading to oxide formation, results in defects and inclusions, heavily affecting the final behaviour of the cast component. The high melting point of titanium leads to further difficulties in achieving an efficient melting process.

Therefore, a casting system for titanium and its alloys has to assure oxygen-free conditions, i.e. inert gas or high vacuum. In this case, the superheating that can be supplied to molten titanium is not very high. Therefore, since the viscosity of the melt is quite high, it is not easy to fill the mould cavity. These preliminary considerations help to understand the strong effort spent in recent years in developing more and more efficient casting processes, as well as in developing engineering approaches aimed at improving each stage of manufacturing (Okabe et al., 1998; Suzuki, 1998).

6.3.1 Investment casting

Investment casting, or lost wax, process can be adopted for other dental materials as well as for titanium alloys (ASM Metals Handbook, 1988; Okabe et al., 1998; Suzuki, 1998). This process (Figure 6.5) was one of the first used to make metal castings.

The basic steps of the investment casting process are: production of heat-disposable wax or plastic patterns;

* assembly of these patterns onto a gating system;
* "investing," or covering the pattern assembly with ceramic to produce a monolithic mould;
* melting the pattern assembly to leave a precise mould cavity;
* firing the ceramic mould to remove the last traces of the pattern material while developing the high-temperature bond and preheating the mould ready for casting;

Table 6.3 Oxides formed in various titanium-based materials

Material	Oxide				
	TiO_2	Al_2O_3	Nb_2O_5	MoO_3/MoO_2	Zr_2O_3
cp Ti	•				
Ti-6Al-4V	•	•			
Ti-5Al-2.5Fe	•	•			
Ti-6Al-7Nb	•	•	•		
Ti-15Mo-5Zr-3Al	•	•		•	•

- pouring;
- knockout, cut-off and finishing.

Some of the advantages of investment casting are excellent surface finishes, tight dimensional tolerances (an accuracy of 0.05 per cent is feasible), and the reduction or elimination of machining.

A significant research effort has recently been devoted to the use of investment materials which can assure chemical stability and adequate expansion. Oxides with standard free formation energy lower than that of titanium oxides have to be used: Al_2O_3, BeO, CaO, MgO, ThO_2, ZrO_2 and Y_2O_3.

The coefficient of thermal expansion of the investment material, on the other hand, should be able to compensate for the shrinkage of the cast alloy (typically 1.9–2.5 per cent). Silicon oxide, which has a volume-increasing phase transition, is usually used as an investment material for alloys other than titanium alloys. Due to the lower chemical stability of silicon oxide with respect to titanium oxides, it is not suitable in this case. The approaches adopted are:

- use of a spinel compound ($MgO + Al_2O_3 \rightarrow MgO \cdot Al_2O_3$), which forms at 900–1000°C with an irreversible expansion;
- use of spodumene ($LiO_2 \cdot Al_2O_3 \cdot SiO_2$), which expands due to a phase change at 1050°C;
- use of metal powders (zirconium), which oxidise, and thus expand, during heating.

6.3.2 Pressure-assisted casting of titanium

The set up of an industrial casting device for titanium and its alloys has led to the development of many types of patented machines and equipment (Okabe et al., 1998). These

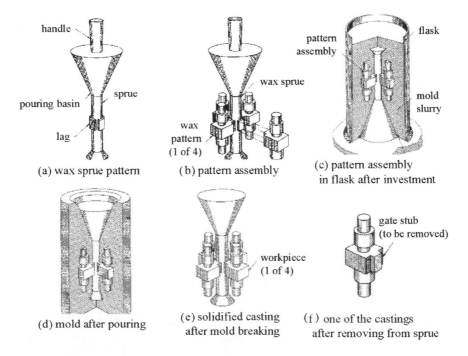

Figure 6.5 Stages of the investment casting process.

machines can be classified according to the way of melting the titanium and the kind of external force used for filling the cavity.

The melting can be carried out by means of:

* argon/arc melting with a non-consumable tungsten electrode;
* high frequency induction melting.

Crucibles are typically made of copper, magnesium oxide or graphite.

To force the molten titanium into the mould cavity, the following can be used:

* centrifugal force;
* pressure difference;
* gas pressure;
* a combination of the above.

Figure 6.6 presents a schematic view of a process based on the horizontal centrifugal force concept. Titanium is melted using the argon arc-melting device, in the upper part of the chamber. The mould, in the bottom of the chamber, is placed close to the periphery of the turntable. A titanium ingot is inserted into a graphite crucible which is placed at the centre of rotation.

First the chamber is evacuated, and then the titanium ingot is arc-melted. The crucible is placed over a graphite runner which the molten titanium is poured onto simply by tilting the crucible. From the runner, the titanium flows into the cavity of the mould. During this operation, the turntable imposes a rotation speed which can reach 3000 rpm. The high centrifugal force which is established leads to a sound casting.

The production unit shown in Figure 6.7, based on the pressure difference approach, is divided into two chambers. The upper one is devoted to the melting operation, while the casting operation is performed in the lower one. After the the titanium ingot has been placed in a copper crucible, the two chambers are evacuated. Then argon is introduced in the upper chamber, with a pressure typically ranging from 0.3 to 0.4 MPa. The titanium, once melted, drops into the mould, thanks to the pressure difference established between the two chambers, and starts to fill the cavity.

The gas pressure approach uses a device made up of a single chamber, as shown in Figure 6.8. After evacuation, argon is introduced into the chamber.

The titanium ingot is then arc-melted into a copper crucible, which is subsequently tilted, allowing the melt to be poured into the mould. When the molten alloy reaches the sprue, pressurisation of the chamber takes place due to the introduction of argon gas (about 0.7–0.8 MPa). Thus, the titanium is forced to fill the cavity of the mould.

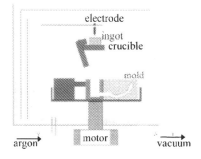

Figure 6.6 Schematic view of the horizontal centrifugal force casting process.

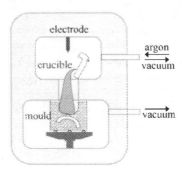

Figure 6.7 Schematic view of the differential pressure casting process.

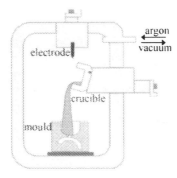

Figure 6.8 Schematic view of the gas pressure casting process.

6.4 EFFECTS OF PROCESSING ON THE QUALITY OF CASTINGS

The main methods for producing titanium castings were briefly described in the previous section. This section focuses on evaluating the level of quality that can be achieved using these methods. In a work by Suzuki (Suzuki, 1998), the defects detected in titanium castings produced by gravity casting, i.e. with the conditions of the investment casting process, or by centrifugal casting, using centrifugal forces up to 40 g, where g is gravity acceleration, were compared qualitatively and quantitatively.

Defects with a smooth internal surface were detected in the upper part of castings when no or little force was used. This is due to the entrapment of gaseous bubbles during the early stages of solidification. They can reach up to ten per cent of the volume of the castings and are caused by the evaporation of water which has originally been absorbed by the mould walls. Porosity with an irregular internal surface was also observed, due to the interdendritic shrinkage phenomena.

The size and number of defects were significantly reduced by increasing the centrifugal force applied. This can be seen in Figure 6.9 where the relative density of the specimens, which is directly related to the number of defects, is plotted as a function of the centrifugal force applied. The density, when 20–40 g forces are applied, is very close to the theoretical one.

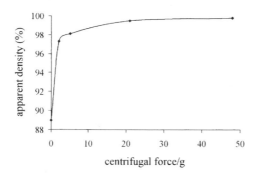

Figure 6.9 Apparent density of titanium castings as a function of the centrifugal force applied.

Table 6.4 Comparison between the characteristics of centrifugally and statically cast titanium specimens

	Centrifugal casting	*Static casting*
Minimum thickness filled [μm]	27	190
Diameter of gaseous defects [μm]	24	90
Diameter of shrinkage porosity [μm]	21	32
Critical liquid fraction for feeding [$-$]	0.15	0.33

In more detail, the effect of the centrifugal force was evaluated using a microfocus X-ray measurement system carried out both on statically cast, with a melt head of 20 cm, and on centrifugally (20 g) cast specimens (Table 6.4).

If the molten alloy does not wet the mould wall enough, as is typical of these casting systems, the increase in the internal pressure of the liquid generated by centrifugal casting gives the mould cavity filling a thickness which is about one-sixth that of static conditions. Another positive effect is achieved by reducing the size of gaseous defects, from 90 to 24 μm. The formation of shrinkage porosity is limited by the capability of the molten alloy to flow between the dendrite arms to feed the cavities which form in the solidifying metal. In static casting, the flow channels consist of a bundle of capillary tubes with a diameter of 32 μm. A critical fraction of the liquid, i.e. the amount of liquid needed for feeding through the bundle, is about 0.33. In centrifugal casting, these two values decrease respectively to 21 μm and 0.15 because of the pressure supplied. This clearly results in less shrinkage porosity in a centrifugally cast part.

6.5 A CASE HISTORY: MANUFACTURING A TITANIUM FRAMEWORK

6.5.1 The framework and the casting process

The object to be manufactured was a titanium framework to connect the different implants of a mandible (Figure 6.10). Grade two titanium was chosen to be the casting material because of its high biocompatibility, even if its mechanical properties, as previously described, are lower than those of other titanium alloys adopted in the biomedical field.

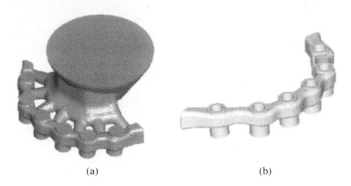

(a)   (b)

Figure 6.10 Geometry of the whole casting configuration (a) and of the titanium framework to be produced by casting (b).

The mould was made up of a ceramic coating inside a steel cylinder (Bonollo et al., 2001a; Natali et al., 2001). A ceramic coating was used because of its thermal stability and non-reactivity with respect to titanium. Moreover, the permeability of ceramic coating is suitable to allow the dispersion of the gas produced during the process.

Six titanium inserts were drowned inside the mould to make it possible to then connect the framework and abutments. The inserts and ceramic coatings were pre-heated at a temperature of 500°C. Argon was used because of its non-reactivity. The atmosphere inside the casting chamber was held under a constant pressure of 3.5 MPa during the tilt filling phase. The mould was initially in a horizontal position. A fast (time 1/18 s) 90° rotation of the casting system started the filling phase of the mould.

Figure 6.11 shows the framework produced.

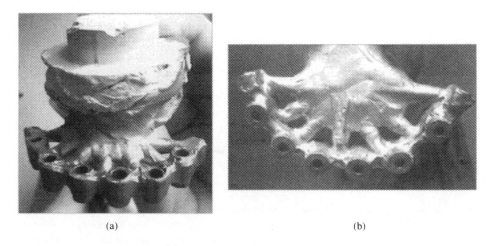

(a)   (b)

Figure 6.11 Upper (a) and lower (b) view of a titanium cast framework.

6.5.2 VISUALISING THE PROCESS BY MEANS OF NUMERICAL SIMULATION

Generally speaking, a casting process can be considered to be made up of five different stages:

- pouring the liquid metal/alloy into the mould;
- filling the mould cavity;
- cooling the alloy from the pouring temperature to the solidification interval;
- solidification;
- cooling to room temperature with (possible) solid state transformations.

The fluid dynamics (Navier-Stokes) and thermal (Fourier) laws make it possible to describe the evolution of the system in terms of mass, temperature and momentum distributions (Bird et al., 1966; Brodkey and Hershey, 1988). The computational tools and numerical methods currently available make it possible to visualise these distributions, i.e. describe the fluid-dynamics and thermal fields induced during a casting process. A thorough description of these approaches can be found elsewhere (Dusinberre, 1961; Nichols et al., 1980; Patankar, 1980; Sahm and Hansen, 1984; Berry and Pehlke, 1988; Desai and Pagalthivarthi, 1988; Hwang and Stoehr, 1988; Raithby and Schneider, 1988; Bonollo et al., 1999; Bonollo and Odorizzi, 2001b; Hattel et al., 2001). As an introduction to the numerical approach, it is enough to recall that all the differential equations expressing the above mentioned laws are taken into account in every elementary volume in which the domain is divided. The way of evaluating these equations and the kind of elementary volumes are related to the numerical method used. In the present case, the Control Volume Method (Patankar, 1980) was adopted. To correctly define the thermal and fluid-dynamics fields, boundary conditions and transport effects between adjacent volumes have to be considered. During solidification, the path of the heat flow was from the titanium framework to the ceramic coating, then to the steel cylinder and finally to the external environment. For each of these materials, the values of the thermophysical properties (density, thermal conductivity, specific heat, viscosity of molten titanium) were specified, together with their dependence on temperature. The values of the heat transfer coefficients at the interfaces between the different regions of the model (framework, coating, cylinder, environment), also had to be defined and implemented into the model (Sahm and Hansen, 1984; Berry and Pehlke, 1988; Bonollo et al., 1999; Bonollo and Odorizzi, 2001b; Hattel et al., 2001). The initial temperature of molten titanium was set at 2000°C.

Various codes which perform these calculations, some of which are available commercially, have been developed. For the case history presented, the MAGMASOFT® code was used. A precise definition of the three-dimensional geometry of the mould and feeders was obviously needed to ensure a correct description of the real phenomenon. The geometry of the cast, in the case here presented, was obtained by a process of reverse-engineering starting with a titanium framework produced in a trial casting. In Figure 6.12 the geometric model (after enmeshment) of the six-implant framework is presented with a detail of the gating system.

In order to describe how the molten alloy fills the cavity, the distribution of the velocity, temperature and pressure of the molten alloy was evaluated. In addition, it was neccessary to verify if the geometry of the cavity was suitable for its total filling, considering the cooling of the fluid front as well. Another aspect that was verified pertains

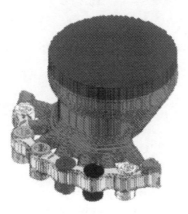

Figure 6.12 Control volume mesh of the titanium framework (including inserts) and of the casting configuration.

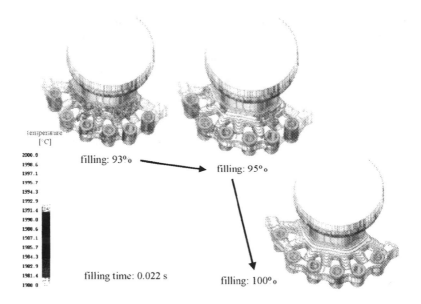

Figure 6.13 Distribution of mass and temperature during the last stages of filling.

to the presence of turbulence in some regions of the cavity because the cavity itself had a complex shape.

Since the results of the simulation can be presented in a colour or gray scale, the description of the process under investigation is clearer and more impressive. In this case, Figure 6.13 shows the distribution of mass and temperature at the final stages of the filling of the mould cavity. The values of the filling time (0.022 s) were also calculated.

The solidification of the framework took place very quickly. About 5 s after casting, the framework was totally solidified. It has already been mentioned that the presence of porosity defects is related to the entrapment of gaseous bubbles or to shrinkage phenomena, both of which happen during solidification. Therefore, the visualisation of the thermal field was fundamental in identifying the presence of the so-called hot spot regions (i.e. the last regions of the casting to solidify, with a significant risk of shrinkage phenomena). The gating and feeding system should be designed in order to ensure as efficient a supply as possible of molten metal to the solidifying (and shrinking) regions.

The results of the thermal field computations can be presented in different ways. Figure 6.14 shows the distribution of the solidification time; the path of solidification seems quite regular. About two seconds were needed to solidify the insert region, while the gates solidified in 4–5 seconds and the massive region presented a solidification time of more than nine seconds.

In fact, this part of the casting presented a noticeable shrinkage macro-porosity, as was observed after sectioning the framework (Figures 6.15–6.16). The computational code was used to evaluate the results regarding the thermal field in order to determine the risk of porosity. This elaboration is generally called "solidification criteria". On the basis of

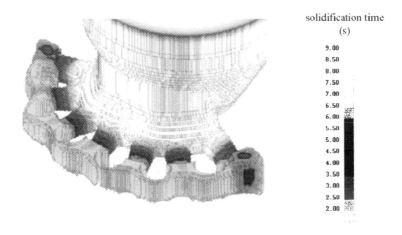

Figure 6.14 Distribution of solidification time.

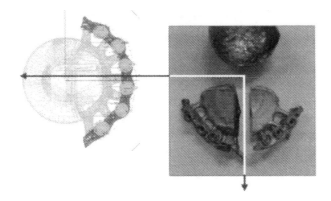

Figure 6.15 Scheme of how the casting was sectioned.

temperature evolution and critical values of the liquid fraction for feeding (Table 6.4), this elaboration makes it possible to identify the regions in which the feeding action of the liquid is not effective or insufficient, thus compensating for solidification shrinkage.

Figure 6.16 shows the visualisation of these criteria and the agreement with experimental results. With reference to the example shown, significant defects were localised in the feeder neck (Figure 6.16) and in the region connecting the feeder neck to the framework ingates (Figure 6.17). Porosity was, however, only localised in parts of the casting that had to be cut and removed; the final component was defect-free. In other words, the positive effect of the argon pressure application is very evident and no other significant solidification defects were observed.

Thermal field prediction provided another interesting kind of information. It is well known that cooling conditions heavily affect the final size of grains. Generally speaking, a law has been verified which correlates solidification time to Secondary Dendrite Arm Spacing (SDAS): $SDAS = k \bullet t_s^n$, where t_s is the solidification time and k and n the material-related constants. The meaning of this correlation is clear: as solidification becomes more

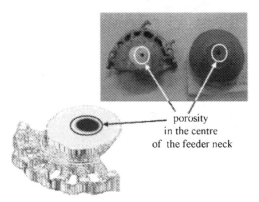

porosity
in the centre
of the feeder neck

Figure 6.16 Comparison between experimentally detected and numerically predicted porosity.

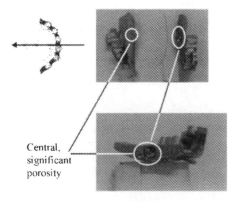

Central,
significant
porosity

Figure 6.17 Porosity in the region connecting the feeder neck to the framework ingates.

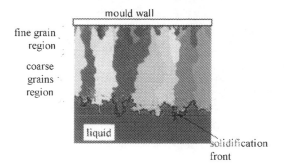

Figure 6.18 Schematic view of the microstructural evolution from the mould wall to the central region of the casting.

rapid, the microstructure becomes finer. Low values of SDAS and small grains lead to a fine microstrucure which is generally associated with increased mechanical properties. Small grains can be achieved in the fast-cooling regions (e.g. near the surface of the casting, see Figure 6.18). This fact can be well understood by observing the microhardness profiles from the surface to the centre of the component (it is probably useful to remember that, for metallic alloys, hardness is quite a good indicator of UTS and YS). In the literature (Figure 6.19) the behaviour of microhardness profiles for different kinds of titanium alloys clearly shows the change in mechanical properties from the surface to the centre of pieces. For cp titanium, a surface hardness of about 650 VHN was measured, rapidly going down to about 200 VHN at 200 μm from the surface.

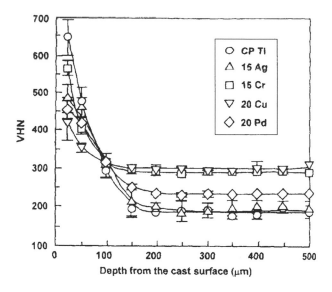

Figure 6.19 Typical hardness profiles (from the surface to the centre of the casting) for different titanium alloys (Okabe et al., 1998).

In the present case, the microhardness profiles were obtained experimentally both in the region preceeding the ingates (Figure 6.20) and in the region surrounding the titanium inserts (profiles one and two shown in Figure 6.21). The behaviour of hardness, displayed in Figures 6.20–6.21, is in perfect agreement with the profiles reported in Figure 6.19.

The experimental microhardness values can be directly correlated to the distribution of cooling rates in the framework, shown in Figure 6.22. The surface of the casting typically presents cooling rates noticeably higher than the internal and massive regions. The consequence is that, in the surface region, for a thickness of about 0.2 mm, microhardness values up to 600 $HV_{0.05}$ were detected.

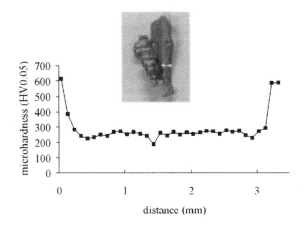

Figure 6.20 Microhardness profile in the region evidenced by the arrow.

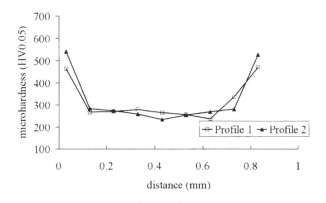

Figure 6.21 Microhardness profiles in the region surrounding the inserts.

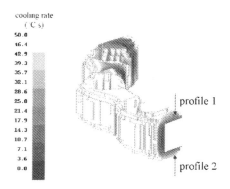

Figure 6.22 Distribution of the calculated cooling rate in the region surrounding the inserts.

6.6 MECHANICAL ANALYSIS OF TITANIUM BARS

In addition to being a helpful way of improving foundry procedures, the use of numerical methods in the simulation of the casting process also makes it possible to estimate the characteristics of the final structure of a titanium device, as far its mechanical performance is concerned. In fact, the necessary thermal treatment of titanium during the different phases of the manufacturing process causes an obvious modification of its mechanical properties. This has a direct impact on the response of the dental devices, under the application of typical loading related to the functional activity of the patient.

In particular, the cooling rate is one of the factors which determines the final microstructure of titanium, and thus the strength of the material to static and cyclic loading. It is particularly important to use empirical formulas of correlation between micro-hardness and elastic limits to determine the strength properties of a titanium bar in order to properly define the mechanical characteristics and to provide for a reliable estimation of the risk of failure.

The simulation of the mechanical response of the bar (or, better, of the whole bar-implants-mandible system) is usually performed using FE methods since they are particularly suitable for complex geometry (Figure 6.23).

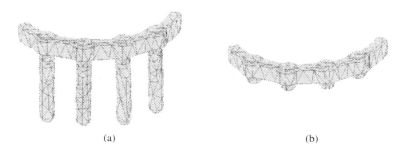

(a)   (b)

Figure 6.23 Finite element model of implants and bar (a) and detail of the bar (b).

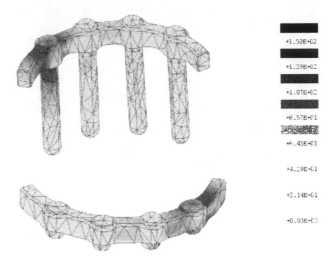

Figure 6.24 Distribution of the Von Mises stress in the implant-bar system under the application of a vertical force at the end of the cantilever: general view of the framework and the bar.

The use of FE methods is aimed at verifying the structure under the application of high magnitude loads in order to estimate the ultimate load bearing capacity, or to evaluate the structure's behaviour for the application of a cyclic loading. It then becomes possible to represent the real conditions during the life of dental devices.

By way of illustration, Figure 6.24 shows the stress field induced by the application of a vertical point-wise force (200 N) at the end of the cantilever of the bar. The stress field in the bar reveals the maximum values near the inserts, at the surface of the bar itself. This fact is particularly important since the surfaces of the bar also represent the regions in which the thermal treatments have the most appreciable effects on the characteristics of the material. The maximum stresses are compared with respect to the strength limit or to the fatigue limit, leading to an estimation of the risk factor of the structure.

6.7 CONCLUSIONS

The role of biomedical devices in terms of quality of life, requires, much more than in the past, the use of an improved and multidisciplinary approach. The manufacturing process has to be seen in connection with the material's peculiarities and with the properties that can be achieved, which, in turn, have to be correctly taken into account in designing the devices and in implanting them into the human body.

This chapter aimed to present a "working example" of this new approach, which consists in the biomechanical, processing and metallurgical evaluation of a titanium framework. It has been shown that this inter-disciplinary approach can lead to increasingly reliable production and application of dental devices. In particular the possibility of joining and comparing analyses and results both of specific manufacturing process and of the biomechanics of the titanium devices leads to greater reliability of the presented methodology.

REFERENCES

ASM Metals Handbook, 9th ed., Vol. 15: Casting, ASM – Metals Park, Ohio, 1988.

J.T. Berry, R.D. Pehlke, Modeling of solidification heat transfer, in ASM Metals Handbook, 9th ed., Vol. 15: Casting (1988), ASM – Metals Park, Ohio, pp. 858–866, 1998.

R.B. Bird, W.E. Stewart, E.N. Lightfoot, Transport Phenomena, J. Wiley and Sons, New York, 1966.

J. Black, Biological performance of materials – Fundamentals of biocompatibility, 2nd edn., Marcel Dekker Inc., New York, 1992.

R.R. Boyer, J.A. Hall, Microstructure-property relationships in titanium alloys (critical review), in Froes FH, Caplan I, editors, Titanium '92 – Science and Technology, The Mineral, Metals & Materials Society, Warrendale, PA, pp. 77–88, 1993.

F. Bonollo, N. Gramegna, S. Odorizzi, La pressocolata delle leghe di alluminio: simulazione numerica del processo, EDIMET, Brescia, 1999.

F. Bonollo, N. Gramegna, A. Natali and P. Pavan, La simulazione di processo nella realizzazione di componenti in titanio per implantologia dentale, Titanium Industry, Vol. 1, pp. 16–19, 2001a.

F. Bonollo, S. Odorizzi, Numerical Simulation of Foundry Processes, SGE, Padova, 2001b.

R.S. Brodkey, H.C. Hershey, Transport Phenomena: A Unified Approach, McGraw-Hill Int.Book Co., New York, 1988.

J.B. Brunski, Classes of materials used in medicine. Metals, in Biomaterials Science, An Introduction to Materials in Medicine, Edited by B. Rutner, A. Hoffman, F. Schoen, J. Lemons, Academic Press, San Diego, CA, 1996.

E.W. Collings, The physical metallurgy of titanium alloys, ASM Series in Metal Processing. Gegel HL, editor, American Society for Metals, Cleveland, Metals Park, OH, 1984.

P.V. Desai, K.V. Pagalthivarthi, Modeling of combined fluid flow and heat/mass transfer, in ASM Metals Handbook, 9th ed., Vol. 15: Casting (1988), ASM – Metals Park, Ohio, pp. 877–882, 1998.

G.M. Dusinberre, Heat-Transfer Calculations by Finite Differences. Int. Textbook Co., Scranton Pa., USA, 1961.

J. Hattel et al. (eds.), Numerical Modelling of Casting Processes, Nova Science Publ. (in preparation).

N.L. Hernandez de Gatica, G.L. Jones, J.A. Gardella, Surface characterization of titanium alloys sterilized for biomedical applications, Appl Surface Sci, Vol. 68, pp. 107–121, 1993.

W.S. Hwang, R.A. Stoehr, Modeling of fluid flow, in ASM Metals Handbook, 9th ed., Vol. 15: Casting (1988), ASM – Metals Park, Ohio, pp. 867–876, 1998.

E. Kobayashi, S. Matsumoto, H. Doi, T. Yoneyama, H. Hamanaka, Mechanical properties of the binary titanium-zirconium alloys and their potential for biomedical materials, J Biomed Mater Res, Vol. 29, pp. 943–950, 1995.

P. Kovacs, J.A. Davidson, The electrochemical behavior of a new titanium alloy with superior biocompatibility, in Titanium '92 – Science and Technology, The Minerals, Metals and Materials Society, Warrendale, pp. 2705–2712, 1993.

S. Lampman, Wrought titanium and titanium alloy, in ASM Metals Handbook, 10th ed., Vol. 2, Non-ferrous alloys, ASM – Metals Park, Ohio, 1994.

M. Long, H.J. Rack, Titanium alloys in total joint replacement. A materials science perspective, Biomaterials, Vol. 19, pp. 1621–1639, 1998.

P.A. Manusli, S.G. Steineman, J.P. Simpson, Properties of surface oxides on titanium and some titanium alloys in 6th World Conference on Titanium, les editions de physique, Les Ulis Cedex, France, part IV, pp. 1759–1764, 1988.

A.K. Mishra, J.A. Davidson, P. Kovacs, R.A. Poggie, Ti-13Nb-13Zr: a new low modulus, high strength, corrosion resistant near-beta alloy for orthopaedic implants, in Beta Titanium in the 1990s, The Minerals, Metals & Materials Society, Warrendale, pp. 61–72, 1993.

P.H. Morton, T. Bell, Surface engineering of titanium, Memoires et Etudes Scientifiques Revue de Metallurgie, Vol. 86, pp. 639–646, 1989.

A. Natali, P. Pavan, F. Bonollo, N. Gramegna, "Numerical analysis of titanium cast devices for dental implantology", Computer Methods in Biomechanics and Biomedical Engineering, Vol. 5, Issue 2, pp. 615–623, 2002.

B.D. Nichols, C.W. Hirt, R.S. Hotchkiss, SOLA-VOF: A Solution Algorithm for Transient Fluid Flow with Multiple Free Boundaries, Rep. LA-8355, Los Alamos Scientific Lab., Los Alamos, NM, 1980.

M. Niinomi, Mechanical properties of biomedical titanium alloys, Materials Science and Engineering, Vol. A243, pp. 231–236, 1998.

T. Okabe, C. Ohkubo, I. Watanabe, O. Okuno, Y. Takada, The present status of dental titanium casting, Journal of Metals, Vol. 50, Issue 9, 24–29, 1998.

Y. Okazaki, Y. Ito, A. Ito, T. Tateishi, Effect of alloying elements on mechanical properties of titanium alloys for medical implants, Mater. Trans. JIM, Vol. 34, pp. 1217–1222, 1993.

J.B. Park R.S. Lakes, Biomaterials – An introduction, 2nd edn., Plenum Press, New York, 1992.

S.V. Patankar, Numerical heat transfer and fluid flow, Hemisphere Publ., Washington D.C., 1980.

J.J. Polmear, Titanium alloys, in Light alloys, Chapter 6, Edward Arnold Publ, London, 1981.

N.G. Raikar, J. Gregory, J.L. Ong, L.C. Lucas, J.E. Lemons, D. Kawahara, M. Nakamura, Surface characterization of titanium implants, J Vac Sci Technol, Vol. 13A, pp. 2633–2637, 1995.

G.D. Raithby, G.E. Schneider, in Minkowycz W.J. et al. (eds.), Handbook of Numerical Heat Transfer, Chap. 7, J. Wiley, New York, pp. 241–291, 1988.

K. Rundinger, D. Fischer, Relationship between primary alpha content, tensile properties and high cycle fatigue behavior of Ti-6Al-4V, in Luntjering G, Zwicker U, Bunk W, editors. Titanium '84 – Science and technology, Vol. 4. Deutsche Gesellschaft Fur Metallkunde EV, Munich, pp. 2123–2130, 1985.

P.R. Sahm, P.N. Hansen, "Numerical Simulation and Modelling of Casting and Solidification Processes for Foundry and Cast-House", CIATF, 1984.

R.W. Schutz, An overview of beta titanium alloy environmental behavior, in Eylon D, Boyer RR, Koss DA, editors. Beta Titanium Alloys in the 1990's, The Mineral, Metals & Materials Society, Warrendale, pp. 75–91, 1993.

S.G. Steinemann, Corrosion of titanium and titanium alloys for surgical implants, in Titanium '84 – Science and Technology, Vol. 2, Deutsche Gesellschaft Fur Metallkunde EV, Munich, pp. 1373–1379, 1985.

K. Suzuki, The high quality precision casting of Titanium alloys, Journal of Metals, Vol. 50, 9, pp. 23–34, 1998.

A. Vassel, Microstructural instabilities in beta titanium alloys, in Eylon D, Boyer RR, Koss DA, editors, Beta Titanium Alloys in the 1990s, The Mineral, Metals and Materials Society, Warrendale, pp. 173–185, 1993.

K. Wang, L. Gustavson, J. Dumbleton, Low modulus, high strength, biocompatible titanium alloy for medical implants, in Titanium '92 – Science and Technology, The Minerals, Metals and Materials Society, Warrendale, pp. 2696–2704, 1993a.

K. Wang, L. Gustavson and J. Dumbleton, The characterization of Ti-12Mo-6Zr-2Fe, a new biocompatible titanium alloy developed for surgical implants, in Beta Titanium in the 1990s, The Minerals, Metals & Materials Society, Warrendale, pp. 49–60, 1993b.

D.N. Williams, R.A. Wood, Effects of surface condition on the mechanical properties of titanium and its alloys. MCIC-71–01 Report. Metals and Ceramics Information Center, Battelle Columbus Laboratories, OH, 1971.

7 Testing the reliability of dental implant devices

*M Soncini, RP Pietrabissa, AN Natali, PG Pavan,
KR Williams*

7.1 INTRODUCTION

It is generally recognized that the majority of implant designs can successfully transmit occlusal forces to the supporting tissue without systematic failure. Indeed, a review of the implant literature suggests it is difficult to find a truly novel implant configuration. The problem of the implant fixity in bone tissue essentially determines the design and hence geometry of implants and associated bridgework. The fixity mainly depends on osseointegration, which according to Branemark (Branemark et al., 1985) is defined as 'a direct structural and functional connection between ordered living bone and the surface of a load carrying implant'. Different techniques can be adopted to carry out implant osseointegration, guiding or favouring the bone ingrowth around the implant up to its mechanical fixation. Macro-interlock mechanical fixation to bone is obtained by arranging for the implant to be threaded or by creating holes to run through the material. Surface roughness on a finer scale, such as plasma-sprayed coatings of metals or the chemical deposition of ceramics, allow bone to grow into small ridges or asperities; this type of fixation is by micro-interlocking. It is possible to provide for a bioactive surface so that the developing bone may bond chemically with the implant. Typically implants can be coated with hydroxyapatite which essentially has a chemical composition similar to bone. The bone formation can also be guided by using specific peptides that favour the adhesion and growth of the new bone tissue around the implant, reducing the healing time after the surgical insertion. The experimental activity in this field has lead to promising results for further applications of these techniques on a larger scale.

It's worth pointing out, however, that implants were not initially designed according to engineering principles. This was essentially due to the lack of good information on implant loading, bone-implant contact area, boundary conditions, bone properties and several other factors. Although the current interest in the use of the finite element method for design purposes is becoming established, researchers still have to deal with largely unknown parameters. To quote from reviews, the history of dental implants reveals that implant research and development represent a design problem in the true sense of the word. It is necessary to set design objectives, formulate a rational solution strategy, and then evaluate the extent to which the design objectives are achieved. Through this approach, it is also possible to arrive at quantitative measures of implant success or failure.

However, there are a significant number of biomechanical design objectives that still need to be clarified for dental implants. While everyone recognizes that the goal is to solve the biomechanical fixation problem, questions remain about exactly how best to accomplish this. In addressing these questions, the nature of implant loading, interfacial stress transfer and interfacial tissue response will all be of primary importance.

Methods to estimate the reliability of dental implants by means of both experimental tests and numerical simulation must be investigated. Integration and comparison of information coming from both approaches reveals to be probably the best method for a deep understanding of the biomechanics of dental implants. An introduction to the experimental testing of dental implants and a short note on numerical analysis are presented. It is not possible to report an adequate amount of data from different experimental and numerical analyses, and so this chapter simply presents a description of some procedures.

7.2 MECHANICAL RELIABILITY OF DENTAL IMPLANTS

One of the most interesting aspects of the biomechanics of dental implants regards determining the loading acting on the implant and how the loading is transmitted to the periimplant bone tissue through the implant itself. Though these aspects have been studied for years, they are still far from being completely defined. Functional activity induces a complex configuration of loading, mainly characterized by vertical and transversal forces. These loads induce a consequent distribution of stress in both the implant itself and the surrounding bone. The type of loading, shape and dimension of the implant, implant surface, configuration of the prosthetic superstructure and quantity and quality of the bone tissue around the implant are all factors affecting the load bearing capacity of the system.

In the following paragraphs, attention is focused on the mechanics of the implant and its components, i.e. fixture, abutment and connecting screw. The materials and surface treatments affecting the strength of the implant and the bone-implant interaction are briefly recalled. The results of experimental testing under different loading conditions are discussed. These results can serve as basic information for the evaluation of the reliability of the implant-bone system as a load bearing structure.

7.2.1 Dental implant configuration

There are two typical surgical procedures for the insertion of dental implants: one is based on the one-stage technique (Buser et al., 1998; Buser et al., 1999; Weber et al., 2000); the other is based on the two-stage technique (Adell et al., 1981; Albrektsson and Sennerby, 1991; van Steenberghe and Naert, 1998). A one-stage implant is inserted in the jaw bone with only one surgical intervention; once it has been inserted, it protrudes through the gingival tissue and is not covered up with soft tissues. On the contrary, during the first phase of a two-stage procedure, the implant is surgically placed in the anatomical site and totally covered by the gingival tissue. Once the implant is fixed, the gingival tissue is opened and an abutment is connected to the endosseus system on top of the fixture and the whole system emerges from the soft tissue. The endosseous implants adopted in this type of surgical procedure consist of a fixture, abutment and connection screw between the fixture and abutment.

Prosthetic superstructures are defined on the basis of the specific morphometry of the patient and their construction must be based on a custom made procedure. For example, metal alloy dental bars are manufactured through a sequence of technological steps that may entail different phases such as impression of the patient's mouth, preparation of the master model, waxing, casting, etc. (Jemt, 1995; Natali et al., 2002).

Experience in the field of dental implant biomechanics and surgical practice, from the early applications to the present, has lead to the development of different types of implants, adopting specific shapes and surfaces, as reported for example in Figure 7.1. Nowadays, threaded implants are the most common type of implant. Many studies have been carried out on the shapes of the fixtures, in order to optimise the transmission of the loads from the fixture to the periimplant bone tissue.

Ensuring the optimal conditions for the growth of the bone around the implant and osseointegration is the key factor for the long-term stability of the implant-bone system. These conditions can be favoured by optimising the mechanical behaviour at the bone-implant interface, as well as guiding the biological process of bone regeneration, for example by using adhesion and growth factors (Ferris et al., 1999; Shah et al., 1999; Sykaras et al., 2001; Dettin et al., 2002). Implant length has a significant influence on the transmission of the loads to the surrounding implant. The configuration of the implant and the number and placement of implants supporting the prosthetic superstructure also influence how much the loads affect the overall structure and bone. Several studies have used numerical analysis to compare the distribution of stress in the bone tissue around different types of dental implants (Siegele and Soltész, 1989; Lum, 1992; Natali et al., 1998; Natali, 1999; Joos et al., 2000; Meyer et al., 2001). It has been recognized that threaded and non-threaded cylindrical implants lead to very different distributions of stress in the periimplant bone.

The position of the fixture in the anatomical site and its inclination often require the use of angulated abutments. This procedure is the only way to overcome aesthetic problems and to ensure full functionality of the prosthetic device in patients that have complex anatomical configurations. The use of angulated abutments also has a direct effect on the transmission of the loads to the fixture and on the stress state induced. An important characteristic of dental implants is the configuration of the coupling between implant and abutment.

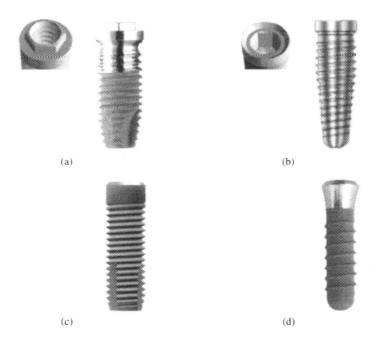

(a)   (b)

(c)   (d)

Figure 7.1 Different types of threaded implants.

7.2.2 Materials and surface treatments

The characteristics of the titanium based materials commonly adopted in dental implantology are dealt with in detail in chapter five. Hence, this topic is only briefly treated here. The main favourable properties of titanium devices are their excellent resistance to corrosion in physiological environments and their high biocompatibility, which is necessary for the growth of bone around the endosseus components (Kasemo, 1983; Kasemo and Lausmaa, 1986; Buser et al., 1991). Commercialy pure titanium is adopted for all the components of dental implants that come into direct contact with bone. The alloy TiAl6V4 is often adopted for the other components, such as abutments, since they have better mechanical properties.

In order to guarantee the long-term reliability of dental implants, the surface characteristics should be improved to enhance the fatigue strength. This can be carried out using surface hardening technologies, such as ion implantation (Pillar and Weatherly, 1986). The mechanical properties of the bone-implant system strongly depend on the interaction phenomena at the interface. In particular, the roughness and porosity of the fixture surface have a significant influence on the bone in-growth. Roughness and porosity of about 80 μm favour bone tissue in-growth, while individual cells are directly influenced by surface structural features which are in the range of 1–10 μm (Brunette, 1988; Quirynen and Bollen, 1996). Different treatments can be adopted to obtain modifications of the surface, which can lead to favourable conditions for bone growth. The surface area of the fixture can be increased by a titanium plasma spray treatment, allowing for better microretention. Implant surfaces can be treated by using sandblasting, electro-deposition or electro-erosion treatments or by adopting hydroxyapatite coating (Leimola-Virtanen et al., 1995; Wheeler, 1996; Cochran et al., 1998; Lincks et al., 1998; Mustafa et al., 2001; Bigerelle et al., 2002). The use of hydroxyapatite coating favours bone adaptation, reduces the healing time and inhibits the formation of fibrous tissues in the periimplant region (Klein et al., 1991; Gottlander, 1992; Kay, 1992; Sendax, 1992; Dhert, 1993; Klein et al., 1994). Therefore, coating treatments can actually lead to a general improvement in the stability of the implant, even if the reliability over time of these techniques has not yet been properly assessed.

7.2.3 Loading conditions

Evaluating the loads acting on implants or natural teeth during the functional activity of a patient is not an easy task. Since there are still no fully reliable testing devices, it is difficult to gather exhaustive data about the type and amount of loads. Many efforts have been made in the investigation of forces in the case of dental implants, fixed and removable prostheses, as well as natural teeth.

Experimental data by different authors varies quite a bit, and this aspect can be partially justified by the fact that the values depend on many different factors, for example, the specific masticatory conditions. (Craig, 1980; Ludgren et al., 1987; Brunski, 1992; Brunski, 1995; Paphangkorakit and Osborn, 1998). This is, obviously, also due to the significant differentiation of the anatomy from patient to patient. The loading conditions related to chewing activity are mainly a combination of forces. The loading conditions induce different stress distributions within the implant itself and in the surrounding bone tissue (Rangert et al., 1989; Weinberg, 1993), and can also lead to the failure of the system, e.g. a fracture of the implant components or marginal bone loss (Quirynen et al., 1992; Hoshaw et al., 1994; Rangert et al., 1995).

The loads related to functional activity are not the only source of stress on implants and bone. In fact, in multi-implant configurations, if one or more implants are misfit with the dental bar, a pre-load can be induced when the bar is forced on the abutments causing stress at the bone-implant interface (Pietrabissa et al., 2000). The intensity of the pre-load depends on the size of the misfit (Jemt, 1991; Jemt et al., 1992; Jemt and Book, 1996). In the case of a multi-implant system, the effects of pre-loads can be particularly evident when there are framework distortions (Carr et al., 1993). The consequent additional stress is summed to the one induced by functional activity, giving rise to possible critical conditions.

The mean intrusive forces acting on single implants are usually in the order of 200 N, while the transversal forces are about ten percent of the vertical component. These are just the indicative values referring to the general case of masticatory activity. However, experimental testing and numerical analysis take into account larger forces, in order to estimate the limit load bearing capacity of the implant system and thus evaluate its safety condition.

7.3 MECHANICAL TESTING OF DENTAL IMPLANTS

The reliability of dental implant-retained prostheses is related to how well the prostheses can replace the natural functions of a patient. It is obviously essential that the functional capability of a prosthetic system be maintained for a long-term period. At present, the success rates of prosthetic systems based on edosseus implants is quite high. This can mostly be considered to be the result of empirical methods and the experience of several years of clinical activity. Nonetheless, it is important to investigate the problem of the biomechanical reliability of implant systems in order to reduce the risk of failure. Engineering methods, both experimental and numerical, can give a significant contribution in this sense.

During the functional activity of a patient, the dental implant system is subjected to various conditions. These can induce cycling stresses both in the different components of the prosthesis and in the bone around the implant. The value of these stresses depends on several terms, such as specific anatomy of the patient and the functional activity, as well as on the conditions of the periimplant bone tissue. The latter aspect can largely affect the constraint of the implant. The type of overstructure is another factor that greatly influences functional behaviour. The boundary and loading conditions of a dental implant system are far from be precisely specified. It is essential that the experimental testing be carried out by simulating, as well as possible, the critical conditions that an implant system can experience. The experimental procedure must be repeatable and allow a comparative analysis of the mechanical response of different types of implants, undergoing the same loading and boundary conditions.

A typical experimental procedure aimed at evaluating the mechanical strength of dental implants is proposed in the following paragraphs. Ultimate strength and fatigue strength tests of titanium implants are described, together with an experimental procedure aimed at evaluating the load bearing capacity of the bone-implant system. The numerical simulation of the mechanical response of the dental implant, to support experimental activity, is also shown. Some of the quantitative results reported are obviously related to the very specific conditions considered and cannot be generalised to other types of dental implants. Nonetheless, the experimental and numerical tests presented can be considered as an example of a general procedure.

7.3.1 Experimental tests for evaluating ultimate load

Figure 7.2 shows the set up for the compression test of a typical commercial double-stage titanium dental system. The fixtures tested were 13 mm long and 3.75 mm in diameter with a 25° pre-angled abutment connected to the fixture by a screw. In each implant, the connecting screw was tightened with a torque of 20 Ncm, the value that is usually recommended by the manufacturer. The way the compressive force was applied, at the top of the abutment, gave rise to bending moments, which were summed to the compressive state of the fixture. This represents the worst-case condition for an implant. The testing was carried out by using a MTS 858 Mini Bionix machine equipped with a MTS 661.19F-02 10 kN load cell, aligned with the actuator. The implants were inserted in a cylindrical aluminium support and placed to have the fixture axis parallel to the loading direction. The force-displacement tests were carried out with displacement control and a rate of 1 mm/min, up to the failure of the system.

The implants were tested under different boundary and loading conditions. Two types of constraints were considered inserting the implant completely or only partially into the cylindrical support. The second case aimed at simulating the behaviour of an implant with the neck not fully inserted in the jawbone. The different behaviour of the two systems, completely and partially inserted, is shown in Figure 7.3.

The system failure occurred at the level of the abutment-fixture connecting screw. In fact, the connecting screw is usually the weakest component in an implant system. This is due not only to the small cross section but also to the pre-load induced by tightening, which causes tensile stresses in the body of the screw from the neck through the threaded area. A significant reduction in the load bearing capacity of the implant system was found when it was partially inserted in the support. The ultimate load for a fully inserted implant was measured in the range of 2014 N ÷ 2346 N, while for a partially inserted implant in the range of 1251 N ÷ 1850 N.

In a second test on the same type of implant, two configurations of compressive loads were applied, acting parallel to the abutment axis or the fixture axis. The load bearing capacity was much lower for the case of the compressive force acting parallel to the fixture axis. In this case, the ultimate load was 1190 N, but this value was almost doubled for a load acting parallel to the abutment axis.

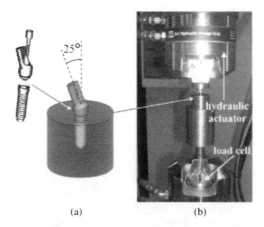

(a)   (b)

Figure 7.2 Details of the implant and support (a) and machine used for the compression tests (b).

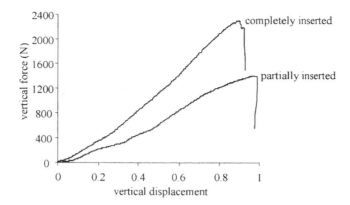

Figure 7.3 Effect of the different types of constraint on the load bearing capacity of a two-stage dental implant.

This confirms the importance of a careful evaluation of the geometrical configuration of implants and loadings to properly define the most critical conditions. The data presented above should serve just as an example to emphasize the significance of the insertion length and loading conditions on the implant response. In fact, in reality the loads associated to the functional activity of a patient are smaller than the loads used in the tests, and the boundary conditions of the experimental tests can differ from the ones induced by the cortical and trabecular bone in the jaw. For the case presented above, the implant can be considered mechanically resistant if its ultimate load is larger than 800 N, even if this limit is greater than the usual forces caused by masticatory activity. Clearly many different loading and boundary conditions must be investigated to offer a complete characterisation of the specific implant response.

7.3.1.1 Analysis of the post-elastic behaviour of dental implants

An interesting aspect concerning the response of dental implants is the limit strength behaviour and strength hierarchy of the implant components. An analysis of this aspect can make it possible to evaluate the type of failure of the system and identify its weakest elements.

Figures 7.4 (a) and 7.4 (b) refer to a compression-bending test carried out on two types of titanium dental implants. The implants were completely inserted in a polymethylmethacrylate cylindrical support, which simulated the elastic constraint of the surrounding bone. The compressive force was parallel to the fixture axis, as shown in Figure 7.4 (b), and applied at the end of the cantilever connected to the top of the abutment. The loading also induced a bending moment in the implant. The tests were carried out using displacement control in order to properly keep track of the post-elastic phase. The maximum eccentricity of the point of application of the load was 18 mm. A maximum compressive force of about 200 N was recorded during the test.

The two types of implants showed different behaviour in the post-elastic phase. Both of them showed significant ductility and were thus able to experience plastic deformation before failure. The first type showed the ultimate brittle failure of the screw connecting the abutment and fixture, as depicted in Figure 7.4 (a), while a progressive deformation occurred in the second type (Figure 7.4 (b)), once again at the fixture-bone connection, but without a final brittle failure of the components.

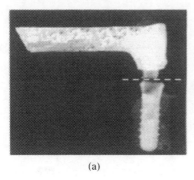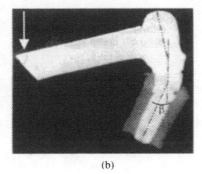

(a)   (b)

Figure 7.4 Two examples of implant failure caused by failure of the connecting screw (a) or a large plastic strain (b).

It must be pointed out that the load bearing capacity appeared very small, if compared with previous cases reported. In fact, in this test the length of the cantilever caused a much larger bending moment on the implants than in the test described in paragraph 2.1. In addition, the use of a polymethylmethacrylate cylindrical support determined very different boundary conditions from those in the case of an aluminium support, thus affecting the overall behaviour of the implant system. These data are reported to recall the relevance of loading configurations and boundary conditions on the overall biomechanical response of implants.

7.3.2 Numerical simulation of experimental tests

The stress and strain acting on implant structures under different loading conditions can be conveniently studied by means of numerical techniques, such as the finite element method. Computational methods, if validated by experimental testing, have proven to be a useful tool for simulating the real behaviour of the system. This makes it possible to partially overcome the well-known limits of experimental procedures and provide information about internal structures, which otherwise remain inaccessible. Because of the lack of adequate data gathering devices, it is extremely difficult to carry out experimental activity in the field of biomechanics to evaluate stress and strain states in biological tissues.

Due to these difficulties, researchers have spent much effort using numerical methods to evaluate stress states in the bone tissue around dental implants, as well as in the implants and their components (Lozada et al., 1994; van Zyl et al., 1995; Baiamonte et al., 1996; Papavasiliou et al., 1996b; Williams and Williams, 1997; Natali and Pavan, 2002). Two-dimensional finite elements models have been used to study the effects of tightening the screws retaining abutments and crowns. The same approach has been adopted to verify the effects of masticatory loads (Papavasiliou et al., 1996a) and similar procedures have been used to study the mechanical performance of different types of implant-abutment connections (Merz et al., 2000). It is important to recall that only a three-dimensional model can provide a realistic interpretation of the phenomena investigated.

The mechanical reliability of a double-stage dental implant system was evaluated to exemplify the use of the numerical approach and its possibilities. The three-dimensional finite element model adopted for the analysis is reported in Figure 7.5. The model includes the three components: the fixture, abutment and connecting screw. For simplicity's sake, the external thread of the fixture was not considered in the model, and the thread of the connecting screw was assumed to be axial-symmetric. The implant was considered to be inserted in an aluminium cylindrical support, simulating the actual conditions of experimental tests. Table 7.1 reports the material properties assumed for the different parts of the model. The post-elastic behaviour of titanium was described using a rate-independent metal-plasticity model. In this way it was possible to evaluate the plastic response of the fixture neck for the application of a load applied on the top of the abutment.

Since the connecting screw has proven to be the weakest structural component of the implant system, particular attention was paid to representing the actual conditions at the fixture-abutment interface. There was assumed to be a sliding contact with a 0.3 friction coefficient (Sakaguchi and Borgersen, 1995) in three regions of the implant system: between the screw head surface and the abutment surface, in the flaring between the fixture neck and the abutment, between the external surface of the abutment hexagon and the surface of the hexagonal seat in the fixture.

All the other surfaces of the different components in reciprocal contact were considered to be tied. The boundary conditions of the external surface simulate the constraint of the testing device.

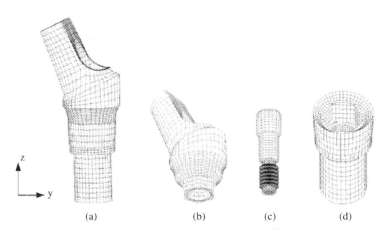

(a)   (b)   (c)   (d)

Figure 7.5 Finite element model of the assembled implant components (a) detail of the abutment (b) connecting screw (c) and smoothed fixture (d).

Table 7.1 Material properties for the different components of the finite element model represented in Figure 7.5. E is the Young elastic modulus, v is Poisson's ratio, σ_y is the yield stress and σ_u is the ultimate stress.

Component	Material	E[GPa]	v	σ_y[Mpa]	σ_u[Mpa]
Fixture	Titanium c.p.	110	0.28	380	450
Abutment	Titanium alloy	110	0.28	790	860
Connecting screw	Titanium alloy	110	0.28	790	860
Cylindrical support	Aluminium	63	0.28	178	230

A 280 N pre-load was applied on the connecting screw, in order to simulate its initial torque of 20 Ncm. The loading condition refers to the experimental testing described in paragraph 2.1. A compressive vertical load corresponding to the ultimate compressive force was applied on top of the abutment. The loading condition induces the compression and the bending on the implant, due to the eccentricity of the load axis with respect to the fixture axis.

Figure 7.6 (a) shows the normal stress in vertical direction σ_z induced by tightening the connecting screw. The Von Mises stress field determined by adding a vertical compressive load of 1190 N is shown in Figure 7.6 (b), at the middle longitudinal section of the implant.

Further analyses must be performed to have an exhaustive investigation, which takes into account different loadings or boundary conditions.

7.3.3 Fatigue tests for evaluating the long-term reliability of dental implants

Any structure subjected to time-variable loading can show a cycle-dependent strength. The load bearing capacity of the structure can be much lower than the ultimate loading recorded during a static test. Furthermore, there can be structure failure even if the stress that occurred during the loading history is very far from the elastic limit of the material. This type of failure is due to a progressive degradation of the micro-structure, with the formation of voids and cracks, and is known as fatigue failure. It is extremely important to identify the parameters affecting the life of a structure under cyclical loading, i.e. the estimation of its fatigue life, in order to achieve a long-term reliability of the implants.

To establish the fatigue limit of the implants it is essential to identify the loading spectra that represent a reasonable loading history. This is probably the most difficult aspect, since it is very hard to completely estimate the loading conditions with regard to magnitude, direction, etc. If one excludes environmental factors, such as high temperature or chemicals, the parameters influencing the fatigue life of a structure are the total number of loading cycles, maximum and minimum stress. These parameters define the stress history if constant stress amplitude is assumed. The adoption of a loading spectrum with constant amplitude is usually conservative. As for the ultimate strength tests, the whole implant system is tested

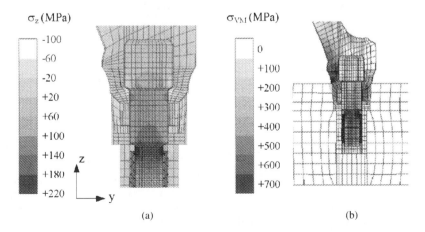

(a)   (b)

Figure 7.6 Stress field σ_z in the central longitudinal section of the implant system due to the tightening of 20 Ncm (a) and the Von Mises stress field σ_{VM} (b) for the combination of the tightening with a vertical compressive force.

in order to get information about the single components and their coupling. The load applying devices should be able to generate compression and bending, a typical loading combination on the implant.

An experimental procedure adopted for the evaluation of the fatigue strength of titanium implants is presented here. The fatigue tests were carried out using the device represented in Figure 7.7. The apparatus can test four implants at the same time, with a consequent time and cost saving.

The tests were carried out in a non-aggressive environment with a temperature of $22 \pm 2°C$ and humidity of 60 ± 5 per cent. A sine wave shaped load was applied with a maximum value of 500 N and a minimum value of 20 N. The frequency of the loading history was in the range of 5 and 7 Hz. The maximum value of the load applied in the fatigue tests was fixed at about 60 per cent of the maximum load recorded in the molar region during masticatory activity. The tests were considered to have been completed successfully if the implant survived up to 5×10^6 loading cycles.

The maximum number of cycles should be fixed on the basis of the severity of the loading conditions applied, in comparison with the actual loading history. If an implant fails before the maximum number of cycles, it can be interesting to study the source of the failure, by using, for example, scanning electron microscope (SEM) analysis. Possible defects in the system, such as inclusions or surface defects caused by mechanical processing can thus be identified. In Figure 7.8 four images found with an SEM analysis on a double stage implant, which failed at 63,557 cycles of the fatigue test presented above. The failure involved the first thread level of the screw connecting the fixture and abutment. In Figures 7.8 (a) and 7.8 (b) it is possible to identify the region where the fracture arose, and details of the surface in Figures 7.8 (c) and 7.8 (d).

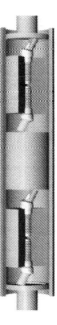

Figure 7.7 Representation of a typical device adopted for fatigue testing. The device is capable of testing four implants at the same time.

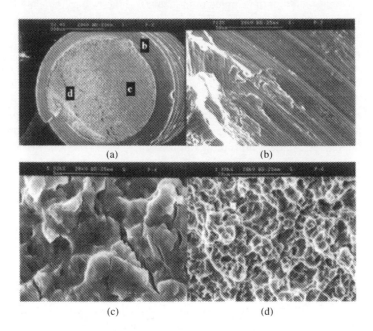

Figure 7.8 Scanning electron microscopy of an implant failed during a fatigue test: fracture surface of the connecting screw (a) fracture starting point zone (b) fracture zone with different magnification factors as (c) and (d).

7.4 EXPERIMENTAL TESTS TO EVALUATE THE EFFICIENCY OF BONE-IMPLANT INTERACTION

One of the factors that deeply affects the long-term success of dental implants is the mechanical reliability of the bone-fixture system, affected by the level of osseointegration, as well as by the mechanical properties of the periimplant bone tissue. The experimental tests usually adopted to investigate the bone-fixture interaction are torque tests, push-in tests, pull-out tests and resonance frequency tests. Torque tests are suitable for estimating the percentage of the fixture surface integrated with the bone tissue, while push-in tests are used to verify the load bearing capacity of the bone region surrounding the implant, i.e. the bone as a constraint.

Much effort has been spent in the scientific community to evaluate these tests. Torque tests have been carried out on implants inserted in the dyaphyses and methaphyses of animal femur and tibia (Carlsson et al., 1991; Johanson et al., 1991; Brånemark et al., 1997). The same procedure has also been adopted using mastoid human cadaver bone (Tjellström et al., 1988) or mastoid and temporal human cadaver bone (Ueda et al., 1991). Attempts have been made to relate the torsional strength of screw-shaped implants in baboon mandibles to implant position, type of biomaterials and healing time (Carr et al., 1995). Pull-out tests for evaluating the bone-fixture interface strength have also been carried out (Kraut et al., 1991; Ivanoff et al., 1995; Berzins et al., 1997). Finally, resonance frequency analysis represents an indirect quantitative method to evaluate bone-fixture stability. This method can be very interesting because of the field of resulting data and its non-destructive characteristics (Meredith, 1998; Sennersby and Meredith, 1998; Friberg et al., 1999).

7.4.1 The experimental procedure

The experimental procedure described below was carried out to evaluate the mechanical properties of the bone-implant interaction. The characteristic of the bone region that extends 2 mm around the external surface of a titanium dental fixture is investigated (Soncini et al., 2002), as a function of different factors, such as surgical technique and healing time. It is worth pointing out that the aim of the following description is to define the procedure rather than offer a complete set of results. The experimental procedure basically consisted in three steps. The first step was represented by the surgical insertion of the fixtures in animal tibia, in order to prepare the specimens. The second step was pull-in mechanical testing. The last step was a microradiographic analysis of the bone surrounding the fixture, to relate the mechanical properties of bone tissue to its morphology.

Ten self tapping titanium fixtures were inserted in the tibial proximal sites of two 80 kg 18 month-old sheep, i.e. five fixtures for each sheep. The fixtures were inserted in trabecular bone avoiding the medullary channel, as well as any distal contact with cortical tissue. The fixtures were titanium made with a 3.5 mm diameter and titanium dioxide blasted surface. The animals were anaesthetized and the tibia exposed for the bone site preparation. A countersink was used to create some defects in the periimplant bone tissue of the coronal region and the consequent gaps were filled with deantigenate bovine bone particles. The surgical site was then covered with a reabsorbable polyglactin membrane. The fixtures were then inserted into the tibia and the healing cap applied. A total of six fixtures were inserted into the same number of surgically prepared 3.2 mm diameter sites with coronal implant defects filled with biomaterial, while the four other fixtures were inserted into sites without defects. One sheep was sacrified after 24 days with an intrapulmonary injection, while the other one was sacrified after 45 days to obtain specimens with different healing times. After the removal of soft tissues, the specimens, made up of the fixture and surrounding bone tissue, were cut and stored in four per cent paraformaldehyde. Six specimens were used for the mechanical testing, while the other ones were used for microradiographic analyses.

A cylindrical support was used to position the specimens correctly in the testing device, by using glass-ionomer cement. The specimens had to be kept in place in order to ensure the alignment between the axis of the fixture and the axis of application of the load. The specimens were attached to the testing machine through an abutment, which was screwed into the fixture and glued to the seat of the load-applying device, as depicted in Figure 7.9. The testing machine was a MTS 858 MiniBionix, equipped with a 10 kN load cell. The tests were performed with displacement control in order to record the force-displacement curve even in the presence of softening behaviour. A rate of 0.25 mm/min was applied. The maximum load recorded during the test was considered to be the ultimate load.

The value of the ultimate load was then used to estimate the mechanical properties of the periimplant bone tissue under different conditions of healing time and for different surgical techniques. Numerical simulations of similar bone-fixture systems show that the application of a vertical intrusive load induces a stress on the bone tissue with peak values in the regions close to the coronal part of the fixture.

In order to evaluate the microstructure of the periimplant bone tissue, a microradiographic analysis was performed for the other fixtures. These fixtures were inserted next to the ones used for the mechanical testing. Assuming that the periimplant tissue has the same configuration around the adjacent fixtures, this type of analysis can be used to correlate the mechanical properties of the bone around the implant with its structural configuration.

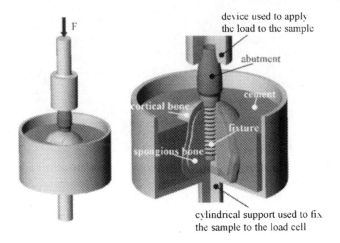

Figure 7.9 Details of the testing machine. The specimen is placed in and cemented into a cylindrical support. The fixture is assembled with its abutment and connected to the load cell.

7.4.2 The mechanical test results

Table 7.2 reports the values of the ultimate load recorded during the push-in experimental tests in addition to other data, e.g. healing time and the use of restorative biomaterials. Table 7.3 reports the characteristics of the specimens used for the microradiographic analysis.

The force-displacement curves obtained with data from the push-in test on the specimens with a healing time of 24 days are depicted in Figure 7.10. The different behaviour of specimens with the fixture inserted using standard techniques and those inserted in sites with surgical defects filled with bone regenerative material can be seen in this Figure.

It is evident that the latter specimens have much lower ultimate loads than the ultimate load measured for the specimen without surgical defects. This obviously means that after 24 days of healing time the mechanical properties of the bone formed starting from regenerative materials are poor if compared with those of healthy bone.

Figure 7.11 shows the difference found for specimens with defects filled with restorative material at different times during the healing process. Specimens at 45 days of healing time

Table 7.2 Specimen data for the push-in tests.

Specimen code	Type of surgery	Regenerative material	Vycril membrane	Healing time (days)	Ultimate load (N)
M1	No defect	No	No	24	2200
M2	Coronal defect	Yes	Yes	24	370
M3	Coronal defect	Yes	Yes	24	420
M4	No defect	No	No	45	5700
M5	Coronal defect	Yes	Yes	45	2390
M6	Coronal defect	Yes	Yes	45	2940

Table 7.3 Specimen data for the microradiographic tests.

Specimen code	Type of surgery	Regenerative material	Vycril membrane	Healing time (days)
R1	Coronal defect	Yes	Yes	24
R2	No defect	No	Yes	24
R3	Coronal defect	Yes	Yes	45
R4	No defect	No	Yes	45

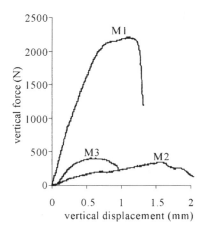

Figure 7.10 Load-displacement curves for the specimens at 24 days of healing time. Specimen M1 was inserted using the standard procedure while specimens M2 and M3 were inserted in sites with surgical defects filled with substitute biomaterial.

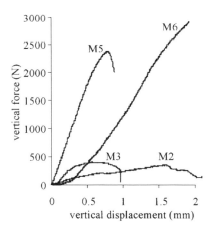

Figure 7.11 Comparison of load-displacement curves for specimens at 24 days of healing time (M2, M3) and load-displacement curves for specimens with 45 days healing time (M5, M6). All these specimens were inserted in sites with surgical defects filled with regenerative biomaterial.

have much better mechanical properties, with an ultimate load which is up to six times higher than the ultimate load of specimens at 24 days of healing time. Mechanical testing makes it clear that healing time largely affects the mechanical properties of regenerated bone. The investigation of the load bearing capacity of the bone-fixture system and its evolutionary behaviour during healing after surgical insertion is, obviously, of fundamental importance.

Because of the specific methodology applied in a push-in test, the ultimate load must be primarily related to the mechanical properties of the bone tissue in the region around the implant. In fact, the main inelastic phenomena, which can also lead to failure, occur in this region. The osseointegration of the fixture can be estimated also by using torque tests. The behaviour of the bone-fixture system under torsional loading can give data about the percentage of the fixture surface resulting anchored to the bone tissue because of the osseointegration process.

The reliability of this testing procedure is affected by different uncertainties. For example, one pertains to the contact of the fixture with the cortical portion of bone in the apical region, contact which can affect the ultimate load recorded. This depends on the anatomy of the tibia but even more so on clinical practice. Attention should be paid to keeping the right direction of the fixture during its insertion, avoiding the contact between parts of the fixture with the cortical bone of the lower layer. Another problematic aspect is the risk of a misalignment between the fixture axis and the load application axis.

7.4.3 Morphological aspects of the bone surrounding implants

An interesting aspect of experimental activity is the possibility of correlating information about the microstructure and morphology of periimplant bone tissue with the ultimate load recorded for a specimen. The microradiographic analysis of a specimen treated with restorative material and having a healing time of 24 days showed newly-formed trabeculae spread over the surface of the fixture, especially around the apical part of the fixture. The regions close to the grooves show some thin trabeculae in contact with the fixture. At 45 days of healing, the same type of specimen presented newly-formed bone in contact with the surface of the fixture, ensuring its osseointegration. The newly-formed bone started forming itself from regions of pre-existing bone or, in the proximity of the defect, from ipercalcified cementing surface, which represents a separation between the pre-existing and newly-formed bone. Most of the restorative material grains were wrapped by fibrous tissue, while few granules proved to be in contact with the newly-formed bone. Significant differences were found between the condition at 24 and 45 days after the insertion of the fixtures. In the first case, the new formation of bone is in the initial phase, while at 45 days the defects are reduced by about 50 per cent. In particular, the areas of direct contact between the surface of the implant and the newly-formed trabeculae are very well distributed in all the portions of the implant, i.e. the apex, grooves, threads and neck.

7.5 CONCLUSIONS

The reliability of dental implant systems depends on several factors. Some of these are related to the specific clinical situation of the patient, others depend on the manufacturing technologies, which may largely affect the mechanical properties of the materials and the geometrical precision of the different prosthetic components. As a consequence, the experimental activity is very extensive since it must be aimed at investigating the effect of every factor, and their potential combinations, on the overall behaviour of the systems. The present chapter has offered only a few examples of experimental activity carried out to test the reliability of single implants and their components. Many aspects have been left out of consideration, e.g. the experimental testing of multi-implant systems, which show further complications with respect to the cases presented here. This chapter has simply tried to offer a general overview of the possible activities that can be performed. The aim of the chapter was to help the reader understand the significance of experimental activity and the capacity of experimental methods to offer a general improvement of the techniques in dental implantology.

Numerical methods are a useful support to experimental activity, because of the limitations of experimental activity make it difficult to completely define implant functional response. As has been partially demonstrated by the example presented above, the numerical approach is a powerful tool for investigating the biomechanics of dental implants. Numerical methods, such as the finite element method and experimental tests can lead to a reciprocal validation. The coupling of the two different approaches offers the greatest possibilities of effectively and properly evaluating the biomechanical reliability of dental devices.

REFERENCES

R. Adell, U. Lehkolm, B. Rockler, P.I. Brånemark, A 15 years study of osseointegrated implants in the treatment of edentulous yaws. International Journal of Oral Surgery, Vol. 6, pp. 387–416, 1981.

T. Albrektsson, L. Sennerby, State of the art in oral implants, Journal of Clinical Periodontology, Vol. 18, pp. 474–481, 1991.

T. Baiamonte, M.F. Abbate, F. Pizzarello, J. Lozada, R. James, The experimental verification of the efficacy of finite element modeling to dental implant systems, Journal of Oral Implantology, Vol. 22, pp. 104–110, 1996.

A. Berzins, B. Shah, H. Weinans, D.R. Sumner, Nondestructive measurements of implant-bone interface shear modulus and effects of implant geometry in pull-out tests, J Biomed Mater Res, Vol. 34, pp. 337–340, 1997.

M. Bigerelle, K. Anselme, B. Noël, I. Ruderman, P. Hardouin, A. Iost, Improvement in the morphology of Ti-based surfaces: a new process to increase *in vitro* human osteoblats response, Biomaterials, Vol. 23, pp. 1563–1577, 2002.

R. Brånemark, L.O. Ohrnell, P. Nilsson, P. Thomsen, Biomechanical characterization of osseointegration during healing: an experimental in vivo study in the rat, Biomaterials, Vol. 18, 969–978, 1997.

P.I. Brånemark, G. Zarb, T. Albrektsson (eds), Tissue Integrated Prostheses, Quintessence, Chicago, 1985.

D.M. Brunette, The effect of surface topography on the behaviour of cells, International Journal of Oral Maxillofacial Implants, Vol. 3, pp. 231–246, 1988.

J.B. Brunski, Biomechanical forces affecting the bone-dental implant interface, Dent. Mats., Vol. 10, 153–201,1992.

J.B. Brunski, Biomechanics of dental implants. In Endosseous Implants for Maxillofacial Reconstruction. M.S. Block, J.N. Kent (ed). Philadelphia, Sounders, pp. 22–39, 1995.

D. Buser, U.C. Belser, N.P. Lang, The original one-stage dental implant system and its clinical application, Periodontology 2000, Vol. 17, pp. 106–118, 1998.

D. Buser, R.K. Shenk, S. Steinemann, J.P. Fiorellini, C.H. Fox, H. Stich, Influence of surface characteristics on bone integration of titanium implants. A histomorphometric study in miniature pigs, Journal of Biomedical Materials Research, Vol. 25, pp. 889–902, 1991.

D. Buser, R. Mericske-Stern, K. Dula, N.P. Lang, Clinical experience with one-stage, non-submerged dental implants, Advances in Dental Research, Vol. 13, pp. 153–161, 1999.

L.V. Carlsson, T. Albrektsson, C. Berman, Bone response to plasma-cleaned titanium implants, Int J Oral Maxillofac Implants, Vol. 4, pp. 199–204, 1991.

A.B. Carr, J.B. Brunski, I. Labishak, B. Bagley, Pre-load comparison between as-received and cast-to implant cylinders, Journal of Dental Research, IADR Abstract, Vol. 72, pp. 695, 1993.

A.B. Carr, P.E. Larsen, E. Papazoglou, E. McGlumphy, Reverse torque failure of screw shaped implants in baboons: baseline data for abutment torque application, Int J Oral Maxillofac Implants, Vol. 10, pp. 167–174, 1995.

D.L. Cochran, R.K. Schenk, A. Lussi, F. Higginbottom, D. Buser, Bone response to unloaded and loaded titanium implants with sandblasted and acid-etched surface: a histometric study in the canine mandible, Journal of Biomedical Materials Research, Vol. 40, pp. 1–11, 1998.

R.G. Craig, Restorative dental materials (6th edn). St. Louis, MO, Mosby C.V., pp. 60–61, 1980.

M. Dettin, M.T. Conconi, R. Gambaretto, A. Pasquato, M. Folin, C. Di Bello, P.P. Parnigotto, Novel osteoblast-adhesive peptides for dental/orthopedic biomaterials, Journal of Biomedical Materials Research, Vol. 60, pp. 466–471, 2002.

W.J.A., Dhert, C.P.A.T. Klein, J.A. Jansen, E.A. van der Velde, R.C. Vriesde, P.M.K. Rozing, de Groot, A histological and histomorphometrical investigation of fluorapatite, magnesium whitlockite and Hydroxyapatite plasma-sprayed coatings in goats, Journal of Biomedical Material research, Vol. 27, pp. 127–138, 1993.

D.M. Ferris, G.D. Moodie, P.M. Dimond, C.W.D. Gioranni, M.G. Ehrlich, R.F. Valentini, RGD-coated titanium implants stimulate increased bone formation in vivo, Biomaterials, Vol. 20, pp. 2323–2331, 1999.

B. Friberg, L. Sennerby, N. Meredith, U. Lekholm, A comparison between cutting torque and resonance frequency measurements of maxillary implants. A 20-month clinical study, Int. J. Oral Maxillofac. Surg., Vol. 28, Issue 4, pp. 297–303, 1999.

M. Gottlander, T. Albrektsson, L.V. Carlason, A histomorphometric study of unthreaded hydroxyapatite-coated and titanium-coated implants in rabbit bone, International Journal of Oral and Maxillofacial Implants, Vol. 7, pp. 485–490, 1992.

S.J. Hoshaw, J.B. Brunski, G.V.B. Coebran, Mechanical loading of Brånemark implants affects interfacial bone modeling and remodeling, International Journal of Oral and Maxillofacial Implants, Vol. 9, pp. 345–360, 1994.

C.J. Ivanoff, L. Sennerby, C. Johansson, B. Rangert, U. Lekholm, Influence of implant diameters on the integration of screw implants. An experimental study in rabbits, J Oral Maxillofac Surg, Vol. 26, pp. 141–148, 1997.

T. Jemt, Failures and complications in 391 cosecutively inserted fixed prostheses supported by Brånemark implants in the edentulous jaw: a study of a treatment from the time of prosthesis placement to the first annual annual check-up, International Journal of Oral and Maxillofacial Implants, Vol. 6, pp. 270–276, 1991.

T. Jemt, B. Lindèn, U. Lekholm, Failures and complications in 127 consecutively placed fixed partial prostheses supported by Brånemark implants: from prosthetic treatment to first annual check-up, International Journal of Oral and Maxillofacial Implants, Vol. 7, pp. 40–44, 1992.

T. Jemt, Three dimensional distortion of gold alloy castings and welded titanium frameworks. Measurements of the precision of fit between completed implant prostheses and master casts in routine edentulous situations, Journal of Oral Rehabilitation, Vol. 22, pp. 557–564, 1995.

T. Jemt, K. Book, Prosthesis misfit and marginal bone loss in edentulous implant patients, International Journal of Oral and Maxillofacial Implants, Vol. 11, pp. 620–625, 1996.

C.B. Johanson, L. Sennerby, T. Albrektsson, A removal torque and histomorphometric study of bone tissue reactions to commercially pure titanium and vitallium implants, Int J Oral Maxillofac Implants, Vol. 6, pp. 437–441, 1991.

U. Joos, D. Vollmer, J. Kleinheinz, Effect of implant geometry on strain distribution in periimplant bone, Mund-, Kiefer-Und Gesichtschirirurgie: MKG, Vol. 4, pp. 143–147, 2000.

B. Kasemo, Biocompatibility of titanium implants: surface science aspects, Journal of Prosthetic Dentistry, Vol. 49, pp. 832–837, 1983.

B. Kasemo, J. Lausmaa, Surface science aspects of inorganic biomaterials, CRC Crit Rev Biocompat, Vol. 2, pp. 335–380, 1986.

J.F. Kay, Calcium phosphate coatings for dental implants: current status and future potential. In Hydroxyapatite-coated implants. Sendax V.I. (ed). Philadelphia, Sounders, pp. 1–18, 1992.

C.P.A.T. Klein, P. Patka, H.B.M. van der Lubbe, J.G.C. Wolke, K. de Groot, Plasma-sprayed coatings of tetracalcium-phosphate, hydroxylapatite and a TCP on titanium alloy: an interface study, Journal of Biomedical Material Research, Vol. 25, pp. 53–65, 1991.

C.P.A.T. Klein, P. Patka, J.G.C. Wolke, J.M.A. de Blieck-Hogervorst, K. de Groot, Long-term *in vivo* study of plasma-sprayed coatings in titanium alloys of tetracalcium-phosphate, hydroxyapatite, and a-tricalcium-phosphate, Biomaterials, Vol. 15, pp. 146–150, 1994.

R.A. Kraut, J. Dootson, A. McCullen, Biomechanical analysis of osseointegration of IMZ implants in goats mandibles and maxillae, Int J Oral Maxillofac Implants, Vol. 6, pp. 187–194, 1991.

R. Leimola-Virtanen, J. Peltola, E. Oksala, H. Helenius, ITI titanium plasma-sprayed screw implants in the Treatment of edentulous mandibles: a follow-up study of 39 patients, International Journal of Oral Maxillofacial Implants, Vol. 10, pp. 373–378, 1995.

J. Lincks, B.D. Boyan, C.R. Blanchard, C.H. Lohmann, Y. Liu, D.L. Cochran, D.D. Dean, Z. Schwartz, Response of MG63 osteoblast-like cells to titanium and titanium alloy is dependent on surface roughness and composition, Biomaterials, Vol. 19, pp. 2219–2232, 1998.

J.L. Lozada, M.F. Abbate, F.A. Pizzarello, R.A. James, Comparative three-dimensional analysis of two finite-element endosseous implant designs, Journal of Oral Implantology, Vol. 20, pp. 315–321, 1994.

D. Ludgren, L. Laurell, H. Falk, T. Bergendal, Occlusal force pattern during mastication in dentitions with mandibular fixed partial dentures supported on oseeointegrated implants, Journal Prosthetic Dentistry, Vol. 58, pp. 197–203, 1987.

L.B. Lum, A biomechanical rationale for the use of short implants, Journal of Oral Implantology, Vol. 17, 126–131, 1992.

N. Meredith, Assessment of implant stability as a prognostic determinant, Int J Prosthodont, Vol. 11, pp. 491–501, 1998.

B.R. Merz, S. Hunenbart, U.C. Belser, Mechanics of the implant-abutment connection: an 8-degree taper compared to a butt joint connection, International Journal of Oral and Maxillofacial Implants, Vol. 15, pp. 519–26, 2000.

U. Meyer, D. Vollmer, C. Runte, C. Bourauel, U. Joos, Bone loading pattern around implants in average and atrophic edentulous maxillae: a finite-element analysis, Journal of Cranio-Maxillo-Facial Surgery, Vol. 29, pp. 100–105, 2001.

K. Mustafa, A. Wennerberg, J. Wroblewski, K. Hultenby, B.S. Lopez, K. Arvidson, Determining optimal surface roughness of TiO_2 blasted titanium implant material for attachment, proliferation and differentiation of cells derived from human mandibular alveolar bone, Clinical Oral Implants Research, Vol. 5, pp. 515–525, 2001.

A.N. Natali, E.A. Meroi, S.A. Donà, Tissue-implant interaction process of dental implant: a numerical approach, Ceramics, Cells and Tissues, pp. 93–100, 1998.

A.N. Natali, The simulation of load bearing capacity of dental implants, Computer Technology in Biomaterials Science and Engineering, 132–148, J. Wiley and Sons, 1999.

A.N. Natali, P.G. Pavan, A comparative analysis based on different strength criteria for evaluation of risk factor for dental implants, Computer Methods in Biomechanics and Biomedical Engineering, Vol. 5, Issue 1, 511–523, 2002.

A. Natali, P. Pavan, F. Bonollo, N. Gramegna, "Numerical analysis of titanium cast devices for dental implantology", Computer Methods in Biomechanics and Biomedical Engineering, Vol. 5, Issue 2, 615–623, 2002.

G. Papavasiliou, A.P. Tripodakis, P. Kamposiora, J.R. Strub, S.C. Bayne, Finite element analysis of ceramic abutment-restoration combinations for osseointegrated implants, International Journal of Prosthodontics, Vol. 9, pp. 254–260, 1996a.

G. Papavasiliou, P. Kamposiora, S.C. Bayne, D.A. Felton, Three-dimensional finite element analysis of stress-distribution around single tooth implants as a function of bony support, prosthesis type, and loading during function, Journal of Prosthetic Dentistry, Vol. 76, pp. 633–640, 1996b.

J. Paphangkorakit, J.W. Osborn, Effects on human maximum bite force of biting on a softer or harder object, Archives or Oral Biology, Vol. 43, pp. 833–839, 1998.

R. Pietrabissa, R. Contro, V. Quaglini, M. Soncini, L. Gionso, M. Simion, Experimental and computational approach for the evaluation of the biomechanical effects of dental bridge misfit, Journal of Biomechanics, Vol. 33, pp. 1489–1495, 2000.

M.N. Pillar, G.C. Weatherly, Developments in implant alloys, CRC Crit Rev Biocompat, Vol. 1, pp. 371–403, 1986.

M. Quirynen, I. Naer, D. van Sttenberghe, Fixture design and overload influence marginal bone loss and fixture success in the Brånemark system, Clinical Oral Implants Research, Vol. 3, pp. 104–111, 1992.

M. Quirynen, C.M. Bollen, The influence of titanium abutment surface roughness on plaque accumulation and gingivitis: short-term observation, International Journal of Oral Maxillofacial Implants, Vol. 11, pp. 169–78, 1996.

B. Rangert, R. Jemt, L. Jörneus, Forces and moments on Brånemark implants, International Journal of Oral and Maxillofacial Implants, Vol. 4, pp. 241–247, 1989.

E. Rangert, P.H.J. Krogh, B. Langer, N. Van Roekel, Bending overload and implant fracture: a retrospective clinical analysis, International Journal of Oral and Maxillofacial Implants, Vol. 10, pp. 326–334, 1995.

R.L. Sakaguchi, S.E. Borgersen, Nonlinear contact analysis of pre-load in dental implant screws, International Journal of Oral and Maxillofacial Implants, Vol. 10, pp. 295–302, 1995.

V.I. Sendax, Hydroxyapatite-coated implants. Philadelphia, Sounders, pp. 1–277, 1992.

L. Sennerby, N. Meredith, Resonance frequency analysis: measuring implant stability and osseointegration, Compendium of Continuing Education in Dentistry, Vol. 19, pp. 493–498, 1998.

A.K. Shah, J. Lazatin, R.K. Sinha, T. Lennox, N.J. Hickok, R.S. Tuan, Mechanism of BMP-2 stimulated adhesion of osteoblastic cells to titanium alloy, Biology of the Cell, Vol. 91, pp. 131–142, 1999.

D. Siegele, U. Soltész, Numerical investigations of the influence of implant shape on stress distribution in the jaw bone, International Journal of Oral and Maxillofacial Implants, Vol. 4, pp. 333–340, 1989.

M. Soncini, R. Rodriguez y Baena, R. Pietrabissa, V. Quaglini, S. Rizzo, D. Zaffe, Experimental procedure for the evaluation of the mechanical properties of the bone surrounding dental implants, Biomaterials, Vol. 23, pp. 11–19, 2002.

N. Sykaras, R.G. Triplett, M.E. Nunn, A.M. Iacopino, L.A. Opperman, Effect of recombinant human bone morphogenetic protein-2 on bone regeneration and osseointegration of dental implants, Clinical Oral Implants Research, Vol. 12, pp. 339–349, 2001.

A. Tjellström, M. Jacobsson, T. Albrektsson, Removal torque of osseointegrated craniofacial implants: a clinical study, Int J Oral Maxillofacial Implants, Vol. 3, pp. 287–289, 1988.

M. Ueda, M. Matsuky, M. Jacobsson, A. Tjellström, The relationship between insertion torque and removal torque analysed in fresh temporal bone, Int J Oral Maxillofac Implants, Vol. 6, pp. 442–447, 1991.

D. van Steenberghe, I. Naert, The first two-stage dental implant system and its clinical application, Periodontology 2000, Vol. 17, pp. 89–95, 1998.

P.P. van Zyl, N.L. Grundling, C.H. Jooste, E. Terblanche, Three-dimensional finite element model of a human mandible incorporating six osseointegrated implants for stress analysis of mandibular cantilever prostheses, International Journal of Oral and Maxillofacial Implants, Vol. 10, pp. 51–57, 1995.

H.P. Weber, C.C. Crohin, J.P. Fiorellini, A 5-year prospective clinical and radiographic study of non-submerged dental implants, Clinical Oral Implants Research, Vol. 11, pp. 144–153, 2000.

L.A. Weinberg, The biomechanics of force distribution in implant-supported prostheses, International Journal of Oral and Maxillofacial Implants, Vol. 8, pp. 19–31, 1993.

S.L. Wheeler, Eight-year clinical retrospective study of titanium plasma-sprayed and hydroxiapatite-coated cylinder implants, International Journal of Oral Maxillofacial Implants, Vol. 11, Issue 3, pp. 340–50, 1996.

K.R. Williams, A.D. Williams, Impulse response of a dental implant in bone by numerical analysis, Biomaterials, Vol. 18, pp. 715–719, 1997.

8 On the mechanics of superelastic orthodontic appliances

FA Auricchio, VC Cacciafesta, LP Petrini, RP Pietrabissa

8.1 INTRODUCTION

Historical background

The first scientific attempt to move teeth occurred in 1728 when the French physician, Pierre Fauchard, used a flat strip of metal, pierced with holes suitably placed. The strip was formed into an arch. Teeth were secured to it by means of threads passing around them and through the holes. The threads were then tied to apply a force to the teeth. Such appliance accomplished only tipping movements and lacked stability (Angle, 1907). For more than hundred years several removable appliances were made, until in 1870 it was invented the first dental cement. At the end of the 19th century Edward Angle, the father of modern orthodontics, designed a standard appliance (Angle System) consisting of basic components: attachment tubes, jack screws, lever wires, band material, and archwire. This system enabled practitioners to treat more patients and to reach a higher level of excellence, with less expense. In 1907, Angle developed the E Arch Appliance, which consisted of an ideal, heavy, expansion arch attached by solder to two first molar clamp bands. It employed crown movements of teeth and simple anchorage. Brass ligature wires were used to expand all the teeth into normal alignment and occlusion (Angle, 1907). In order to produce root movements, Angle developed a few years later the Pin and Tube Appliance. It consisted of pins which had to be soldered, fitted perfectly into the tubes of the bands, removed, moved along the archwire and soldered again. This precise and delicate operation had to be carried out with each appointment (Steiner, 1933). Because the Pin and Tube Appliance was difficult to use, Angle, in 1915, developed the Ribbon Arch Appliance. Brackets were introduced with this new appliance. It was much simpler to construct and activate. It was characterized by brackets with vertical slots. The archwire was held in place in the brackets by brass pins. Based on this experience, Angle changed the form of the brackets by locating the slot in the centre and by placing it in a horizontal plane, instead of in a vertical plane. In 1928 he developed the Edgewise Appliance System. The archwire was held in position first by a brass ligature and later by a stainless steel wire ligature. The new edgewise bracket consisted of a rectangular box with three walls within the bracket, 0.022 inch by 0.028 inch in dimensions. The slot was open horizontally. This new design provided more accuracy and thus a more efficient torquing mechanism (Steiner, 1933).

Contemporary fixed appliances

Contemporary fixed appliances are mostly variations of the Edgewise Appliance System developed by Angle in 1928. They consist of an archwire, that is inserted into the slots of the brackets which are generally bonded directly to the teeth or soldered to steel bands. Usually, brackets have a rectangular slot which can engage either round or rectangular archwires.

Bands

The pioneer orthodontists of the early 1900 used clamp bands, which were tightened around molar teeth by screw attachments. Preformed steel bands came into widespread use during the 1960s and are now available in anatomically correct shapes for all the teeth. Bands are cemented to the teeth by means of different adhesive systems, such as composites, resin-modified glass ionomers or compomers. The inner surface of the bands can be microetched for a better adhesion to the tooth structure. Indications for the use of bands rather than a bonded attachment include (Graber and Vanarsdall, 1994):

- teeth that will receive heavy intermittent forces against the attachments; a common example is an upper first molar to which an extraoral force will be applied by means of an headgear;
- teeth that will need both labial and lingual attachments; a common example is again the upper or lower first molar to which a transpalatal arch or a lingual arch will be applied;
- teeth with short clinical crowns;
- teeth incompatible with successful bonding, as for example teeth affected by fluorosis.

In order to properly seat a band, some device to separate the teeth must usually be used before banding. There are several methods that can be used to separate the teeth: the most commonly used are the elastomeric separators, the separating springs, and the brass wire. Those devices must be left in place for maximum one week before the banding procedure can start. After final seating, the bands are usually cemented using resin-modified glass ionomers or compomers, which are able to release fluoride ions to the enamel surface in an attempt to reduce enamel surface decalcifications which can often develop around the margins of the band or underneath (Wilson and Donley, 2001).

Brackets

Bonded brackets became available in the mid 1970s. They have several advantages over conventional bands (Graber and Vanarsdall, 1994):

- they have no interproximal component; thus no separation is required before bonding;
- they are easier to be placed and to be removed;
- they can be placed more precisely than bands;
- they are more aesthetic and more hygienic;
- they allow interproximal strippings or build-ups already during treatment;
- they can also be applied to partially erupted or fractured teeth.

Direct bonding of orthodontic attachments is based on the mechanical locking of an adhesive to irregularities of the enamel surface of the tooth, and to mechanical locks formed in the bracket base. Successful bonding, therefore, requires careful attention to three essential components: the tooth surface and its preparation, the design of the bracket base, and the bonding agent.

Before bonding brackets, it is necessary to remove the organic pellicle and to create irregularities in the enamel surface. This is accomplished by cleaning the enamel surface using a mix of pumice and water with a rubber cup mounted on a low-speed hand-piece. The tooth is subsequently rinsed with water to remove any pumice debris, thoroughly dried with a stream of oil-free air, and then etched with orthophosphoric acid for about 15–30 seconds. The tooth surface must not be contaminated with saliva, which promotes immediate remineralization, until bonding is completed; otherwise, re-etching is required. After rinsing again the enamel in order to completely remove the etching, the tooth surface must be thoroughly dried and then a liquid resin is applied on it. The resin is able to penetrate into the irregularities created in the etched enamel surface, allowing the bonding material to mechanically interlock with the tooth surface. After application of the resin to the tooth, a small quantity of adhesive is applied to the bracket base, which is then pressed against the enamel. Depending on the type of bonding material, it can set either by a self-curing process or by light-curing.

The development of appliances which would combine both acceptable and aesthetics for the patient and adequate technical performance for the orthodontist has remained an elusive goal. Three methods of achieving these criteria have been attempted:

- altering the appearance of or reducing the size of stainless steel brackets;
- repositioning the appliance on to the lingual surfaces of the teeth;
- changing the material from which brackets are made.

Early attempts to coat metal brackets with a tooth coloured coating were unsuccessful due to failure of the coating to adhere and its translucence. Smaller brackets offer only a limited aesthetic advantage over conventionally sized appliances. Lingual orthodontics satisfies aesthetic criteria by positioning the fixed appliance on the lingual surfaces of the teeth, but in doing so produces a significant decrease in the performance of the appliance. Early attempts to produce brackets of different materials included the use of polycarbonate. These brackets, while aesthetically satisfactory in the early stages of treatment, deteriorated in appearance with time and were insufficiently strong to withstand long treatments or transmit torque (Reynolds, 1975). In 1986, ceramic brackets became available. The ceramic material used in almost all orthodontic brackets is alumina, either in its polycrystalline or monocrystalline form. A few brackets are made from the chemically similar zirconia. The advantage of using alumina for orthodontic brackets is that its appearance is very good, its chemical resistance is excellent, and it is both hard and, in certain respect, very strong. The disadvantages are that it lacks ductility, and is difficult and expensive to manufacture (Swartz, 1988). The mechanical properties of ceramic brackets which give rise to potential clinical problems are low fracture toughness, lack of ductility and hardness. Ceramic brackets are much harder than enamel and rapidly cause wear if occlusal interferences are present (Swartz, 1988). The low fracture toughness leads to a higher rate of bracket breakage than with stainless steel brackets. Placement of additional torque in the archwires may cause tie-wing fractures (Scott, 1988). Moreover, ceramic brackets produce more friction than stainless steel brackets (Angolkar et al., 1990; Pratten et al., 1990). More recently, ceramic brackets with metal slots have been introduce on the market. This new design should reduce friction during sliding mechanics. Another disadvantage of ceramic brackets is the risk of enamel damage during debonding, as the very high bond strength can cause enamel cracks when removing those brackets at the end of treatment (Winchester, 1991).

Orthodontic wires

Orthodontic wires are available as either straight pieces or preformed archwires. Preformed archwires are usually inserted in all the bracket slots and ligated by means of elastomeric or stainless steel ligatures. The straight pieces of wires can be bent, thus producing for example cantilevers or loops. Loops can have different shapes. The simplest design is represented by the vertical (V) loop, which is generally used for tooth retraction and space closure. The limit of such loop is its height: usually it can not be longer than 10–12 mm, otherwise it will be uncomfortable for the patient. In order to reduce the load/deflection rate, more wire can be added to either one of both sides of the V loop. By doing so, it is possible to fabricate either the L loop or the T loop. The L loop is generally used for tooth alignment, whereas the T loop is generally used for tooth retraction and space closure. Another type of loop is represented by the rectangular (or box) loop, which is mainly used for tooth alignment. Each loop can be of course fabricated in different alloys, depending on the clinical situation. It is therefore important to understand the mechanical properties of the different alloys used in orthodontics, so that the best alloy can be employed in each particular clinical situation.

Stainless steel wires

Up until the 1930s, the only orthodontic wires available were made of gold. Austenitic stainless steel (SS) was introduced as an orthodontic wire in 1929, and shortly afterwards gained popularity over gold (Wilkinson, 1962). Since then, several other alloys with desirable properties have been adopted in orthodontics. Carbon interstitial hardening and cold working contribute to the high yield strength and modulus of elasticity of SS wires. High stiffness is advantageous in resisting deformation caused by extra- and intraoral tractional forces. SS wires show lower springback and less stored energy compared with those of beta-titanium and nickel-titanium wires (Drake et al., 1982). This means that SS wires produce higher forces which dissipate over shorter periods of time than either beta-titanium or nickel-titanium wires, thus requiring more frequent reactivations and monitoring. SS wires can be fused together by welding and they present a good resistance to corrosion. Moreover, they offer lower resistance to tooth movement than other alloys (Frank and Nikolai, 1980). Clinically, rectangular SS wires are commonly used for reinforcing the anchorage of reactive units, and as main working archwires for sliding mechanics or when Class II or III elastics are used. Round SS wires are often used during the finishing phase of treatment.

Cobalt-chromium wires

In most respects, the mechanical properties of Co-Cr wires are very similar to those of SS wires.

Beta-titanium wires

Beta-titanium wires have a modulus of elasticity which is less than that of SS and about twice that of nickel-titanium wires. This makes its use ideal when forces less than those of SS are necessary and in instances in which a lower modulus material such as nickel-titanium is inadequate to produce the desired force magnitudes. The springback is superior to that of stainless steel: this means that such wire can be deflected almost twice as much as SS wires without permanent deformation (Burstone and Goldberg, 1980). Beta-titanium wires also deliver about half the amount of force as do comparable SS wires (Burstone and Goldberg, 1980). The good formability allows stops and loops to be bent into the wire and it can easily be welded together. The corrosion resistance is comparable to that of SS and Co-Cr wires, however, they produce higher levels of frictional resistance (Angolkar et al., 1990). Clinically, the use of rectangular beta-titanium wires is indicated when fabricating the active component of an appliance, as for example utility arches or cantilevers, which demonstrate a wide range of deactivation and do not require frequent monitoring.

Nickel-titanium wires

Nitinol, the first nickel-titanium wire, was introduced in 1971. Nowadays, there are several different types of nickel-titanium (Ni-Ti) wires which demonstrate differences in some properties. The most advantageous properties of Ni-Ti wires are the good springback and flexibility, which allow for large elastic deflections. For a given amount of activation, Ni-Ti wires produce more constant forces on teeth than SS wires. Clinically, their use is indicated during the initial phases of orthodontic treatment for tooth alignment and levelling.

8.2 SHAPE-MEMORY MATERIALS

Shape-memory alloys (SMA) are "materials with an intrinsic ability to remember an initial configuration". This memory is revealed at the macroscopic level in two main unusual behaviours, the superelastic effect (SE) and the shape-memory effect (SME). In particular, the superelastic effect indicates the material ability to undergo large deformations – up to 10–15 per cent strains – in mechanical loading-unloading cycles without showing permanent deformations (Figure 8.1); the shape-memory effect indicates the material ability to present inelastic deformations during mechanical loading-unloading cycles, which can be recovered through thermal cycles (Figure 8.2).

As usual, the macro-behaviour finds its explanation and justification in the underlying micro-mechanics. From a crystallographic point of view, shape-memory alloys may in general present two different structures, one characterized by a more ordered unit cell, the

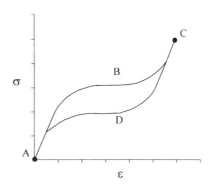

Figure 8.1 Superelasticity effect. At a constant high temperature the material is able to undergo large deformations with zero final permanent strain.

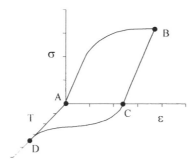

Figure 8.2 Shape-memory effect. At the end of a mechanical loading-unloading path (*ABC*) performed at a constant low temperature, the material presents residual deformation (*AC*), which can be recovered through a thermal cycle (*CDA*).

austenite (A), the other characterized by a less ordered unit cell the martensite. Moreover, the martensite may have a global structure where the unit cells have a variable orientation minimizing the misfit with the surrounding material, or a global structure where the unit cells follow a preferred orientation given by an external field such as stress; in the former case we talk of twinned or multiple-variant martensite (M), in the latter case of detwinned or single-variant martensite (S).

From a micro-mechanical point of view, the presence of two different crystallographic structures is the base for a reversible solid-solid phase transformation between the austenite and the martensite. The phase transformation is in general function of temperature and stress. In particular, for the case of a stress-free material, we may distinguish two reference temperatures, A_f and M_f, with $A_f > M_f$ such that: the austenite is the only phase stable at temperatures above A_f; the martensite is the only phase stable at temperatures below M_f; an austenite-martensite mixture is possible in the temperature interval between A_f and M_f. In general, both A_f and M_f depend on the material composition as well as on the thermo-mechanical treatment. For the case of a stressed material, a similar situation occurs, with the difference that the reference temperatures are monotonic (approximatively linear) function of the loading level.

From a macro-mechanical point of view, as mentioned above, the reversible martensitic phase transformation results in two unique effects, the superelasticity (SE) and the shape memory effect (SME). At temperatures above A_f, if loaded the material shows non-linear large deformations, which are recovered during the unloading, describing an hysteretic loop in terms of stress and strain (Figure 8.1). This response can be explained noting that the load induces a transformation from austenite to single-variant martensite; however, since the austenite is the only phase stable above A_f, the reverse transformation occurs during the unloading.

At temperatures below A_f, if loaded the material shows non-linear large deformations, which are partially retained during the unloading; however, this residual strain can be recovered heating the material above A_f (Figure 8.2).

This response can be explained noting that the load induces a transformation from austenite or multiple-variant martensite to single-variant martensite and that both type of martensite are stable for temperature below A_f in the case of unstressed material. However, since the martensite is unstable above A_f, heating the material, a transformation from martensite to austenite occurs and the material recovers the initial shape; moreover, such a shape is retained also during the cooling at the initial temperature.

As a consequence of these two behaviours, in general not present in traditional materials, shape-memory alloys lend themselves to be used in innovative applications relative to many different fields, ranging from cardiovascular non-invasive surgery to micro-actuator for endoscopy, and in particular relative to orthodontics, as discussed in the following section.

8.3 SMA IN DENTISTRY: STATE OF THE ART

Due to a combination of good material biocompatibility (Shabalovskaya, 1996; Ryhänen, 1999) and of the unique mechanical properties, there are several applications exploiting the unusual SMA response in medicine, in general, and in dentistry, in particular (Duerig et al., 1996; Gil and Planell, 1998; Van Humbeeck et al., 1998; Torrisi, 1999; Chu et al., 2000; Pelton et al., 2000).

In the following we briefly review the three major applications in the field of dentistry as well as the state of the art both from an experimental and a numerical perspective.

8.3.1 Applications

This work concerns the use of SMA in orthodontics, as already cited in the Introduction, but we remember that SMA are also widely used in implantology and endodontics, as briefly discussed in the following.

Orthodontics

Dental movement during orthodontic therapy is achieved by applying forces to teeth, resulting in a bone remodelling process. The optimal tooth movement is in general achieved applying forces which are low in magnitude and continuous in time; in fact, light constant forces are optimal to induce physiological dental movements without damaging the underlying tissues as well as to minimize patient discomfort. In contrast, forces with high magnitude encourage hyalinization of the periodontal ligament and they may cause irreversible tissue damage and root resorption.

Accordingly, SMA appliances, such as archwires or retraction loops, are more effective compared to appliances made of classical alloys, since they take advantage of the material ability to exert light constant springback forces over a large range of deformations (Duerig et al., 1996). Moreover, they are particularly suitable in situations requiring large deflections such as the preliminary alignment stage, in most cases resulting also in a limited mobility at the end of the therapy.

It is interesting to observe that a large variety of situations can occur, depending on the archwire geometrical parameters, on the material properties as well as on the specific loading conditions. Moreover, the oral cavity temperature varies during the day, for example due to the intake of cold or hot drink; henceforth, the springback force may also vary and it would be important to control the variation range in terms of therapy effectiveness and patient comfort.

Implantology

A dental implant is an artificial system connected to the mandibular bone to replace one or more damaged teeth. A classical problem with standard dental implants is how to obtain an effective and lasting fixation of the artificial element, the implant, to the mandibular bone.

The problem can be solved using an artificial tooth root made of SMA and inserted in a deformed shape; using the shape-memory effect, the tooth root can return to its original shape after reaching body temperature, such to tighten itself to the mandible (Gil and Planell, 1998). Compared with ordinary implants, SMA-based implants are in general characterized by good fixation properties, an easy installing procedure and a good stress distribution in the surrounding bone.

Endodontics

Endodontic instruments are constituted by small conical files useful for the restorative preparation of dental root channels. The new generations of such devices are realized in Ni-Ti alloys; in fact, thanks to the superior flexibility and torquability of superelastic material compared to stainless steel, SMA files can be inserted easily in bent dental channels. Moreover, once inserted, the application of a torsional state due to the file rotation and to the friction against the canal inner walls, induce the superelastic effect and a transformation from austenite to martensite. Henceforth, the file works with a constant cutting stress, also in the case of highly bent channels, eroding them uniformly without modifying the overall canal shape. Finally, the risk of file rupture is reduced in martensitic phase and the device can be plastically deformed rather than broken.

On the other hand, it is not possible to use stainless steel files to model the dental channel in combination with a motorized rotation, because the risk of file rupture becomes too high and the erosion of the channel becomes uncontrollable. The high strength of the steel and the high erosion yield, in fact, does not permit a correct use of files inside bent channels. The steel files may change the canal shapes, are too fragile and produce wall steps (Torrisi, 1999; Torrisi and Di Marco, 2000).

8.3.2 Experimental investigations

As discussed above, SMA orthodontic applications exploit both the superelastic and the shape-memory effect. However, the application which has been more investigated from an mechanical experimental point of view is the one relative to the orthodontic archwires, probably as a natural consequence of a greater commercial interest as well as of the major difficulties involved in experimental investigations relative to the other cited applications.

Accordingly, in the following we limit our presentation only to orthodontic archwires, reviewing the experimental investigations discussed in the literature.

The properties of orthodontic wires are commonly determined through a variety of mechanical laboratory tests. In particular, tensile, bending and torsional loading conditions are considered; in fact, although these testing conditions do not reflect specific clinical situations, they provide a basis for a comparison between different wires as well as simple clinical situations.

In our knowledge Drake et al., 1982, are the first to present a SMA archwire investigation in tension, bending and torsion as well as a comparison between stainless steel, nickel titanium and titanium-molybdenum archwires. Due also to the fact that they consider three different sizes for each type of wires, the authors focus on some simple parameters to characterize the mechanical response of the investigated wires.

Miura et al., 1986, 1988a, 1988b, provide a review on the Japanese activities in the area of orthodontic appliances up to the 90s; in particular they investigate orthodontic wires as well as closed and open coil springs, showing how the load value of the super-elastic activity can be effectively controlled by changing the diameter of the wire, the size of the lumen, the martensite transformation temperature and the pitch of the coil springs.

Kapila and Sachdeva, 1989, provide a good review on the wire requirements from a clinical perspective and compare mechanical properties as well as clinical implications for groups of stainless steel, cobalt-chromium, nickel-titanium, beta-titanium and multi-stranded wires.

Hudgins et al., 1990, investigate the effect of long-term deflection on permanent deformation of Ni-Ti archwires, reporting also a literature review of previous works on the same subject.

Nardi et al., 1993, comment on the effectiveness of superelastic wires in specific clinical situations, in particular claiming that the use of superelastic wires should be avoided in the case of brachy facial patients, i.e. when the masticatory action may induce particularly high stresses in the wire since cyclic high loading conditions may cause fractures into the wire.

Sabrià et al., 1996, investigate the cyclic response of SMA orthodontic archwires in the superelastic range. In particular, the authors consider the variation of the plateau stress and the variation of the residual deformation with the number of cycles, up to a maximum of 200 cycles.

Airoldi and Riva, 1996, investigate the effects of the oral cavity temperature changes throughout the day as a consequence of hot/cold drink intakes; accordingly, the developed recovery stress can vary depending on temperature. Therefore, the authors consider a three-point bending situation as reproducing a therapy state and, at fixed deflection, they experimentally investigated the modification of the recovery force level with temperature. In particular, reference (Airoldi and Riva, 1996) consider the temperature cycles described in Table 8.1, highlighting the expected temperature dependency.

Among others interesting work on the area we wish to cite reference (Evans et al., 1998). Finally, we recall that Laino et al., 1990, comments on the so-called "archmate wire bender", produced by GAC and able to modify the archwire geometry without changing the wire superelastic properties.

8.3.3 Constitutive law and numerical modelling

The more and more frequent use of SMA in commercially valuable applications have stimulated a vivid interest not only on the experimental investigation but also on the modelling.

In particular, the literature presents several examples of macroscopic constitutive models able to reproduce the shape-memory alloy response. However, only in few cases such modelling attempts have been devoted to the analysis of orthodontic appliances. In particular, to our knowledge we have the following references:

Table 8.1 Thermal loading

Case 1	37 °C →	5 °C	→	37 °C → 55 °C
Case 2	37 °C →	55 °C	→ 5 °C	→55 °C →	37 °C

Auricchio and Sacco present a one-dimensional small-deformation constitutive equation, able to reproduce either the superelastic response (Auricchio and Sacco, 1997b) or both the superelastic and the shape-memory effect (Auricchio and Sacco, 1999). Both models are developed in combination with a beam finite-element and used to study several problems, some of them similar to classical test conditions for orthodontic appliances. In particular, Reference (Auricchio and Sacco, 1997b) consider a three-point bending situation in the superelastic range investigating the loading-unloading pattern; Reference (Auricchio and Sacco, 1999) consider a three-point bending situation in the superelastic range investigating the loading-unloading pattern as well as the change in recovery force due to thermal cycles as proposed in Reference (Airoldi and Riva, 1996) (Table 8.1).

Auricchio et al. (Auricchio and Taylor, 1997; Auricchio et al., 1997; Auricchio, 2000) present a three-dimensional finite-deformation constitutive equation, able to reproduce the superelastic response. Using such an approach the authors study a wire subject to a three-point bending test and the response of an orthodontic vertical loop.

Raboud, 1998, adopts a resultant moment-curvature constitutive equation in a finite-rotation beam element and simulate the response of a cantilever beam, a three-point bending test, a vertical loop and a T-loop retraction appliance.

Glendenning et al., 2000, adopt the uniaxial superelastic model proposed in Reference (Auricchio and Sacco, 1997b) and, using a beam finite-element, investigate the mechanical response of the following superelastic elements: a wire under three-point bending, a vertical closing loop and a T-shaped closing loop. In particular, they compare the results obtained from the numerical scheme with experimental data and obtaining an excellent correlation.

8.4 A NEW EXPERIMENTAL INVESTIGATION

To investigate the effective material properties of commercial orthodontic archwires and to properly calibrate the constitutive model described in Section A, a new experimental campaign is in progress at LABS (Laboratory of Biological Structure Mechanics) of Politecnico di Milano, Italy.

As usual, mechanical properties should be investigated through a set of simple tests, such as tensile, compression and torsion tests. However, due to the difficulty in performing compressions on thin wires, we plan to run tension and torsion tests, corresponding to simple loading conditions, and bending tests, corresponding to combined tension-compression loading conditions.

In the following we present and discuss only the initial part of the experimental campaign, i.e. a part relative to the tension tests, since torsion and bending tests are in progress.

8.4.1 Materials and methods

We focus on two producers, 3M/Unitek (Monrovia, CA, USA) and ORMCO (Glendora, CA, USA). For each producer we consider two types of wires, i.e. a wire with a circular cross-section of diameter 0.41 mm and a wire with a rectangular cross-section with dimensions 0.48 mm $\times$ 0.64 mm; accordingly, we investigate a total of four superelastic Ni-Ti archwires.

The wires are subject to isothermal tensile tests under displacement control using a MTS 858 Table 8.1. Top machine, imposing a 40 MPa pre-stress as a lower limit. In particular, for each wire we perform the following tensile tests:

- monotonic loading at different strain rates;
- cyclic loading at slow rate.

The results are in general described through a stress–strain σ–ε curve, where:

$\sigma = F/A_0$ is the nominal stress, i.e. the ratio between the applied force (F) and the initial wire section area (A_0)

$\varepsilon = \Delta L/L_0$ is the ratio between the change in length (ΔL) and the initial length (L_0)

The force F and the change in length ΔL are measured directly by the machine, while the initial length L_0 and the initial area A_0 are measured using a gauge before starting the test.

8.4.2 Cyclic loading at slow rate

To investigate the influence of strain histories on the material behavior, we perform some cyclic loading tests at strain rate $\dot{\varepsilon} = 2.\ 10^{-4}\ \text{sec}^{-1}$. In particular, we consider the following three cyclic histories:

history 1:   a total of 40 cycles, divided in four groups of ten cycles each, respectively up to eight per cent, six per cent, four per cent and two per cent strain.

history 2:   a total of 70 cycles, divided in seven groups of ten cycles each, respectively up to two per cent, four per cent, six per cent, eight per cent, six per cent, four per cent and two per cent strain.

history 3:   a total of 200 cycles, with constant six per cent strain amplitude.

Figure 8.3 presents single cycles at six per cent strain taken at different stages of the considered loading histories. In particular, we report the 20th cycle of history one, that is, after a set of cycles at eight per cent, and the 50th cycle of history two, that is, after sets of cycles at two per cent, four per cent, six per cent and eight per cent.

Figure 8.4 presents single cycles at two per cent strain taken at different stages of the considered loading histories. In particular, we report the 40th cycle of history one, that is, after sets of cycles at eight per cent, six per cent and four per cent, and the 70th cycle of history two, that is, after sets of cycles at two per cent, four per cent, six per cent, eight per cent, six per cent and four per cent.

Figure 8.5 presents single cycles at six per cent strain taken at different stages of the considered loading histories. In particular, we report the first and the 50th cycle of history three, cycles at six per cent constant amplitude, for the circular wires and for the rectangular wires.

Figure 8.6 presents single cycles at six per cent strain taken at different stages of the considered loading histories. In particular, we report the first, tenth, 100th and 200th cycle of history three, cycles at six per cent constant amplitude, for the ORMCO rectangular wire and for the 3M rectangular wire.

In general, we may note the strong influence of the loading history on the wire behaviours.

8.4.3 Comments on experimental results

We present the first results of an experimental campaign devoted to investigate the mechanical properties of Ni-Ti super-elastic alloy archwires employed in the orthodontic therapy.

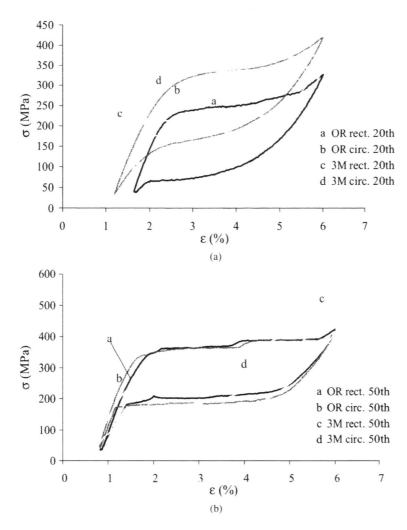

Figure 8.3 Cyclic loading at slow rate. The figure presents single cycles at 6 per cent strain taken at different stages of the considered loading histories. In particular, the 20th cycle of history 1 (that is, after a set of cycles at 8 per cent) (a) and the 50th cycle of history 2 (that is, after sets of cycles at 2 per cent, 4 per cent, 6 per cent and 8 per cent) (b).

The tests point out some interesting differences, between theoretically similar wires, which can not be neglected in the design of an effective orthodontic therapy. In particular, during tensile test up to failure, the ORMCO and the 3M/Unitek wires show different elastic modulus as well as different forward and reverse transformation slopes. During cyclic tests, after an initial inelastic strain accumulation, all the wires show a good spring-back as well as a wide transformation plateau at constant stress, up to six per cent strain; in particular, the transformation region is quite stable in the case of ORMCO wires, while it is more sensible to the strain history and to the number of cycles in the case of 3M/Unitek wires.

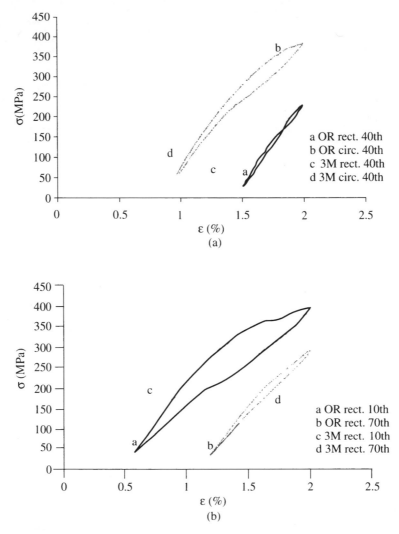

Figure 8.4 Cyclic loading at slow rate. The figure presents single cycles at two per cent strain taken at different stages of the considered loading histories. In particular, the 40th cycle of history one (that is, after sets of cycles at eight per cent, six per cent and four per cent) for the four wires (a); the tenth and the 70th cycle of history two (that is, after a set of cycles at two per cent and after sets of cycles at two per cent, four per cent, six per cent, eight per cent, six per cent and four per cent) for the rectangular wires only (b).

These initial experimental observations seem to point out the greater stability of the ORMCO products, hence their better capacity to satisfy the requirements of an ideal arch-wire for fixed appliance treatment. At the same time, the experimental results emphasize the interest toward parametric analysis able to take into account easily the effective dispersion of possible therapy parameters.

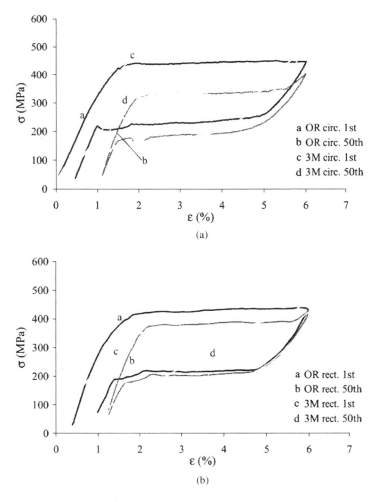

Figure 8.5 Cyclic loading at slow rate. The figure presents single cycles at 6 per cent strain taken at different stages of the considered loading histories. In particular, the 1st and the 50th cycle of history 3 (cycles at 6 per cent constant amplitude) for the circular wires (a) and for the rectangular wires (b).

8.5 ORTHODONTIC SIMULATION

As extensively commented in Section three, SMA superelastic elements are very effective for the correction of teeth malocclusions in orthodontics, allowing to obtain an optimal teeth movement as well as to control and drastically shorten the therapy (Sachdeva and Miyazaki, 1990).

However, the investigation of orthodontic appliances can be very intricate, not only as a consequence of the geometric parameter randomness but also, for example, as a consequence of the frequent temperature modifications in the oral cavity, due to possible food/drink intakes. These aspects lead to complex loading patterns and, in general, to

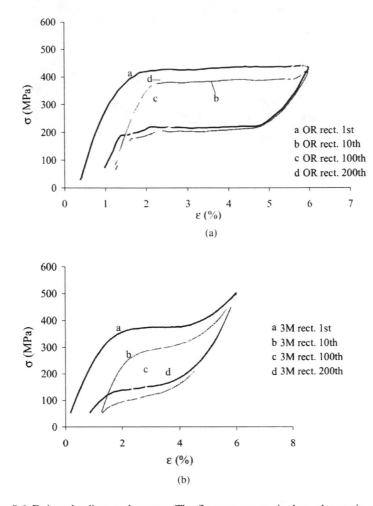

Figure 8.6 Fatigue loading at slow rate. The figure presents single cycles at six per cent strain taken at different stages of the considered loading histories. In particular, the first, tenth, 100th and 200th cycle of history three (cycles at six per cent constant amplitude) for the ORMCO rectangular wire (a) and for the 3M rectangular wire (b).

a variable range for the recovery forces acting on the tooth, with possible consequent painful sensations as well as with an influence on the therapy effectiveness.

According to these considerations, the role of numerical simulations can be of non-negligible interest, as shown in the following. Herein, we focus on three different SMA orthodontic applications:

- archwire;
- retraction T-loop;
- retraction V-loop.

For each problem we assume to start the simulation from an initial temperature T_0 (with $T_0 = 37$ °C), corresponding to an unstrained, unstressed and fully austenitic state. Moreover, we study the appliance response under a mechanical loading followed by a thermal cyclic loading, the former attempting to reproduce the implantation procedure, the latter attempting to reproduce a possible food/drink intake.

The mechanical loading is imposed while keeping fixed the appliance temperature ($T = T_0 = 37$ °C) and controlling the displacement d of some significative cross section; in particular, we distinguish between two different mechanical histories:

L: the displacement d of the significative cross section goes from zero up to a value d_{mec} (loading type history)

U: the displacement d of the significative cross section goes from zero up to a value d_{max} and then from the value d_{max} down to a value d_{mec}, with $d_{mec} < d_{max}$ (loading-unloading type history)

Moreover, the thermal loading is imposed while keeping fixed the displacement of the significative cross section ($d = d_{mec}$) and controlling the appliance temperature (T); in particular, we distinguish between two different thermal histories:

HC: the appliance temperature T goes from the initial value T_0 up to a value T_{max}, down to a value T_{min} and then back to the initial value T_0 (heating-cooling type history)

CH: the appliance temperature T goes from the initial value T_0 down to a value T_{min}, up to a value T_{max} and then back to the initial value T_0 (cooling-heating type history)

Accordingly, in the following we may have at most one of the following four possible loading combinations:

L-HC: mechanical loading followed by an heating-cooling thermal cycle
L-CH: mechanical loading followed by an cooling-heating thermal cycle
U-HC: mechanical loading-unloading followed by an heating-cooling thermal cycle
U-CH: mechanical loading-unloading followed by an cooling-heating thermal cycle

In the following, all the thermal cycles are characterized by the following temperature range:

$$T_{max} = 55 \text{ °C} \quad T_{min} = 5 \text{ °C}$$

Finally, recalling Auricchio and Sacco (1999), we set for all the forthcoming investigations:

E_A	=	55000 MPa	;	E_S	=	25000 MPa
$\sigma_s^{AS,+}$	=	$\sigma_f^{AS,+} = 130$ MPa	;	$\sigma^{SS,+}$	=	30 MPa
$C^{AS,+}$	=	6 MPa/°C	;	$C^{SA,+}$	=	9 MPa/°C
T_s^{AM}	=	10°C	;	T_f^{AM}	=	5°C
T_s^{SA}	=	$T_f^{SA} = 25$°C	;	ε_L	=	0.08 per cent
$\sigma_s^{AS,-}$	=	$\sigma_f^{AS,-} = 190$ MPa	;	$\sigma^{SS,-}$	=	40 MPa
$C^{AS,-}$	=	8.2 MPa/°C	;	$C^{SA,-}$	=	11.4 MPa/°C
ε_L^-	=	0.06 per cent	;	γ	=	1 MPa/sec

8.5.1 Archwire

To investigate the response of a superelastic archwire, we first consider a simplifying case, i.e. a three-point bending state, analyzing then the complete dental implant. It is interesting to observe that the three-point bending situation has been often explored experimentally and some data are available in the literature; on the other hand, the study of the more realistic complete dental implant has always been neglected, possibly as a consequence of the problem greater complexity.

For both cases we consider a rectangular 0.558 mm × 0.406 mm cross-section.

3-point bending test

Following the experimental investigations reported by Airoldi and coworkers (Airoldi et al., 1995), we study the behaviour of a simply supported beam subjected to a pointwise central force, three-point bending test, under the thermo-mechanical loading combination U-CH. In particular, the mechanical load is applied controlling the mid-span cross-section displacement with:

$$d_{max} = 8 \text{ mm} \qquad d_{mec} = 4 \text{ mm}$$

The beam has length $L = 14$ mm and, due to symmetry conditions, only half of the beam is discretized using a mesh of ten elements.

As output parameter, we consider the reaction force at the beam mid-span and Figure 8.7 shows the force variation in terms of deflection and temperature. It is interesting to observe how the numerical solution is able to reproduce the experimentally observed changes in the recovery force as a consequence of the intake of hot/cold quantities (Airoldi et al., 1995), predicting a force on the teeth in the range of few newtons.

Complete implant

We now consider the complete archwire sketched in Figure 8.8.

The geometrical parameters are:

$$A = R = 30 \text{ mm} \qquad B = 22.5 \text{ mm}$$

The mechanical load is applied controlling the displacement of a teeth (canine) in the direction orthogonal to the wire with:

$$d_{max} = 8 \text{ mm} \qquad d_{mec} = 4 \text{ mm}$$

The archwire is modeled using ten beam elements between each couple of tooth. The interaction between the archwire and the single teeth is described with different boundary conditions (bc); in particular, we consider:

* clamped or sliding roller for the molar teeth
* roller or hinge or sliding roller or clamped boundary conditions for the remaining teeth

As output parameters we consider the reaction forces and moments on the canine, for which we control the displacement, and on the molar, closer to the former canine. In particular, we distinguish between force components orthogonal to the wire ($F_\perp$) and force components parallel to the wire ($F_\parallel$).

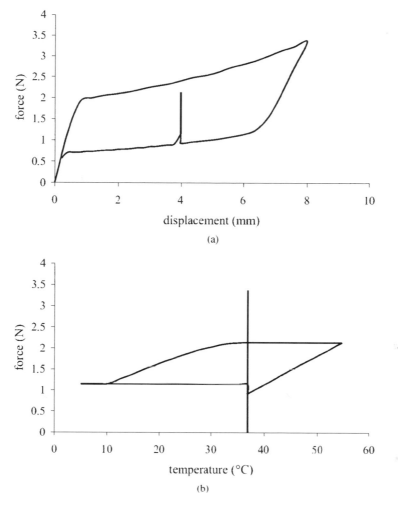

Figure 8.7 Orthodontic wire. Applied force versus midspan deflection (a) and temperature (b). The temperature cycle performed at fixed deflection ($d = 4.0$ mm) induces a change in the recovery force.

Tables 8.2 and 8.3 report the output parameters for all the thermo-mechanical loading and all the boundary conditions under investigations.

It is interesting to observe that the only situation which predicts actions on the canine in the possible physiological range corresponds to sliding roller for all boundary conditions; this condition is also the one considered as the most consistent with effective practice.

As a final example, Figure 8.9 reports some deformed configuration at the end of the mechanical-thermal loading (U-CH) in comparison with the undeformed configuration (dotted line).

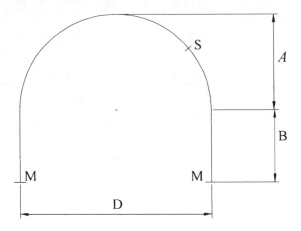

Figure 8.8 Orthodontic archwire: geometric parameters.

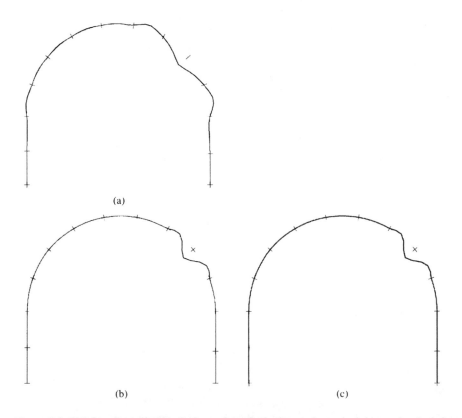

(a)

(b)   (c)

Figure 8.9 Orthodontic archwire: Deformed configuration at the end of the mechanical-thermal
loading (U-CH) and undeformed configuration (dotted line) for the following boundary conditions: clamped bc for the molar teeth and roller bc for the remaining teeth (a)
clamped bc for the molar teeth and hinge bc for the remaining teeth (b) clamped bc
for the molar teeth and clamped bc for the remaining teeth (c).

Table 8.2 Archwire: sliding roller boundary conditions for the molars. Appliance response on the canine for different thermo-mechanical loading histories and for different boundary conditions on the tooth (except the molars)

		$F^i_\perp$ [N]	$F^i_\parallel$ [N]	M^i [Nmm]	$F^f_\perp$ [N]	$F^f_\parallel$ [N]	M^f [Nmm]
Roller	L-HC	3.20	—	—	2.06	—	—
	L-CH	4.66	—	—	4.16	—	—
	U-HC	1.79	—	—	2.25	—	—
	U-HC	1.79	—	—	4.16	—	—
Hinge	L-HC	33.5	0.00	—	23.8	0.03	—
	L-CH	33.5	0.00	—	29.9	0.00	—
	U-HC	18.4	0.00	—	23.3	0.02	—
	U-HC	18.4	0.00	—	29.8	0.00	—
Sl.roller	L-HC	4.95	—	0.63	2.60	—	0.42
	L-CH	4.95	—	0.63	4.60	—	0.53
	U-HC	2.00	—	0.13	2.50	—	0.41
	U-HC	2.00	—	0.13	4.60	—	0.54
Clamped	L-HC	34.4	0.00	0.00	23.7	0.00	0.00
	L-CH	33.5	0.00	0.00	29.8	0.00	0.00
	U-HC	18.4	0.00	0.00	22.9	0.00	0.00
	U-HC	18.4	0.00	0.00	30.1	0.00	0.00

Table 8.3 Archwire: clamped boundary conditions for the molars. Appliance response on the canine for different thermo-mechanical loading histories and for different boundary conditions on the tooth (except the molars)

		$F^i_\perp$ [N]	$F^i_\parallel$ [N]	M^i [Nmm]	$F^f_\perp$ [N]	$F^f_\parallel$ [N]	M^f [Nmm]
Roller	L-HC	17.7	—	—	10.4	—	—
	L-CH	17.7	—	—	14.8	—	—
	U-HC	6.88	—	—	10.2	—	—
	U-HC	6.88	—	—	14.8	—	—
Hinge	L-HC	33.5	0.00	—	23.8	0.03	0.00
	L-CH	33.5	0.00	—	29.9	0.00	—
	U-HC	18.4	0.00	—	23.3	0.02	—
	U-HC	18.4	0.00	0.00	29.8	0.00	—
Sl.roller	L-HC	20.9	—	0.67	12.5	—	0.67
	L-CH	20.9	—	0.67	17.7	—	0.60
	U-HC	11.1	—	1.73	12.2	—	0.68
	U-HC	11.1	—	1.74	18.1	—	0.38
Clamped	L-HC	34.4	0.00	0.00	23.7	0.00	0.00
	L-CH	33.5	0.00	0.00	29.8	0.00	0.00
	U-HC	18.4	0.00	0.00	22.9	0.00	0.00
	U-HC	18.4	0.00	0.00	30.1	0.00	0.00

8.5.2 Retraction T-loop

We now investigate the response of a retraction appliance in the form of a T-loop, sketched in Figure 8.10. Following Reference (Raboud, 1998), the geometrical parameters are set equal to:

$A = 8$ mm $B = 2$ mm $C = 2.5$ mm
$D = 9$ mm $R = 1$ mm

Moreover, we assume a rectangular 0.635 mm × 0.432 mm cross-section.

The appliance is mechanically loaded imposing outward displacements, equal in magnitude, on section S_c (Figure 8.10), assuming for the same sections no vertical displacements and no rotations (clamped boundary conditions). In particular, we set:

$$d_{max} = 20 \text{ mm} \qquad d_{mec} = 10 \text{ mm}$$

As output parameters, we consider the horizontal reaction force and moment in section S_c; in general, we also report the moment/force ratio, since it represents the effective position of the applied force, hence a parameter of particular interest from the applicative perspective. The vertical reaction force is clearly equal to zero for symmetry reasons.

Table 8.4 reports the output parameters for all the investigated thermo-mechanical loadings. It is interesting to observe that:

- the force and the moment produced by the appliance varies in a quite small interval depending on the specific thermo-mechanical loading considered; however, all the values obtained are contained within the possible physiological range;
- the ratio moment/force produced by the appliance is almost constant independently from the specific thermo-mechanical loading considered.

Finally, we consider a parametric analysis for the T-loop rectraction appliance to investigate the effects induced by changes in the geometric parameters. The parametric analysis is expressed in terms of the following non-dimensional parameters:

$$A^* = \frac{A}{A_0} \quad B^* = \frac{B}{B_0} \quad C^* = \frac{C}{C_0} \quad D^* = \frac{D}{D_0} \quad R^* = \frac{R}{R_0}$$

$$F_i^* = \frac{F^i}{F_0^i} \quad M_i^* = \frac{M^i}{M_0^i} \quad F_f^* = \frac{F^f}{F_0^f} \quad M_f^* = \frac{M^f}{M_0^f}$$

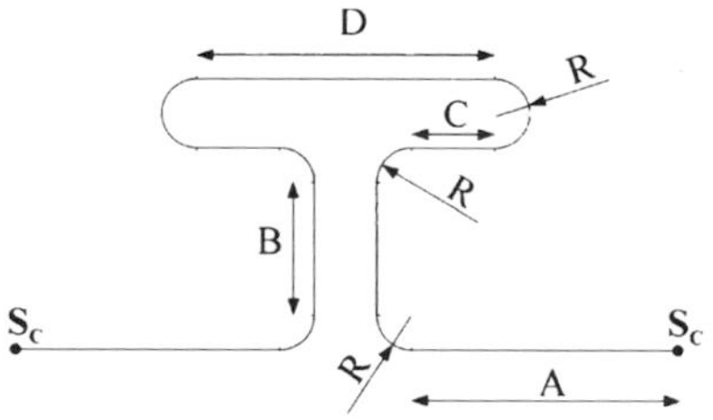

Figure 8.10 T-loop retraction appliance: geometric data.

Table 8.4 Retraction T-loop: standard geometry. Appliance response for different thermo-mechanical loading histories

	F_0^i [N]	M_0^i [Nmm]	F_0^f [N]	M_0^f [Nmm]	M_0^i/F_0^i [mm]	M_0^f/F_0^f [mm]
L-HC	3.19	9.48	1.53	4.57	2.97	2.99
L-CH	1.17	3.51	1.46	4.38	3.00	3.00
U-HC	3.19	9.48	2.85	8.50	2.97	2.98
U-HC	1.17	3.51	2.85	8.51	3.00	2.99

where the subscript 0 indicated the geometric and the output parameters relative to the appliance so far considered and in the following referred as "standard appliance". Accordingly, for the case of the "standard appliance" all the geometric and output non-dimensional parameters are equal to one.

Table 8.5 reports the results relative to output parameters at the end of the thermo-mechanical loadings U-CH and U-HC, where we vary single geometric parameters.

It is interesting to observe that:

- the geometric parameter A^*, C^* and D^* have a small influence on the appliance response
- the geometric parameters B^* and R^* have a greater influence on the appliance response; in fact, increasing B and R increases the appliance flexibility, in particular, reducing only the horizontal stiffness (i.e. decreasing the horizontal force while keeping almost constant the moment), hence resulting in an increase of ratio moment/force.

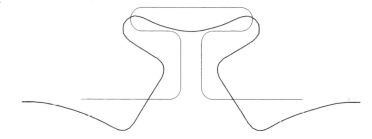

Figure 8.11 T-loop retraction appliance: deformed configuration at the end of the mechanical-thermal loading (U-CH) and undeformed configuration (dotted line)

Table 8.5 Retraction T-loop: parametric analysis for thermo-mechanical loading U-CH and U-HC

A^* [−]	B^* [−]	C^* [−]	D^* [−]	R^* [−]	F_i^* [−]	M_i^* [−]	F_f^* [−]	M_f^* [−]	M_i^*/F_i^* [−]	M_f^*/F_f^* [−]
1.50	1	1	1	1	1.00	1.00	0.99	0.97	1.00	0.98
1	0.50	1	1	1	1.20	1.00	1.20	1.00	0.83	0.83
1	2	1	1	1	0.75	1.01	0.74	0.98	1.34	1.32
1	3	1	1	1	0.61	1.01	0.58	0.95	1.67	1.64
1	4	1	1	1	0.51	1.02	0.46	0.90	1.99	1.96
1	1	2	1.50	1	1.00	1.00	0.99	1.00	1.00	1.01
1	1	0	0.50	1	1.01	1.00	1.00	1.00	0.99	1.00
1	1	1	1.10	1.50	0.75	1.01	0.74	0.98	1.34	1.32
1	2	1	1.10	1.50	0.61	1.01	0.57	0.94	1.67	1.65
1.50	1	1	1	1	1.00	1.00	0.99	0.99	1.00	1.00
1	0.50	1	1	1	1.20	1.00	1.47	1.22	0.83	0.83
1	2	1	1	1	0.75	1.01	0.92	1.22	1.34	1.33
1	3	1	1	1	0.61	1.01	0.73	1.20	1.67	1.66
1	4	1	1	1	0.51	1.02	0.49	0.98	1.99	2.00
1	1	2	1.50	1	1.00	1.00	1.23	1.22	1.00	1.00
1	1	0	0.50	1	1.01	1.00	1.23	1.22	0.99	0.99
1	1	1	1.10	1.50	0.75	1.01	0.92	1.21	1.34	1.32
1	2	1	1.10	1.50	0.61	1.01	0.73	1.20	1.67	1.66

8.5.3 Retraction V-loop

We now investigate the response of a retraction appliance in the form of a V-loop, sketched in Figure 8.12. Following Reference (Raboud, 1998), the geometrical parameters are set equal to:

$$A = 8 \text{ mm} \qquad B = 4 \text{ mm} \qquad R = 1 \text{ mm}$$

Moreover, we assume the same rectangular cross-section as for the T-loop.

The appliance is mechanically loaded imposing outward displacements, equal in magnitude, on section S_c (Figure 8.12), assuming for the same sections no vertical displacements and no rotations (clamped boundary conditions). In particular, we set:

$$d_{max} = 20 \text{ mm} \qquad d_{mec} = 10 \text{ mm}$$

As output parameters, we consider the horizontal reaction force and moment in section S_c; in general, we also report the moment/force ratio, since it represents the effective position of the applied force, hence a parameter of particular interest from the applicative perspective. The vertical reaction force is clearly equal to zero for symmetry reasons.

Table 8.6 reports the output parameters for all the investigated thermo-mechanical loadings. It is interesting to observe that:

- the force and the moment produced by the appliance varies in a quite small interval depending on the specific thermo-mechanical loading considered; however, all the values obtained are contained within the possible physiological range;
- the ratio moment/force produced by the appliance is almost constant independently from the specific thermo-mechanical loading considered.

Finally, we consider a parametric analysis for the V-loop rectraction appliance to investigate the effects induced by changes in the geometric parameters. The parametric analysis is expressed in terms of the following non-dimensional parameters:

$$A^* = \frac{A}{A_0} \qquad B^* = \frac{B}{B_0} \qquad R^* = \frac{R}{R_0}$$

$$F_i^* = \frac{F^i}{F_0^i} \qquad M_i^* = \frac{M^i}{M_0^i} \qquad F_f^* = \frac{F^f}{F_0^f} \qquad M_f^* = \frac{M^f}{M_0^f} \tag{1}$$

Table 8.6 Retraction V-loop: standard geometry. Appliance response for different thermo-mechanical loading histories

	F_0^i [N]	M_0^i [Nmm]	F_0^f [N]	M_0^f [Nmm]	M_0^i/F_0^i [mm]	M_0^f/F_0^f [mm]
L-HC	3.40	9.49	1.68	4.57	2.79	2.72
L-CH	1.30	3.50	1.60	4.37	2.69	2.73
U-HC	3.40	9.48	3.05	8.50	2.79	2.79
U-HC	1.30	3.50	3.05	8.50	3.05	2.79

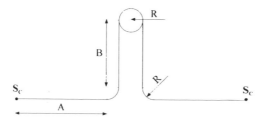

Figure 8.12 V-loop retraction appliance: geometric data.

where the subscript 0 indicated the geometric and the output parameters relative to the appliance so far considered and in the following referred as "standard appliance". Accordingly, for the case of the "standard appliance" all the geometric and output non-dimensional parameters are equal to one.

Table 8.7 reports the results relative to output parameters at the end of the thermo-mechanical loadings U-CH and U-HC, where we vary single geometric parameters. It is interesting to observe that:

- the geometric parameter $A*$ has a small influence on the appliance response
- the geometric parameters $B*$ and $R*$ have a greater influence on the appliance response; in fact, increasing B and R increases the appliance flexibility, in particular, reducing

Table 8.7 Retraction V-loop: parametric analysis for thermo-mechanical loading U-CH and U-HC

$A*$ [−]	$B*$ [−]	$R*$ [−]	F_i* [−]	M_i* [−]	F_f* [−]	M_f* [−]	M_i*/F_i* [−]	M_f*/F_f* [−]
1.50	1	1	1.00	1.00	0.99	0.97	1.00	0.98
0.50	1	1	1.00	1.00	1.01	1.03	1.00	1.02
1	0.50	1	1.88	0.99	0.77	1.00	0.53	0.57
1	1.50	1	0.70	1.01	0.72	0.98	1.44	1.36
1	2	1	0.55	1.01	0.55	0.95	1.83	1.71
1	2.50	1	0.46	1.02	0.45	0.90	2.21	2.01
1	1	1.50	0.82	1.00	0.82	0.99	1.23	1.21
1	1	2	0.68	1.01	0.70	0.98	1.47	1.39
1	1.50	2	0.55	1.01	0.55	0.94	1.83	1.72
1	2	2	0.46	1.02	0.45	0.90	2.22	2.02
1	2.00	3	0.40	1.03	0.35	0.83	2.59	2.37
1.50	1	1	1.00	1.00	1.19	1.21	1.00	1.01
0.50	1	1	1.00	1.00	1.01	1.00	1.00	1.00
1	0.50	1	1.88	0.99	1.83	0.99	0.53	0.54
1	1.50	1	0.70	1.01	0.71	1.00	1.44	1.40
1	2	1	0.55	1.01	0.56	1.00	1.83	1.77
1	2.50	1	0.46	1.02	0.46	0.99	2.22	2.16
1	1	1.50	0.82	1.01	0.83	1.00	1.23	1.20
1	1	2	0.68	1.01	0.69	1.00	1.47	1.44
1	1.50	2	0.55	1.02	0.56	0.99	1.84	1.79
1	2	2	0.46	1.03	0.46	0.98	2.22	2.13
1	2.00	3	0.40	1.04	0.39	0.97	2.59	2.50

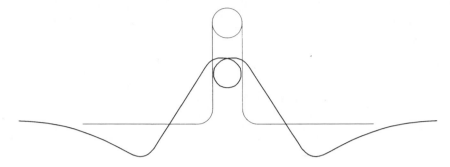

Figure 8.13 V-loop retraction appliance: deformed configuration at the end of the mechanical-thermal loading (U-CH) and undeformed configuration (dotted line).

only the horizontal stiffness (i.e. decreasing the horizontal force while keeping almost constant the moment), hence resulting in an increase of ratio moment/force

8.6 CONCLUSIONS

The present work has focused on the use of shape-memory materials in orthodontics. In particular, after a brief review on the material macroscopic features and on their exploitations in orthodontics, we gave some details on actual experimental and numerical investigations that our research group is carring on such a specific subject.

In both experimental and numerical areas we take advantage of classical mechanical concepts and procedures; however, we hope to have shown how an extensive use of such methodologies may lead to a better understanding, interpretation and justification of typical clinical methodologies.

Accordingly, shape-memory materials are herein used as a innovative example of how biomechanics could be able to build a deep and fruitful connection between the more theoretical mechanics and the more applied and therapy oriented orthodontic world.

REFERENCES

P.V. Angolkar, S. Kapila, M.G. Duncanson and R.S. Nanda, Treatment of malocclusion of teeth, American Journal Orthodontics and Dentofacial Orthopedics, Vol. 98, pp. 499–506, 1990.

E.H. Angle, Treatment of malocclusion of teeth, SS White Dental Manufacturing, 1907.

G. Airoldi and G. Riva Innovative materials: the Ni-Ti orthodontics, Bio-Medical Materials and Engineering, Vol. 6, pp. 299–305, 1996.

G. Airoldi, G. Riva, and M. Vanelli, Superelasticity and shape-memory effect in Ni-Ti orthodontic wires, Proceedings of the International Conference on Martensitic Transformations (ICOMAT), 1995.

F. Auricchio and E. Sacco, A one-dimensional model for superelastic shape-memory alloys with different elastic properties between austenite and martensite, International Journal of Nonlinear Mechanics, Vol. 32, pp. 1101–1114, 1997.

F. Auricchio and E. Sacco, A superelastic shape-memory-alloy beam model, Journal of Intelligent Material Systems and Structures, Vol. 8, pp. 489–501, 1997.

F. Auricchio and E. Sacco, A temperature-driven beam for shape-memory alloys: constitutive modelling, finite-element implementation and numerical simulations, Computer Methods in Applied Mechanics and Engineering, Vol. 174, pp. 171–190, 1999.

F. Auricchio and R.L. Taylor, Shape-memory alloys: modelling and numerical simulations of the finite-strain superelastic behavior, Computer Methods in Applied Mechanics and Engineering, Vol. 143, pp. 175–194, 1997.

F. Auricchio, R.L. Taylor and J. Lubliner, Shape-memory alloys: macromodelling and numerical simulations of the superelastic behavior, Computer Methods in Applied Mechanics and Engineering, Vol. 146, pp. 281–312, 1997.

F. Auricchio, A robust integration-algorithm for a finite-strain shape memory-alloy superelastic model, International Journal of Plasticity, 2000, accepted for publication.

P.H. Adler, W. Yu, A.R. Pelton, R. Zadno, T.W. Duerig and R. Barresi, On the tensile and torsional properties of pseudoelastic Ni-Ti, Scripta Metallurgica et Materialia, Vol. 24, pp. 943–947, 1990.

C.J. Burstone and A.J. Goldberg, Beta-titanium: a new orthodontic alloy, American Journal of Orthodontics, Vol. 77, pp. 121–132, 1980.

L.C. Brinson, One-dimensional constitutive behavior of shape memory alloys: Thermomechanical derivation with non-constant material functions and redefined martensite internal variables, Journal of Intelligent Material Systems and Structures, Vol. 4, pp. 229–242, 1993.

Y. Chu, K. Dai, M. Zhu, and X. Mi, Medical application of NiTi shape memory alloy in China, Proceedings of the International Symposium on Shape Memory Materials, Materials Science Forum, Vol. 327–328, pp. 55–62, 2000.

R.G. Craig, Restorative dental materials, 10th ed., Mosby, St. Louis, MO, 1997.

T.W. Duerig, A.R. Pelton and D. Stökel, The utility of superelasticity in medicine, Bio-Medical Materials and Engineering, Vol. 6, pp. 255–266, 1996.

S.R. Drake, D.M. Wayne, J.M. Powers and K. Asgar, Mechanical properties of orthodontic wires in tension, bending, and torsion, American Journal of Orthodontics, Vol. 82, pp. 206–210, 1982.

T.J.W. Evans, M.L. Jones and R.G. Newcombe, Clinical comparison and perfomance perspective of three aligning arch wires, American Journal of Orthodontics and Dentofacial Orthopedics, Vol. 114, pp. 32–39, 1998.

C.A. Frank and R.J. Nikolai, A comparative study of frictional resistances between orthodontic bracket and archwire, American Journal of Orthodontics, Vol. 78, pp. 593–609, 1980.

R.W. Glendenning, J.A.A. Hood and R.L. Enlow, Orthodontic applications of a superelastic shape-memory alloy model, Proceedings of the International Symposium on Shape Memory Materials, Materials Science Forum, Vol. 327–328, pp. 71–74, 2000.

F.J. Gil and J.A. Planell, Shape memory alloys for medical applications, Proceedings of the institution of mechanical engineers. Part H-Journal of Engineering in Medicine, 212 NH6, pp. 473–488, 1998.

K. Gall, H. Sehitoglu, Y.I. Chumlyakov and I.V. Kireeva, Tension-compression asymmetry of the stress-strain response in aged single crystal and polycristalline NiTi, Acta Materialia, Vol. 47, pp. 1203–1217, 1999.

T.M. Graber and R.L. Vanarsdall, Orthodontics – Current principles and techniques. Mosby, St. Louis, MO, 2nd ed., 1994.

Harcourt, Inc. Academic Press Dictionary of Science and Technology, 2001. http://www.harcourt.com/dictionary/.

J.J. Hudgins, M.D. Bagby and L.C. Erickson, The effect of long-term deflection on permanent deformation of nickel-titanium archwires. The Angle Orthodontist, Vol. 60, pp. 283–288, 1990.

S. Kapila and R. Sachdeva, Mechanical properties and clinical applications of orthodontic wires, American Journal of Orthodontics and dentofacial orthopedics, Vol. 96, pp. 100–109, 1989.

A. Laino, F. Boscaino and A. Michelotti, Considerazioni sui fili super-elastici in ortognatodonzia, Mondo ortodontico, Vol. XV, pp. 707–714, 1990.

T.J. Lim and D.L. McDowell, Mechanical behavior of an Ni-Ti alloy under axial-torsional proportional and non-proportional loading, Journal of Engineering Materials and Technology, Vol. 121, pp. 9–18, 1999.

F. Miura, M. Mogi, Y. Ohura and H. Hamanaka, The super-elastic properties of the Japanese NiTi alloy wire for use in orthodontics, American Journal of Orthodontics and Dentofacial Orthopedics, Vol. 90, pp. 1–10, 1986.

F. Miura, M. Mogi and Y. Ohura Japanese NiTi alloy wire: use of the direct electric resistance heat treatment method, European Journal of Orthodontics, Vol. 10, pp. 187–191, 1988.

F. Miura, M. Mogi, Y. Ohura and M.Karibe, The super-elastic properties of the Japanese NiTi alloy wire for use in orthodontics. Part III. Studies on the Japanese NiTi alloy coil springs, American Journal of Orthodontics and Dentofacial Orthopedics, Vol. 94, pp. 89–96, 1988.

E. Nardi, G. Gambarini and R. Tosti, Archi preformati Ni-Ti a sezione tonda: aspetti meccanici e clinici, Minerva stomatologica, Vol. 42, pp. 217–221, 1993.

L. Orgéas and D. Favier, Stress-induced martensitic transformation of NiTi alloy in isothermal shear, tension and compression, Acta Materialia, Vol. 46, pp. 5579–5591, 1998.

E.P. Popov, Engineering Mechanics of Solids, Prentice Hall, 1990.

D.H. Pratten, K. Popli, N. Germane and J.C. Gunsolley, Frictional resistance of ceramic and stainless steel orthodontic brackets, American Journal Orthodontics and Dentofacial Orthopedics, Vol. 98, pp. 398–403, 1990.

A.R. Pelton, D. Stökel and T.W. Duerig, Medical use of Nitinol, Proceedings of the International Symposium on Shape Memory Materials, Materials Science Forum, Vol. 327–328, pp. 63–70, 2000.

D. Raboud, Simulation of the superelastic response of SMA orthodontic wires, Journal of Biomechanical Engineering, Vol. 120, pp. 676–685, 1998.

I.R. Reynolds, A review of direct orthodontic bonding, British Dental Journal, Vol. 2, pp. 171–178, 1975.

J. Ryhänen, Biocompatibility evaluation of nickel-titanium shape-memory metal alloy, Ph.D. dissertation, University of Oulu, Department of Surgery, 1999.

J. Sabrià, M. Cortada, L. Giner, F.J. Gil, E. Fernández, J.M. Manero and J.A. Planell, A study of load cycling in a Ni-Ti shape memory alloy with pseudoelastic behaviour used in dental prosthesis fixators, Bio-Medical Materials and Engineering, Vol. 6, pp. 153–157, 1996.

G. Scott, Fracture toughness and surface cracks – the key to understanding ceramic brackets. Angle Orthodontist, Vol. 58, pp. 5–8, 1988.

S.A. Shabalovskaya, On the nature of the biocompatibility and on medical applications of Ni-Ti shape memory and superelastic alloys, Bio-Medical Materials and Engineering, Vol. 6, pp. 267–289, 1996.

R.C.L. Sachdeva and S. Miyazaki, Superelastic Ni-Ti alloys in orthodontics, in T.W. Duerig, K.N. Melton, D. Stökel and C.M. Wayman, editors, Engineering aspects of shape memory alloys, pp. 452–469, 1990.

C.C. Steiner, The Angle orthodontist, EH Angle Society of Orthodontia, 1933.

M.L. Swartz, Ceramic brackets, Journal of Clinical Orthodontics, Vol. 24, pp. 91–94, 1988.

L. Torrisi and G. Di Marco, Physical characterization of endodontic instruments in NiTi alloy, Proceedings of the International Symposium on Shape Memory Materials, Materials Science Forum, Vol. 327–328, pp. 75–78, 2000.

L. Torrisi, The Ni-Ti superelastic alloy application to the dentistry field, Bio-Medical Materials and Engineering, Vol. 9, pp. 39–47, 1999.

J. Van Humbeeck, R. Stalmans and P.A. Besselink, Metals as Biomaterials, chapter Shape memory alloys, pp. 73–100, Biomaterials Science and Engineering. John Wiley and Sons, 1998.

C.M. Wayman, Introduction to the crystallography of martensitic transformations. MacMillan, 1964.

J.V. Wilkinson, Some metallurgical aspects of orthodontic stainless steel, Angle Orthodontist, Vol. 48, pp. 192–206, 1962.

R.M. Wilson and K.J. Donley, Demineralization around orthodontic brackets bonded with resin-modified glass ionomer cement and fluoride-releasing resin composite., Pediatr. Dent., Vol. 23, pp. 255–259, 2001.

L.J. Winchester, Bond strengths of five different ceramic brackets: an in vitro study, European Journal of Orthodontics, Vol. 13, pp. 293–305, 1991.

9 Clinical procedures for dental implants

G Vogel, S Abati, E Romeo, M Chiapasco

9.1 INTRODUCTION

Osseointegrated oral implantology could be regarded as the most important achievement of the modern era in the field of rehabilitation of compromised masticatory function and apparatus. To obtain long-term high success rates of osseointegrated implants it is necessary that a progressive series of medical interventions are made in a precise and accurate manner.

This chapter is intended to describe the clinical steps in such a way that the biomechanical implications become apparent.

The following four main steps could be defined:

- diagnostic procedures;
- surgical procedures;
- prosthetic design;
- prognostic evaluation and maintenance.

9.2 DIAGNOSTIC PROCEDURES

As in any other clinical field, a great part of the success of the planned treatment relies in the accuracy of the diagnostic phase. The diagnosis should follow a sequence of clinical steps in which a correct and deep clinical interaction with the patient is fundamental. The diagnostic phase in oral implantology should follow a comprehensive stomatological evaluation schedule, namely:

- medical history;
- extra-oral clinical examination;
- intra-oral clinical examination;
- study models and diagnostic waxing;
- radiographic analysis.

9.2.1 Medical history

The first step in the diagnosis is to assess the general and dental clinical history of the patient. Medical history is addressed to identify those systemic and oral conditions and diseases which could interfere with oral rehabilitation with osseointegrated implants. Two series of absolute and relative main contraindications could be identified, respectively relative to systemic and local conditions. They could be summarized as in the following.

Absolute systemic contraindications

- heart diseases such as recent myocardial infarction, unstable angina pectoris and heart failure;
- diseases of the leukocyte system;
- severe coagulopathies;
- severe platelet diseases;
- severe liver diseases;
- severe kidney diseases;
- neurologic disease such as Parkinson disease, Huntington chorea, Alzheimer disease or cerebral stroke, mental handicaps, Down syndrome, psychosis: a severe physical and mental impairments may jeopardize cooperation or oral hygiene maintenance;
- alcohol or drug abuse.

Relative systemic contraindications

- minor heart diseases: stable angina pectoris;
- endocardial and valvular diseases: the need of an antibiotic prophylaxis should be considered;
- chronic respiratory failure;
- mild liver and kidney failure;
- non controlled diabetes mellitus;
- adrenocortical failure;
- relevant osteoporosis;
- coagulation disorders: patients treated with anticoagulant agents, such as heparin and antagonists of Vitamin K (acenocoumarol, warfarin) or platelet antiaggregants (acetilsalicylic acid, dipyridamole, ticlopidine);
- arterial hypertension;
- radiotherapy in the head and neck area, especially for doses exceeding 48 Gy;
- anxiety, stress;
- patients in evolutionary age to prevent risks of infraocclusion of implants;
- heavy smoking (more than ten cigarettes daily) may cause an increase in the early and late failure rates.

Absolute local contraindications

- xerostomia;
- functional disorders resistant to therapy such as restricted opening of the mouth or microstomia, myoarthropathy or rheumatic pathologies of temporomandibular joint, progressive systemic sclerosis (scleroderma), systemic lupus erythematosus.

Relative local contraindications

- osteoradionecrosis of maxillary bones;
- skeletal maxillary ratio not favourable to the implanto-prosthetic rehabilitation;

- parafunctions: clenching, bruxism;
- acute or chronic inflammatory pathologies of residual teeth;
- cystic lesions of maxillary bones;
- diseases and conditions of oral mucous membranes such as oral lichen planus, pemphigus and benign mucous pemphigoid, erythema multiforme, herpetic and aphthous stomatitis.

9.2.2 Extra-oral clinical examination

Extra-oral clinical examination should establish the assessment of the support given by the natural or prosthetic tooth elements to the upper and lower lip, exposure of teeth or gingiva during smile, the patient's profile and intermaxillary relationships.

9.2.3 Intra-oral clinical examination

Intraoral clinical examination will be addressed to assess the health state of both soft and hard tissues, as well as the periodontal status of residual dentition and type of occlusion (Figures 9.1 (a), (b)).

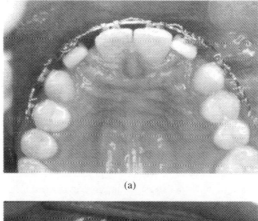

(a)

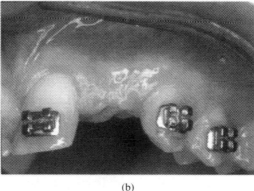

(b)

Figure 9.1 Preoperative situation in a patient presenting agenesia of both upper lateral incisors (a) and detail of vestibular left incisor (b).

9.2.4 Study casts and waxing

This diagnostic step is of a fundamental importance to assess the occlusal relationship for the correct design of the length and morphology of the clinical crown of the prosthetic elements supported by implants and the relations between these latter and the oral soft tissues. In edentulous patients, diagnostic waxing is mandatory to assess the skeletal relationships and the ratio between the ideal position of tooth elements to be reconstructed and the residual alveolar ridge. Moreover, diagnostic waxing enables to fabricate stents and perform accurate tomographic evaluations. These stents may also be converted into surgical stents to optimise implant placement.

9.2.5 Evaluation of implant site

A qualitative and quantitative evaluation of the residual bone and an evaluation of anatomic structures which can interfere with implant placement can be obtained using different diagnostic techniques:

- radiography by means of:
    - intraoral radiograms;
    - panoramic radiograms;
    - profile radiograms of the skull;
    - computed tomography (CT scan);
- torque measurement during implant site preparation and insertion;
- Periotest®;
- resonance frequency.

Ideally, bone volume for reliable implant long-term survival should be enough to embed completely and implant at least 3–4 mm in diameter and 8–10 mm in length (Spiekermann et al., 1995; Adell et al., 1981; Albrektsson et al., 1986). If residual bone volume is less, implants may be employed, but it is necessary to correct the bone deficit with regenerative or reconstructive procedures prior or during implant installation (Breine and Branemark, 1980; Kahnberg et al., 1989; Keller et al., 1987; Lang et al., 1994; Ronchi et al., 1995; Buser et al., 1996; Chiapasco and Ronchi, 1994; Chiapasco et al., 1998–1999; Chiapasco and Romeo, 2001).

The use of tomography (CT scan) should be carefully evaluated as a function of the information which could be obtained and, thus, of the cost/efficacy ratio (Figure 9.2).

The evaluation of bone quality is very important to predict future primary stability of an oral implant. Lekholm and Zarb, 1985, proposed the following classification:

- Class I – Highly corticalized bone;
- Class II – Thick layer of cortical bone surrounding a dense cancellous bone;
- Class III –Thin layer of cortical bone surrounding cancellous bone;
- Class IV – Very thin layer of cortical bone surrounding spongy bone with numerous and large marrow spaces.

Class I and II are normally associated to predictable primary implant stability, whereas class III and IV may expose to a higher risk of lack of stability. In the latter situation implant design (implants with threads) and rough surface preparation (sand-blasted, acid-etched, etc.) are of paramount importance to increase primary stability.

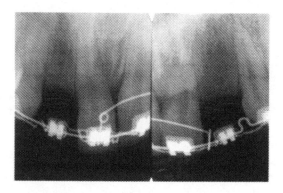

Figure 9.2 Radiographic evaluation with intraoral radiograph.

The bone quality can be evaluated either preoperatively with radiographic examination or intraoperatively (at time of implant site preparation, during implant placement and at the end of the procedure) by means of torque drilling measurements, Periotest® and resonance frequency values.

Tomography could be also used to evaluate the quality of the bone and the data coming from this examination can be used to construct CAD-CAM models of the jaws. In addition these information could help greatly to personalize any geometrical and numerical analysis.

9.3 SURGICAL PROCEDURE IN ORAL IMPLANTOLOGY

The placement of endosseous implants has become a safe and predictable method for the rehabilitation of partially or totally edentulous patients. However, long-term success of implants is connected to the strict application of some rules, which can be summarized as follows (Laney et al., 1986; Branemark et al., 1969; Schroeder et al., 1976; Adell et al., 1981; Albrektsson et al., 1986; Adell et al., 1990; Arvidson et al., 1992; Buser et al., 1997; Lekholm et al., 1994).

9.3.1 Antisepsis and patient preparation

The oral cavity cannot be sterilised: however, a significant reduction of contamination risk can be obtained with correct preparation of the surgical environment, patient and surgeons. Only sterile surgical instruments (including hand pieces, suctioning systems, etc.) must be used. Surgeon and assistants must wear head cap, facemask, sterile gown and gloves. Reduction of intraoral bacteria can be significantly reduced with clorhexidine digluconate mouth rinses, to be started one or two days before surgery and repeated for one minute just before starting the procedure. Iodine and/or clorhexidine solutions should be always used to reduce the perioral skin bacteria. The operating field must be then isolated with sterile towels, leaving exposed only the mouth and nose region. Antibiotic prophylaxis is usually recommended. An oral dose of two grams penicillin V, administered one hour before starting the surgical procedure or an intravenous dose of one million U. penicillin G, immediately preoperatively have demonstrated both effective. Alternative medications include amoxicillin in association with clavulanic acid, two grams per os one hour before surgery.

The initial doses can be repeated 12 hours and 24 hours after surgery (Vecksler et al., 1990; Scharf and Tarnow, 1993; Dent et al., 1997; Lambert et al., 1997; Gynter et al., 1998; Romeo et al., 1998).

The majority of the procedures can be performed under local anaesthesia. Only in case of multiple implant placements or in case of non-cooperating patients, per os or intravenous sedation or general anaesthesia may be indicated.

Profound local anaesthesia is indicated to permit a painless surgical procedure. As far as the mandible is concerned, infiltration anaesthesia is indicated in the interforaminal area, whereas block anaesthesia of the inferior alveolar nerve in association with infiltration anaesthesia is indicated in case of implant placement in areas distal to the mental foramen.

As far as the maxilla is concerned, infiltration anaesthesia is normally sufficient in the anterior part of the maxilla. Close to maxillary midline, block anaesthesia of the nasal-palatine nerves may be indicated as well as imbibition of local anaesthetic of the mucosa of the floor of the nose. In the posterior maxilla local infiltration can be associated to the block of the posterior alveolar nerves. Only in a small number of cases (in particular in case of procedures involving maxillary sinus elevation), block of the infraorbital nerve is indicated.

9.3.2 Atraumatic surgery for implant placement

Any surgical procedure determines a trauma to the hard and soft tissues involved. A reliable result is strictly linked to the minimization of this trauma (Branemark et al., 1969; Schroeder et al., 1976).

Soft tissue incisions

Normally, both for submerged and non-submerged implants, a full-thickness crestal incision is indicated with subperiosteal dissection of the flap obtained. Mesial and/or distal releasing incisions can be performed to increase access to the surgical field. However, it must be remembered that, specially in older patients, vascular supply to the underlying bone is dominantly periosteal, whereas endosteal supply tends to reduce with increasing age of the patients. Therefore, excessive exposure of the bone may determine a reduction of blood supply, with consequent bone ischemia. This can increase postoperative bone resorption and delay osseointegration of implants.

The blades must be kept perpendicular to the bone in order to obtain a precise, sharp incision. The soft tissue flap must be kept retracted during the surgical procedure, avoiding excessive traction which may determine ischemia.

A buccal incision in the mandible or a buccal or palatal incision is normally indicated only in cases where advanced regenerative procedures (guided bone regeneration, bone grafts) are indicated.

In case of surgical procedures close to important anatomical structures (mental foramen, nasal floor, maxillary sinus) flap design should permit direct control of the area to avoid surgical damage.

Preparation of the implant site

Once the flap has been reflected, bone is exposed and all residual soft tissues on the alveolar crest are removed. Irregularly shaped alveolar crests may be carefully smoothed with a bur under constant cooling with sterile saline.

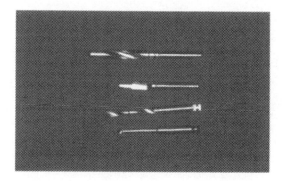

Figure 9.3 The series of surgical burs used for the implant site preparation.

The choice of implant site position should be predetermined according to a prosthetically-driven planification. To obtain a more precise positioning, the use of surgical stents is recommendable. With the aid of stents it is possible to optimise three-dimensionally implant positioning.

Accurate preoperative planning with thorough analysis of preoperative radiographs is fundamental to identify areas at risk (such as the alveolar canal, the nasal floor, the maxillary sinus) in order to avoid surgical damage to these structures (see previous section – preoperative planning).

Implant site preparation is obtained with the use of stainless steel burs of increasing diameters, until the final diameter of the implant site is reached (Figure 9.3).

It has been demonstrated that significant bone necrosis during implant site preparation may occur if the local temperature exceeds 47–50 °C (Eriksson and Albrektsson, 1983). This can jeopardize the further osseointegration in the early phases. The following rules can minimize surgical trauma:

* low-speed (800–2000 rpm), high torque handpieces;
* abundant irrigation with pre-cooled (4 to 10°C) sterile saline;
* use of sharp burs.

The irrigation can be internal, external, or both. No significant difference has been found between bone trauma and internal or external irrigation. Recommendations of the specific implant manufacturer should be followed.

Preparation of implant sites should be performed with an up-and-down intermittent movement of the bur to permit removal of bone fragments from the bur during preparation and adequate cooling. In case of dense bone, it is recommended not to perform high pressures on the handpiece which may determine the development of high temperatures and consequent bone necrosis at the apex of implant site preparation (Figures 9.4–9.8).

According to manufacturer, burs can be disposable or used more than once. However, it must be remembered that prolonged use and multiple sterilization procedures of the burs can determine a reduction in cutting capacity, which leads to higher pressures during implant site preparation and more trauma. In case of threaded non self-tapping cylindrical root shape implants, a final thread preparation may be necessary with very low speed (15–20 rpm).

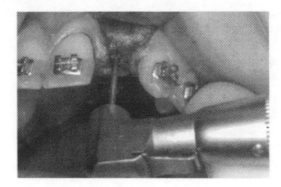

Figure 9.4 After reflection of the flap, the alveolar bone is exposed: a favourable bone volume is found for the placement of one endosseous implant: the first step is represented by perforation of the cortical plate.

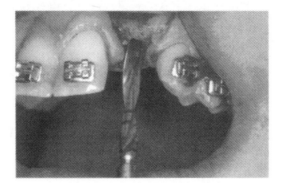

Figure 9.5 Implant site preparation is obtained with a 2 mm wide drill. According to preoperative radiographic evaluation a 15 mm deep preparation is performed.

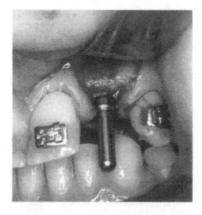

Figure 9.6 The mesio-distal and palatal-buccal direction of implant site is checked with a pin; small correction are still permitted. With the following burs the implant site direction cannot be further modified.

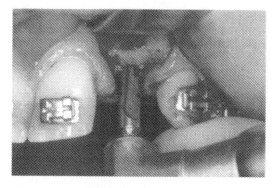

Figure 9.7 Final preparation of the implant site with a 3-mm drill.

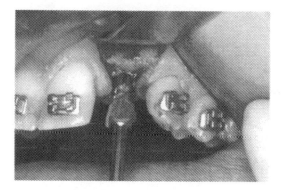

Figure 9.8 Enlargement of the implant site with a countersink bur in order to embed the implant neck which present a larger diameter.

Implant placement

After the programmed depth and diameter of implant site has been obtained, implants are placed. Implants must be inserted at very low speed (15–20 rpm) either manually or with an handpiece. Care must be applied not to contaminate the implant threads with saliva, instruments etc. Once the implants are correctly embedded into bone, cover screws are placed. Irrigation of implants during insertion with sterile saline may be indicated. It is very important to evaluate the final depth of the most coronal part of the implant, in order to optimise prosthetic rehabilitation from a functional and aesthetic viewpoint (Figures 9.9–9.13).

In case of submerged implants, the flap is sutured on the top of the cover screws (Figure 9.14).

A radiographic control at the end of the procedure may be indicated in order to evaluate the correct positioning of implants and to verify the relationship of implants with adjacent anatomical structures. A control radiograph also permits to verify the correct closure of the cover screws (Figure 9.15).

Incomplete screwing may determine, in case of submerged implants, unscrewing of the cover screw during the healing phase or bone formation beneath the cover screw and over the implant shoulder. This can render the following abutment connection very difficult or impossible.

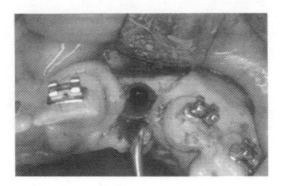

Figure 9.9 Final preparation of the implant site.

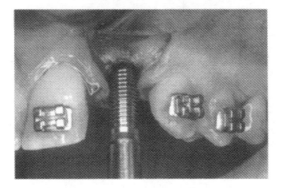

Figure 9.10 Implant placement with a reduced speed hand piece (12–20 rpm).

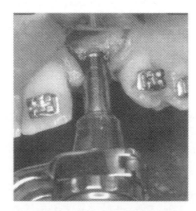

Figure 9.11 Final adjustments of implant placement with a hand wrachet.

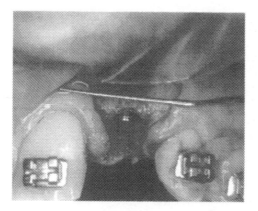

Figure 9.12 Final control of implant shoulder depth: in aesthetic sites the ideal position is generally 2 mm apical to the cement-enamel junction of adjacent teeth.

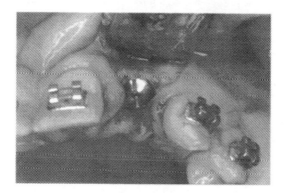

Figure 9.13 Placement of the cover-screw for submerged implant healing.

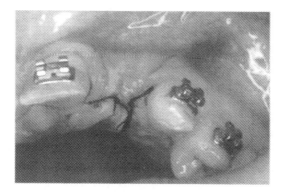

Figure 9.14 Suture of the flap (submerged healing).

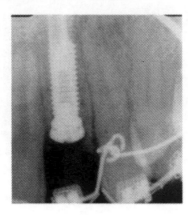

Figure 9.15 Radiographic control at the end of the surgical procedure.

In case of non-submerged implants, the flap is sutured and adapted around the implant neck. An accurate but tension-free suture is indicated.

Postoperative care

At the end of the procedure, the patient is discharged after a thorough explanation of the postoperative recovery and oral hygiene instructions. Postoperative non-steroidal analgesics are usually prescribed for the first days. The maintenance of a good oral hygiene by means of chlorhexidine digluconate mouthrinses, twice a day for two weeks, is normally indicated. A soft and cool diet is indicated for the first postoperative days. Seven to ten days postoperatively, sutures are removed. The patient should not wear removable prostheses which may come in contact with the operated area until the healing of soft tissues has been completed. Thereafter, patients may be allowed to wear prostheses relined with soft liners. In case of regenerative procedures, this waiting period may be prolonged until maturation of the regenerated tissues (six months).

Uncovering of submerged implants

A waiting period between three and six months has been recommended to permit adequate osseointegration of endosseous implants. Three months are usually indicated in areas with dense bone, whereas a longer period is indicated in areas with softer bone. The waiting period is however connected with the type of implant coating and or implant surface treatment (machined, acid etched, sandblasted, etc.). At present, there is a tendency to shorten the healing period in case of "rough" surfaces.

Implants can be uncovered following the same incision performed during the first phase, or with different incisions in case of need of periimplant soft tissue management procedures, such as increasing the quantity of keratinized mucosa around implants on the buccal aspect.

Cover screws are removed and substituted either with healing abutments or with final prosthetic abutments. Obviously, this phase is not necessary in case of non-submerged implants, unless soft tissue recontouring procedures as previously described for submerged implants are necessary.

Following implant uncovering, the prosthetic procedures are started by placing idoneous abutments and prosthetic suprastructures.

9.3.3 Prevention and treatment of surgical complications

A correct preoperative evaluation is the fundamental step to minimize intraoperative and postoperative complications. Nevertheless, also in experienced hands some accidents may occur. Prevention manouvers and treatment modalities of complications are shortly presented in this section.

9.3.3.1 Intraoperative complications

The incidence of complications in correctly planned and performed implant surgery is normally low. The following aspects must be kept in mind to minimize complications:

- correct preoperative evaluation and meticulous surgical and prosthetic planning;
- strict application of antisepsis procedures;
- atraumatic surgery;
- adequate wound closure;
- precise postoperative information to the patients as regards absence of implant load and oral hygiene;
- regular follow-up visits.

Nevertheless, a certain amount of intraoperative and postoperative complications may occur also to experienced surgeons.

Haemorrhage

Causes: Bleeding from the surgical field is unavoidable, but in situations with normal blood pressure and adequate vasoconstriction, bleeding is limited. A relevant haemorrhage is typically consequent to lesions of arterial vessels both from soft tissues or intrabony vessels.

Prevention: Prevention can be obtained with adequate knowledge of the local anatomy and correct preoperative planning. An haemorrhage can occur during flap preparation or during drilling procedure. An accurate subperiosteal dissection normally prevents profuse bleeding.

During the preparation of implant sites with rotating instruments, a relevant bleeding can occur if an arterial or large venous vessel is violated.

Areas at risk are represented by inferior alveolar canal, floor of the mouth, plexus pterigoideus, naso-palatine canal.

Adequate preoperative clinical and radiographic evaluation is important to prevent this situation.

Treatment: An haemorrhage can stop spontaneously due to organization of the blood clot and contraction of the teared vessel. In case of arterial bleeding this event may occur less frequently than in case of venous bleeding. Compression of the bleeding area is the first and simplest way to obtain haemostasis.

Compression can be obtained with gauze or with gauze in association with haemostatic resorbable materials such as oxydated and regenerated cellulose.

In case of persistence of haemorrhage, diathermy of the vessel can be necessary. Caution: do not use diathermy in proximity of important neurologic structures such as the alveolar nerve or the mental nerve. Diathermy can produce haemostasis bur also irreversible damages to the nerves. In case of larger vessels, legation of the vessel may be indicated.

Nerve damage

Causes: the inferior alveolar nerve, the mental nerve, the nasopalatine nerve, and the lingual nerve represent nerves at risk during standard implant surgery.

Prevention: A correct preoperative radiographic evaluation and adequate knowledge of the local anatomy are again the key factors in reducing this complication. Nerves can be teared during flap incision or elevation and more typically during implant site preparation. Nerves can present different levels of damage:

Neuroapraxia: it is a functional disturbance of nerve conduction, but without macroscopic anatomical lesions of the nerve. Recovery will occur spontaneously within hours or days. No treatment is necessary.

Axonotmesis: the nerve damage is represented by interruption of the axon continuity, but with preservation of the external continuity (perinervium is intact). Nerve regeneration may occur within weeks or months. No treatment is necessary.

Neurotmesis: the nerve is completely interrupted. Spontaneous healing is very difficult to occur, and also in case of nerve regeneration complete recovery is rare.

Neurosurgical reconstruction of the nerve continuity may be necessary. It must be remembered that if nerve recovery do not occur within 12 months, the possibilities of spontaneous healing are very low.

Absence of primary stability of implants

Causes: Inadequate quality of the recipient bone and incorrect implant site preparation are typically responsible for absence of primary stability of implants.

Prevention: Prevention is normally achieved with precise implant site preparation and intra-operative evaluation of bone density.

Treatment: In case of very low bone density (which can be frequently felt by the surgeon with excessive ease in implant site preparation) the final preparation of implant site should be underdimensioned in order to obtain more stability immediately after surgery. Another possibility is represented by the use of implants which present a larger diameter. In case of absence of primary stability, removal of the implant may be indicated.

Maxillary sinus penetration

Causes: Maxillary sinus penetration may occur during implant site preparation in the premolar and molar area and is due to incorrect implant site preparation.

Prevention: Again, a thorough preoperative clinical and radiographic evaluation is fundamental in preventing this complication, as well as cautious implant site preparation. Although implant penetration in the maxillary sinus may be followed by normal osseointegration without sinus infection, non-violation of the sinus mucosa is highly recommendable.

Treatment: In the absence of preexisting maxillary sinus infection, a tear of the sinus mucosa do not represent "per se" a contraindication to maintain the implant in situ, if primary stability has been achieved. It is suggested not to penetrate in the sinus with a relevant part of the implant apex, in order to allow spontaneous healing of the sinus mucosa on the top of the implant.

Nasal floor penetration

Causes: Nasal floor penetration can occur during implant site preparation in the anterior maxilla, due to incorrect preoperative planning or to incorrect implant site preparation. A tear of the nasal mucosa can determine infection of the implant starting from its apex, with consequent absence of osseointegration.
Prevention: Prevention is obtained following the same rules followed in prevention of maxillary sinus penetration.
Treatment: A tear of the nasal mucosa during implant site preparation do not represent "per se" a contraindication to implant placement, but the tear should be cleaned very carefully and the mucosa sutured to avoid implant contamination. Penetration of an implant in the nasal floor through the mucosa is not permitted.

Floor of the mouth penetration

Causes: Penetration of burs or implants in the floor of the mouth may occur in case of presence of undercuts in the anterior or posterior mandible, typically due to incorrect planning. Penetration in the floor of the mouth can lead to diffuse haemorrhage due to lesions of branches of the mylohyioid or sublingual arteries. Haemorrhage can cause large haematomas of the floor of the mouth which can lead to obstruction of the upper aerodigestive ways.
Prevention: Prevention can be obtained with adequate preoperative evaluation and intraoperatively with identification of undercuts and protection of the soft tissues after a subperiosteal dissection.
Treatment: For control of the haemorrhage, see the previous sections of this chapter.

9.3.3.2 Postoperative complications

Wound oedema

Causes: Postoperative soft tissue swelling of the surgical field is a very frequent event, but great variations may occur in relation to patients' response to trauma, length of the operation, trauma of soft tissues.
Prevention: Obviously, atraumatic and shorter surgery will reduce the entity of oedema. Medications to control postoperative oedema, such as steroids may be prescribed to the patients.
Treatment: No treatment is normally needed: oedema will reach its peak two to three days postoperatively and normally will be resorbed within one week.

Wound dehiscence

Causes: Wound dehiscence is frequently related to incorrect suturing, with tension of the flap or excessive tightening of the sutures.

Prevention: A primary healing of the surgical soft tissue wound is obtained with a tension-free suture on a well-vascularized bony tissue.

Treatment: As a rule, there is no necessity for secondary sutures when bone is not exposed significantly. The wound will close by secondary intention by granulation and epithelialization.

Flap necrosis

Causes: Excessive tightening of the sutures or incorrect flap design with a too narrow pedicle may cause wound margin necrosis.

Prevention: Adequate flap design with sufficiently wide pedicles and absence of tension during suturing the flap are the general rules for prevention.

Treatment: Because of their tendency to infection, the necrotic tissue should be kept under control or wiped off with frequent irrigations with sterile saline and or with small sterile swabs saturated with 3 per cent hydrogen peroxide solution. If the flap margins are completely necrotic they must be removed.

Haemorrhage and haematoma

Causes: Insufficient haemostasis during or at the end of surgery.
Prevention:

- correct haemostasis intraoperatively;
- avoid medications which can interfere with the function of platelets.

Treatment: Postoperative haemorrhages which do not stop after conventional compression may need reopening of the surgical wound, identification of the bleeding vessel and diathermy or ligation of the vessel. Haematomas may represent a favourable pathway for infection. Drainage is indicated normally only in case of large haematomas. Small haematomas and ecchymosis which frequently may occur do not normally need any treatment; because they undergo spontaneous resorption.

Early infection

Causes: It is a rare complication, but it may occur despite strict observance of asepsis.
Prevention: Strict observance of antisepsis, antibiotic coverage.

Treatment: The abscess must be drained immediately by removing some sutures, rinsing with sterile saline or local antibiotic solution and the wound must be kept open with a drainage until resolution of the infection. Oral antibiotics may be indicated, especially in cases with febrile state. If the implant presents signs of mobility, it is likely that the implant have to be removed soon.

Persistent pain

Causes: persistent postoperative pain is frequently connected to unfavourable healing of tissues around implants and it is considered a sign of implant failure. Possible causes are represented by traumatic surgery, excessive heating of bone during implant site preparation, or compression of the implant on the periimplant bone due to excessive discrepancy between implant diameter and implant site.

Prevention: although some cases of persistent pain can follow a surgical procedure performed correctly, the respect of the general rules for implant surgery reduce significantly this problem.

Treatment: treatment is very difficult and may necessitate implant removal.

Neural disturbances

A transient alteration of function of sensitive nerves (such as the inferior alveolar nerve) in the first postoperative hours or days may be accepted as a possible consequence of surgery, due to traction of a nerve branch during surgery or to postoperative oedema which can compress the neural sheath (neuropraxia) (see previous section for details).

Persistent pain and/or paresthesia-disesthesia time after surgery are related to incorrect surgery with consequent anatomical lesion of the nerve and are a sign of failure. Implants may need to be removed, albeit osseointegrated.

Implant mobility (before prosthetic loading)

Causes: loss of osseointegration can follow an incorrect surgical procedure, but it may also occur in correctly treated patients without any identifiable etiologic factors.

Prevention: respect of the overmentioned basic rules for implant placement (primary stability, absence of early loading, etc.)

Treatment: it is very difficult to obtain re-osseointegration of a mobile implant. In this case, implant removal is normally the only possibility of treatment.

9.4 DESIGNING THE PROSTHETIC REHABILITATION IN ORAL IMPLANTOLOGY

The performance of an implant-supported prosthesis depends on two main factors: implant position and the design of prosthetic splinting. In general, the prosthesis should be designed to avoid high stress concentrations in supporting bone, in order to overcome the different biomechanical characteristics of implant supported prosthetic rehabilitation.

The biomechanical differences between natural teeth and oral implants are mainly related to the absence of a periodontal ligament connecting implants to the supporting bone and of the ligament strain receptors, with different mechanical load transfer to the bone. These differences should influence the fixture positioning and the design of the prosthetic rehabilitation.

Particularly, the absence of periodontal load receptors compromises the adaptive correction of the masticatory neuromuscolar pattern in response to modifications of the masticatory load on prosthetic surfaces. These effects are more evident if the implantoprosthetic rehabilitation involves both opposing jaw, with high risk of damage to the prosthetic structure and/or to the bone-to-implant connection.

The mechanical differences between implants and teeth are responsible of the impairment of the biomechanical characteristics of the implantoprosthetic system with the increase of loading forces and concentration of these in restricted areas of the bone support.

The evaluation of the primary reason for loss of the natural teeth may be an effective way of understanding the occlusal condition of a patient. The magnitude of force during mastication and parafunctional activities each has a proportional impact on the implant load; if these forces are greater than normal, the implant will be subjected to a correspondingly higher load. A history of bruxism or the presence of broken teeth related to heavy occlusal forces, therefore, is an indicator of a load factor risk (Brunski, 1988).

9.4.1 Load factors on implant supported rehabilitations

Dynamic and static forces are generated during the functional activities of implant supported rehabilitations. Dynamic forces mainly exert during masticatory activities, while static forces are prevalent during parafunctional habits. Loading forces should be described using their various characteristics of direction, intensity and type, i.e. axial or lateral, and dynamic or static load. An increased static load on an implant supported rehabilitation is considered potentially more dangerous than the dynamic one.

Various factors increasing the force load on an implant fixture can be defined. These often act independently to each other and, therefore, add geometrically to the load level. A proper term for such parameters could be load factors. Two main reasons for load increase have been defined: the geometric load factors, i.e. the number of implants, their position, and the geometry of the prosthesis, and the occlusal load factors, that includes the direction and type of occlusal force components.

The load level defined by these two groups of factors should be weighed against the bone support capacity, including bone anchorage as well as bone-implant interface load capacity, and against the technological risk factors, such as mechanical strength of the components and prosthesis precision.

9.4.2 Prosthetic framework and prosthetic leverage

Masticatory forces arising in prosthetic occlusal surfaces are transferred to the prosthetic connections devices (abutments and/or screws) and then to the implant fixtures. The mechanical characteristics of the prosthetic framework hence influences the load transfer to the underlying structures. The prosthetic design should favour the functional developing of axial forces reducing the lateral bending components. The morphology of masticatory prosthetic surfaces is the main factor influencing the direction of occlusal forces. The reduction of laterally acting forces is obtained reducing the occlusal surface extension and favouring the position of occlusal contacts inside the implant area. An adequate stiffness of the metallic framework is another essential factor for the duration of the osseointegration.

The presence of cantilevers extending the length of the framework outside of the implant supported area is considered a biomechanical worsening factor. Cantilevers seem to have greater impact in the partially edentulous situation than in complete-arch situations. In principle, cantilevers should not be accepted as a routine arrangement on posterior partial prostheses in the same way as for complete-arch restorations. Prosthesis cantilevers are however accepted by most authors and in some cases their use is mandatory for anatomical, functional and/or economical reasons.

The fitting precision between the prosthetic framework and implants is regarded as a determining factor. The absence of a passive adaptation between them induces a continuous mechanical stress between the two structures with uneven loading of the supporting fixtures and augmented risk of loosing or fracturing the connecting screws (Fredrickson and Gress, 1988; Rangert et al., 1989; Young et al., 1998; Waskewicz et al., 1994; Stergaroiu et al., 1998).

9.4.3 Number and position of implants

The number and position of implants define the geometric support capacity for a prosthesis. The same prosthesis with the same occlusal load may exert entirely different stress levels on the implants and the supporting bone, depending on the number of implants and the configuration in which they are placed. A number of factors influence the number of fixture ideally needed. Among them relevant are the bone quality and amount and the type of prosthetic restoration to be supported. The use of a high number of implants has been advocated by different authors, on the claim that occlusal stress would be distributed on an ample surface. However the ideal number of fixtures should be evaluated on the basis of each patients' characteristics considering the most even distribution of load factors along the framework extent.

The advantage of implant placement in an arch configuration is not possible with less than three implants. If one molar and a premolar are to be restored, the maximum number of implants that can be accommodated is three. In the case of two premolars or a single molar, the maximum number is two. Therefore, if the support value is three or less, the number of implants ideally should be equal to the support value. If this is not the situation, a load factor risk is present.

For larger restorations, the placement of three implants is the ideal minimum number. Combined with a curvature following the alveolar arch form, this situation begins to mimic the complete-arch implant prosthesis regarding load distribution and cross-arch stabiliza-tion. Therefore, if the lost support value is four or more, a load factor risk is at hand if the number of implants is fewer than three.

If the implants are placed along a straight line and the prosthesis is subjected to lateral bending, the implants react with bending rather than axial forces, elevating stresses. The bend-ing moment on a three-implant restoration, however, can be reduced 20 per cent to 60 per cent if there is an offset between the implants of two to three mm. Therefore, in-line implant place-ment leads to a load factor risk. The single-implant restoration may bend in any direction, and a two-implant restoration by definition gives an axis of rotation. Both of these situations imply automatic load factor risks (Tan et al., 1993; Rangert et al., 1989).

9.4.4 Connection to teeth

If the implant support desired is not possible because of anatomic limitations, connection between implants and natural teeth may offer a solution. The reasons for and experience with connecting teeth and implants are diverse; long-term clinical studies supporting the feasibil-ity of connection as a general approach are lacking. Two problematic aspects of connection, however, have been documented. First, if a rigid structure (the implants) is connected to a non rigid structure (the teeth), the more mobile of the two may act like a cantilever, resulting in application of an elevated load to the implant. Second, if a non rigid connector is employed, there is a tendency for teeth to intrude, leaving the implant with an unfavourable cantilevered prosthesis. One way of connecting is to place a stress-breaking attachment on the implant side: potential problems of cement breakage and unpredictable attachment function are however present.

9.5. PROGNOSTIC EVALUATION IN ORAL IMPLANTOLOGY

Success rates of endosseous root-shaped titanium implants, both submerged and non-submerged, are very good. Different success criteria have been proposed in the last years.

Success criteria according to Albrektsson et al., 1986, are as follows:

- that an individual, unattached implant is immobile when tested clinically;
- that a radiograph does not demonstrate any evidence of periimplant radiolucency;
- that vertical bone loss be less than 0.2 mm annually, following the implant's first year of service;
- that individual implant performance be characterized by absence of signs and symptoms such as pain, infection, neuropathies, paresthesia or violation of the mandibular canal.

In the context of the above, 90 per cent or more success rate at the end of a five-year observation period has been demonstrated in the mandible and more then 85 per cent in the maxilla has been demonstrated by several clinical investigations.

Success criteria according to van Steenberghe, 1997, are as follows:

- an implant does not cause allergic, toxic or gross infectious reactions either locally or systemically;
- an implant offers anchorage to a functional prosthesis;
- an implant does not show signs of fracture or bending;
- an implant does not show any mobility when individually tested by tapping or rocking with a hand instrument, or when tested with an electronic tapping device, does not reach improper values of rigidity;
- an implant does not show any signs of radiolucency on an intraoral radiograph using a paralleling technique, strictly perpendicular to the implant bone surface;
- in addition to these criteria, to determine success at a certain time point the prognosis of the implant can be determined by means of a surrogate measurement: the marginal bone loss (on intraoral radiographs) and/or attachment loss (probing depth + recession), which should not jeopardize the anchoring function of the implant or cause discomfort to the patient before 20 years (Chaytor et al., 1991).

It is evident that success rate may vary depending on how strict are the criteria an implant has to meet to be considered successful.

Survival rate, which is the percentage of implants still into the mouth despite the fact that it may not be in an acceptable state of health, is useful but are far less significant then success rate.

Fixed implant bone prostheses in full edentulism

The cumulative survival rates for root-shaped titanium inserted in the maxilla five years after the start of prosthetic load range from 85 per cent to 88 per cent (Adell et al., 1981, 1990;

Arvidson et al., 1998; Buser et al., 1997). The cumulative survival rates five years after the start of prosthetic load in the mandible range from 95 per cent to 99 per cent.

Implant supported overdentures in full edentulism

The cumulative survival rates for mandibular implants five years after the start of the prosthetic load range from 94.5 per cent to 99 per cent (Mericske-Stern, 1990; Bruggenkate et al., 1990; Jemt et al., 1996; Chiapasco et al., 1997–2001; Naert et al., 1998).

The cumulative survival rates for maxillary implants five years after the start of prosthetic load range from 77 per cent to 87 per cent (Wedgwood et al., 1992; Jemt and Lekholm 1995; Versteegh et al., 1995).

Fixed implant-borne prostheses in partial edentulism

The cumulative survival rates for mandibular implants five years after the start of prosthetic load range from 92 per cent to 95 per cent (Lekholm et al., 1994; Buser et al., 1997).

The cumulative survival rates for maxillary implants five years after the start of the prosthetic load is 87 per cent (Lekholm et al., 1994; Buser et al., 1997).

Single tooth replacement with implants

The cumulative survival rates for mandibular implants five years after the start of the prosthetic load range from 95.1 per cent to 100 per cent (Henry et al., 1996; Romeo et al., 2002).

The cumulative survival rates for maxillary implants five years after the start of the prosthetic load range from 97 per cent to 100 per cent (Henry et al., 1996; Romeo et al., in press).

Differences in survival rates between mandibular and maxillary implants is probably connected to the worse quality of the alveolar and basal bone in the maxilla.

9.6. CONCLUSIONS

Retrospective and prospective clinical studies show that osseointegrated oral implants are predictable with high survival and success rates.

Nevertheless, some criticisms must be raised. One of the main problems in performing clinical trials in this field is the impossibility to have uniform samples, being the clinical variables countless. Only recently clinical investigations have been limited to specific clinical situations such as one tooth edentulism, partial or full edentulism. Yet, many variables, like the type of the antagonist, the different implant designs and surfaces, the bone quality and the number and position of the implants used in the prosthetic rehabilitation, are impossible to be taken into consideration in human clinical trials.

Moreover, the same type of prosthetic reconstruction behaves differently according to the number of implants, their position and the quality of bone at the implant site.

Finally, we have to remember that many clinical trials are not allowed in humans and animal studies are not directly transferable to clinical field.

These are the main reasons why biomechanical investigations, both numerical and geometrical, must interact deeply with the clinical ones. Clinical and biological data can help biomechanical research to be more addressed and closed to actual clinical problems.

REFERENCES

R. Adell, U. Lekholm, B. Rockler, P.I. Branemark, A 15 years study of osseointegrated implants in the treatment of edentulous jaws, Int. J Oral Surg., Vol. 10, pp. 387–416, 1981.

R. Adell, B. Eriksson, U. Lekholm, P.I. Brånemark, T. Jemt, A long-term follow-up study of osseo-integrated implants in the treatment of totally edentulous jaws, Int. J. Oral Maxillofac. Implants, Vol. 5, pp. 347–359, 1990.

T. Albrektsson, G.A. Zarb, P. Worthington, A.R. Eriksson, The long-term efficacy of current used dental implants: A review and proposed criteria of success, Int. J. Oral Maxillofac. Implants, Vol. 1, pp. 33–40, 1986.

K. Arvidson, H. Bystedt, A. Frykholm, L. von Konow, E. Lothigius, A 3-year clinical study of Astra dental implants in the treatment of edentulous mandibles, Int. J. Oral Maxillofac. Implants, Vol. 7, pp. 321–329, 1992.

P.I. Branemark, U. Breine, R. Adell, B.O. Hansson, J. Lindström, A. Ohlsson, Intraosseous anchorage of dental prostheses, Scand. J. Plast. Reconstr. Surg., Vol. 3, pp. 81, 1969.

U. Breine, P.I. Branemark, Reconstruction of alveolar jaw bone, Scandinavian Journal of Plastic and Reconstructive Surgery, Vol. 14, pp. 23–48, 1990.

J.B. Brunski, Biomechanics of oral implants: Future research direction, J. Dent. Educ., Vol. 52, pp. 775–787, 1988.

D. Buser, K. Dula, H.P. Hirt, R. Schenk, Lateral ridge augmentation using autografts and barrier membranes: A clinical study with 40 partially edentulous patients, Journal of Oral and Maxillofacial Surgery, Vol. 54, pp. 420–432, 1996.

D. Buser, R. Mericske-Stern, J.P. Bernard, A. Behneke, N. Behneke, H.P. Hirt, U.C. Belser, N.P. Lang, Long term evaluation of non-submerged ITI Implants. Part 1: 8-year life table analysis of a prospective multicenter study with 2359 implants, Clin. Oral Implants Res., Vol. 8, pp. 161–172, 1997.

D.V. Chaytor, G.A. Zarb, A. Schmitt, D.W. Lewis, The longitudinal effectiveness of osseointegrated dental implants. The Toronto study: Bone level changes, Int. J. Periodont Rest. Dent., Vol. 11, pp. 1134–1145, 1991.

M. Chiapasco, P. Ronchi, Sinus lift and endosseous implants, Journal Cranio-maxillo-facial Surgery, Vol. 22 suppl. 1, pp. 73–74, 1994.

M. Chiapasco, C. Gatti, E. Rossi, W. Heafliger, T.H. Markwalder, Implant-retained mandibular overdentures with immediate loading. A retrospective multicenter study on 226 consecutive cases, Clin. Oral Implants Res., Vol. 8, pp. 48–57, 1997.

M. Chiapasco, Reconstruction of residual alveolar cleft defects with one-stage mandibular bone grafts and osseointegrated implants, Journal Oral and Maxillofacial Surgery, Vol. 56, pp. 467, 1998.

M. Chiapasco, Implants for patients with maxillofacial defects and following irradiation, Proceedings III European Workshop on Periodontology. Edited by: NL Lang, T. Karring, J. Lindhe, Quintessence Books, Quintessenz Verlags-GmbH, Berlin, pp. 557–607, 1999.

M. Chiapasco, S. Abati, E. Romeo, G. Vogel, Clinical outcome of autogenous bone blocks or guided bone regeneration with e-PTFE membranes for the reconstruction of narrow edentulous ridges, Clinical Oral Implants Research, Vol. 10, pp. 278–288, 1999.

M. Chiapasco, S. Abati, E. Romeo, G. Vogel, Implant-retained mandibular overdentures with Brånemark system MKII implants: A prospective comparative study between delayed and immediate loading, International Journal Oral Maxillofacial Implants, Vol. 16, Issue 4, pp. 537–546, 2001.

M. Chiapasco, E. Romeo, Vertical Distraction osteogenesis of edentulous ridges for improvement of oral implant positioning: A clinical report of preliminary results, International Journal of Oral and Maxillofacial Implants, Vol. 16, pp. 43–51, 2001.

C.D. Dent, J.W. Olson, S.E. Farish, J. Bellome, A.J. Casino, H.F. Morris, S. Ochi, The influence of postoperative antibiotics on success of endosseous implants up to and including stage II surgery: A study of 2641 implants, J. Oral Maxillofac. Surg., Vol. 55, pp. 19–24, 1997.

A.R. Eriksson, T. Albrektsson, Temperature threshold levels for heat-induced bone tissue injury: a vital microscopic study in the rabbit, J. Prosth, Dent, Vol. 50, p. 101, 1983.

E.J. Fredrickson, M.L. Gress, Laboratory procedures for osseointegrated implant prosthesis, Quint. Dent. Tecnol., pp. 15–37, 1988.

G.W. Gynther, P.A. Kondell, L.E. Moberg, A. Heimdal, Dental implants installation without antibiotic prophylaxis, Oral Surg., Oral Med., Oral Pathol. Radiol. Endodont, Vol. 85, pp. 509–511, 1998.

P.J. Henry, W.R. Laney, T. Jemt, D. Harris, P.H. Krogh, G. Popizzi, G.A. Zarb, I. Hermann, Osseointegrated implants for single-tooth replacement: a retrospective 5-year multicenter study, International J. Oral Maxillofac. Implants, Vol. 11, pp. 450–455, 1996.

T. Jemt, J. Chai, J. Harnett, M.R. Heath, J.E. Hutton, R.B. Johns, S. McKenna, D.C. McNamara, D. van Steeneberge, R. Taylor, R.M. Watson, I. Hermann, A 5-year prospective multicenter follow-up report on overdentures supported by osseointegrated implants, Int J Oral Maxillofac Implants, Vol. 11, pp. 291–298, 1996.

T. Jemt, U. Lekholm, Implant treatment in edentulous maxillae: a 5-year follow-up report on patients with different degrees of bone resorption, Int. J. Oral and Maxillofacial Implants, Vol. 10, pp. 303–311, 1995.

K.E. Kahnberg, E. Nyström, L. Bartholdsson, Combined use of bone grafts and Brånemark fixtures in the treatment of severely resorbed maxillae, International Journal of Oral and Maxillofacial Implants, Vol. 4, pp. 297–304, 1989.

E.E. Keller, N.B. Van Roekel, R.P. Desjardins, D.E. Tolman, Prosthetic-surgical reconstruction of severely resorbed maxilla with iliac bone grafting and tissue-integrated prostheses, International Journal of Oral and Maxillofacial Implants, Vol. 2, pp. 155–165, 1987.

P.M. Lambert, H.F. Morris, S. Ochi, The influence of 0.12 per cent chlorhexidine digluconate rinses on the incidence of infectious complications and implants success, J. Oral Maxillofal. Surg., Vol. 55, pp. 25–30, 1997.

N.P. Lang, C.H.F. Hammerle, U. Bragger, B. Lehmann, S.R. Nyman, Guided tissue regeneration in jawbone defects prior to implant placement, Clinical Oral Implant Research, Vol. 5, pp. 92–97, 1994.

W.R. Laney, D.E. Tolman, E.E. Keller, R.P. Desjardins, N.B. van Roekel, P.I. Brånemark, Dental implants: tissue- integrated prosthesis utilizing the osseointegration concept, Mayo Clin. Proc., Vol. 61, pp. 91–97, 1986.

U. Lekholm, G. Zarb, Patient selection and preparation, Tissue integrated prosthesis: osseointegration in clinical dentistry, Eds. P.I Branemark, G. Zarb , T. Albrektsson, Chicago Quintessence Pub. Co. Inc., pp. 199–209, 1985.

U. Lekholm, D. van Steenberghe, I. Herrmann, C. Bolender, T. Folmer, J. Gunne, P. Henry, K. Higuchi, W.R. Laney, Osseointegrated implants in the treatment of partially edentulous jaws: A prospective 5-year multicenter study, Int. J. Oral Maxillofac. Implants, Vol. 9, pp. 627–635, 1994.

R. Merickse-Stern, Clinical evaluation of overdenture restorations supported by ossointegrated titanium implants: a retrospective study, Int. J. Oral Maxillofac. Implants, Vol. 5, pp. 375–383, 1990.

I. Naert, S. Gizani, D. van Steenberghe, Rigidly splinted implants in the resorbed maxilla to retain a hinging overdenture: a series of clinical reports for up to 4 years, J. Prosthet. Dent., Vol. 79, pp. 156–164, 1998.

B. Rangert, T. Jemt, L. Jörneus, Forces and moments on Brånemark implants, Int. J. Oral Maxillof., Vol. 4, pp. 241–247, 1989.

E. Romeo, A. Restelli, A. Felloni, E. Brambilla, L. Francetti, Clorexidina spray nel controllo della colonizzazione batterica periimplantare. Analisi clinica e morfologica al SEM, Dental Cadmos, Vol. 17, pp. 65–74, 1998.

E. Romeo, M. Chiapasco, M. Ghisolfi, G. Vogel, Long-term clinical effectiveness of oral implants in the treatment of partial edentulism. 7-year life table analysis of a prospective study with ITI dental implants used for single-tooth restorations, Clinical Oral Implants Research, Vol. 13, Issue 2, pp. 133–143, 2002.

P. Ronchi, M. Chiapasco, Endosseous implants for prosthetic rehabilitation in bone grafted alveolar clefts, Journal Cranio-Maxillo-Facial Surgery, Vol. 23, pp. 382–386, 1995.

D.R. Scharf, D.P. Tarnow, Success artes of osseointegration for implants placed under sterile versus clean conditions, J. Periodontol., Vol. 64, pp. 954–956, 1993.

A. Schroeder, O.M. Pohler, F. Sutter, Gewebsreaktion auf ein titan-hohlzylinderimplantat mit titan-Spritzschichoberflache, Schweiz Monatsschr Zahnheilkd, Vol. 85, pp. 713, 1976.

R. Stergaroiu, T. Sato, H. Kusakari, O. Miyakawa, Influence of prosthesis material on stress distribution in bone and implant: a 3-dimensional finite element analysis, Int. J. Oral Maxillofac. Implants, Vol. 13, pp. 781–790, 1998.

K.B. Tan, J.E. Rubestein, J.L. Nicholls, R.A. Yuodelis, Three- dimensional analysis of the casting accuracy of one-piece, osseointegrated implant-retained prostheses, Int. J. Prosthodont., Vol. 6, pp. 346–363, 1993.

D. Van Steenberghe, Outcomes and their measurement in clinical trials of endosseous oral implants, Annals Periodontology, Vol. 2, pp. 291–298, 1997.

A.E. Vecksler, G.A. Kayrouz, M.G. Newman, Chlorhexidine reduces salivary bacteria during scaling and root planing, J. Dent. Res., Vol. 69, pp. 240, 1990.

P.A.M. Versteegh, G.J. van Beek, J. Slagter, J.P. Ottervanger, Clinical evaluation of mandibular over-dentures supported by multiple-bar fabrication: a follow-up study of two implant system, Int. J. of Oral Maxillofac. Implants, Vol. 10, pp. 595–603, 1995.

D. Wedgwood, K.J. Jennings, H.A. Critchlow, A.C. Watkinson, J.P. Shepherd, J.M. Frame, W.R.E. Laird, A.A. Quatle, Experience with ITI osseointegrated implants at five centres in the UK, Brit. J. Oral Maxillofac. Surg., Vol. 30, pp. 377–381, 1992.

G.A. Waskewicz, J.S. Ostrowski, V.J. Parks, Photoelastics analysis of stress distribution transmitted from a fixed prosthesis attached to osseointegrated implants, Int. J. Oral Maxillof., Vol. 9, pp. 405–411, 1994.

F.A. Young, K.R. Williams, R. Draughn, R. Strohaver, Design of prosthetic cantilever bridgework supported by osseointegrated implants using the finite element method, Dent. Mater., Vol. 14, pp. 37–43, 1998.

10 Clinical procedures in orthodontics

G Garattini, MC Meazzini

10.1 INTRODUCTION

Orthodontic treatment aims at obtaining the best possible occlusion, a harmonious bone structure, whilst guaranteeing a pleasant aesthetic effect, and safeguarding the neuromuscular and articular function as well as the stability of the results in time. Therefore, orthodontic treatment does not end with the straightening of teeth after wearing a device, but its objective is to control, guide and correct the dento-facial structure during growth, and/or harmonize it at growth termination in the adult, in order to obtain a good occlusal, functional and aesthetic balance (Nanda, 1997; Proffit, 2000).

To reach these objectives the diagnosis, prevention and early treatment of all malocclusions and associated structural alterations (skeletal and muscular) is essential. This can be obtained by means of various types of corrective devices, according to the problem at hand.

Within what can be termed general orthodontic treatment, there are two big therapeutic categories, these are maxillary orthopaedic treatment and pure orthodontic treatment. This subdivision is elementary since in the vast majority of patients both skeletal and dental problems are present in various measures. This applies both to growing subjects and adults; the fundamental therapeutic difference being the impossibility of correcting the maxillary bones, at the end of growth, without undergoing maxillo-facial surgery, that can in fact modify and normalize the majority of bone alterations.

Considering the great variety of clinical cases that can be encountered and their complexity, it is easy to understand just how important an accurate diagnosis is. The second phase foresees the planning of precise, personal treatment for each single patient, bearing in mind the patient's expectations. This means planning all dento-skeletal movements, according to the orthodontic devices selected for each single case, and programming all the biomechanical phases, if necessary, by simulating treatment. Finally, the feasibility of such a therapeutic project should be verified by an accurate analysis of the cost-benefits ratio, as well as the stability in time of the results obtained.

Only with a formula that considers all the variables is it possible to obtain orthodontic treatment with good, stable results, that satisfy both the orthodontist and the patient.

10.1.1 Diagnosis

Diagnosis in orthodontics, as in other medical disciplines, requires the collection of patient information for each single subject, to allow the compilation of a problem list, i.e. problems to be solved (Nanda, 1997).

The diagnosis is based mainly on an interview/questionnaire, an accurate clinical examination and finally analysis of diagnostic records, mainly X-rays.

The interview is not limited to the recording of medical and orthodontic history of the patient and his family, but it also foresees the evaluation of the patient's (or parents') expectations, level of motivation, compliance and collaboration that derive from socio-cultural and behavioral factors. The patient's or parents' expectations derive from the type of motivation, and this in particular must be borne in mind when treating adults, relative to their aesthetic expectations. The evaluation of the level of collaboration is particularly important in growing subjects, who undergo orthodontic treatment mainly decided upon by their parents.

During the interview, the orthodontist must pay careful attention to patient's answers, and attempt to establish a good relationship to gain his/her confidence from the beginning. The time spent may prove an excellent investment to obtain the best and most satisfactory results for each patient.

Through the clinical examination, the facial characteristics must be recorded, paying particular attention to facial proportions, both frontal and sagittal. Usually, facial disproportions are correlated with underlying discordant hard tissue, that will be investigated at a second stage by means of other tests. The clinical examination of the occlusal characteristics allows the evaluation of the type of occlusion and all the irregularities of the teeth in the arch, as well as the matching between teeth of both arches. Functional characteristics connected to oral cavity functions (mastication, swallowing, speech), and above all temporo-mandibular joint function, in terms of mandibular movement and its characteristics, must be recorded with great attention. From an analysis of these clinical static and dynamic aspects, diagnostic records will be later requested. The large variety of diagnostic records available today, does not mean each single patient must undergo every possible exam. The request for further investigation must reflect a real necessity on behalf of the orthodontist to complete his diagnosis. Unfortunately, very often there is an excessive request of further exams, especially radiographic, that are not always indispensable to complete the diagnostic picture. In the vast majority of cases treated daily, the interview and clinical examination, if carried out properly, can supply a diligent orthodontist with a sufficiently complete picture, that generally calls for very few further exams. The better these two diagnostic phases are carried out, the less ulterior exams become necessary. In any case, all considered, the first clinical evaluation to be carried out is most certainly the general condition of the oral cavity of the patient.

It is a well known fact, to the international scientific community that orthodontic treatment can be performed only when the hard and soft tissues of the oral cavity are in perfectly good health. In other words, a patient candidate to orthodontic treatment must not present caries or other periodontal diseases of any sort. In the case of such a disease, the patient must first undergo treatment to solve these problems, then maintain a suitable state of health of the tissues, by means of scrupulous oral hygiene, before starting any orthodontic treatment. Otherwise it is impossible to start any orthodontic treatment due to the serious complications that might arise. Orthodontic therapy is an elective therapy. Pathological situations where emergency treatment may be called for are inexistent in the orthodontic field. There are also systemic diseases where orthodontic treatment is contraindicated. After recording the patient's case history and clinical examination, we are in a position to request, where necessary, further diagnostic tests. Some of these tests are routine to those candidate to orthodontic treatment and represent the minimal diagnostic records for each case. These usually include the panoramic film, eventually associated with appropriate periapical radiographs, casts of the dental arches with a record of the occlusion so that the casts can be articulated, and facial and intraoral photographs. Another essential exam, in the majority of cases, is the lateral cephalogram with relative cephalometric tracing.

Amongst the other possible X-rays are the periapical and bite-wing radiographs, these, only when greater details are required.

If orthodontic treatment for a significant facial asymmetry is required, a frontal, postero-anterior, cephalometric radiograph with cephalometric analysis is indicated.

In growing patients, a hand-wrist radiograph can be used to establish the child's skeletal age more clearly.

Radiographs of the temporo-mandibular joint (TMJ) should be reserved for patients who have symptoms of TMJ dysfunction or anomalies of the condyle that are suspected from the panoramic film. Individualized tomograms of the TMJ should also be taken in patients at risk of condylar resorption prior to orthognathic surgery. Diagnostic capabilities in orthodontics have improved dramatically in parallel with advances in computer technology. Digital cephalometry, both radiographic and sonic, allows practitioners to have access to extensive measurements designed to reveal an individual patient's subtle deviations from average values. The technology to allow three-dimensional analysis of the facial hard and soft characteristics is available in selected cases.

As well as the above mentioned X-rays, there are other exams available that might contribute, in particular cases, to completing the diagnostic picture.

The casts can be mounted on an articulator in cases where it is necessary to record and quantify the presence of a CO-CR discrepancy, or to record the lateral and excursive paths of the mandible. Thorough clinical examination of facial appearance, occlusal relationships and function, however, remain essential components of the diagnostic process.

Accurate diagnosis is a key element in the design of any successful treatment plan. The diagnostic phase must foresee the collection and analysis of all the pathological aspects present, in a scientifically precise and pragmatic way. Only in this way will it be possible to carry out a personal treatment plan that considers all aspects relative to the single patient, that will lead to the treatment proposal that may not completely correct all the problems present, but will prove the best solution for that patient.

10.1.2 Orthodontic treatment planning

Once an accurate diagnosis considering all the aspects described has been made, an orthodontic problem list in priority index should be compiled. This list allows the formulation of the possible therapies to be followed. At this point, in order to choose the best therapy, it is essential to carry out an accurate analysis that takes into consideration costs and risks versus benefits for the patient. This is the most delicate phase which however, acts as a guide for the whole treatment setup.

The benefits the patient gains from the orthodontic treatment should be: occlusal, aesthetic and functional. All the pathological aspects found during diagnosis should be solved, and it would seem simple to deal with them one by one with 'habito matematico', thus resolve them. In actual fact it is more complex and the choice of therapy must take into consideration numerous variables concerning each patient. In other words, a set therapeutic strategy for all patients presenting the same malocclusive characteristics is inexistent, but each patient may represent a case on its own, when deciding on the best procedure to be adopted.

For example, an adult patient may present significant skeletal alterations with malocclusion and facial disproportions, that calls for occlusal, aesthetic and functional correction by means of orthognathic surgery (Proffit and White, 1991). The proposal of surgery must be based on the evaluation of the many parameters not strictly correlated with the malocclusion, but relative to that particular subject, his motivations, expectations, background, etc., and in some cases a different course may be chosen, without surgery or even without any therapy whatsoever. Another example is represented by a growing subject with a serious mandibular deficiency that requires conspicuous mandibular advancement. The aim is clear, but by means of which treatment is it to be reached? Is it better to suggest orthopaedic treatment using long duration functional devices with an unforeseeable outcome, or is it better to program mandibular surgery at the end of growth? In general, the more complex cases are and the more invasive and lengthy the therapy (surgery, tooth extraction, considerable dental movement, significant orthopaedic stimulation, etc.), the more important it is to scrupulously analyze the costs and risks versus the benefits, as well as all the possible alternatives. When the term 'cost evaluation' is used for a treatment, it does not only mean the actual economic cost, though not negligible, but also possible biological costs that might derive as a consequence of that treatment, for example: the need to extract permanent healthy teeth, maxillo-facial surgery, discomfort, duration of therapy, etc. The risks in orthodontic treatment are multiple. The first is the patient interrupting treatment for lack of compliance. This event is particularly worrying when teeth are extracted in view of orthodontic treatment, or in the case of orthodontic pre-surgical preparation. Another risk is failure to reach or maintain the planned therapeutic results due to lack of compliance on behalf of the patient. Lack of collaboration usually refers to oral hygiene, or incorrect use of devices prescribed (headgear, removable devices, elastics, retainers, frequent breaking of fixed appliances due to inappropriate use), as well as missing programmed appointments. Other risks are connected to the onset of periodontal problems, root resorption, or the appearance of temporo-mandibular joint dysfunction symptoms not present or diagnosed before.

In conclusion, to formulate a proper treatment plan one must be competent, flexible and down to earth.

Once the most suitable orthodontic treatment has been chosen for each patient (objectives to be reached, devices to be used, etc.), the biomechanical sequence should be traced, to obtain tooth or skeletal movements with the devices chosen. When assessing the biomechanical phases, it is essential to define movement direction, phase by phase, to avoid contrasting movements back and forth. If this occurs the treatment time is prolonged, or worse still it can lead to bone destruction with irreversible periodontal damage, or root resorption. The type of force to be employed is also a parameter that should be planned. Optimum orthodontic movement is produced by light and continuous forces. The forces are to be neither too great nor too variable over time. It is particularly important that the light forces do not decrease rapidly, decaying away. Obviously, treatment planning, from a biomechanical point of view, must seriously consider the anatomy of each single patient. This is particularly true in the treatment of adults who have reduced periodontal support, although not affected by inflammatory problems. In conclusion, the proper application of biomechanical principles increases treatment efficiency through improved planning and delivery of care. A section on the choice of mechanotherapy can be found further on in the chapter.

The final phase of treatment planning consists of presenting the patient with an operative program and obtaining informed consensus. In presenting this program, the patient must be informed of the problems to be dealt with, therapeutic possibilities and the various alternatives, including that of no treatment at all. Treatment benefits and connected risks must all be explained. Finally, patient collaboration must be illustrated clearly, i.e. oral hygiene and use of devices (headgear, removable appliances, elastics) as well as a cost estimate.

The patient must also be aware of problems concerning relapse, thus of the possible use of permanent retainers to prevent same. At this stage, the patient should be informed of all the diagnostic-therapeutic factors that have led to the proposed treatment plan. He has every right to know all the details and check the type of the treatment he is to receive. The patient must also be informed of all the possible therapeutic alternatives, including, as already stressed, that of not undergoing treatment at all. Possible long-term complications deriving from each alternative should be outlined so the best possible choice can be made.

10.2 COMPONENTS OF ORTHODONTIC APPLIANCES AND THEIR ACTION

The basis of orthodontic treatment lies in the clinical application of biomechanical concepts. Orthodontic treatment applies forces to the teeth and/or skeletal structures through the teeth themselves.

The forces are generated by a variety of orthodontic appliances. An analogy is the use of pharmaceutical agents in medicine. To carry out orthodontic treatment, we use appliances that represent, for analogy in medicine our drugs, specific for the single malocclusion or group of alterations. An accurate diagnosis and treatment plan are the key elements in the design of any successful treatment. The choice of the best appliance for any single patient is a pure consequence of the diagnostic and treatment process.

Obviously, the clinician needs to know every single appliance regarding biomechanical properties and effects on both teeth and skeletal structures.

A typical subdivision can be made between fixed and removable orthodontic devices. These are two big categories of appliances, within which there are several therapeutic devices, all with different functions.

Apart from the obvious differences in construction, the division into these two groups derives from their historical characteristics. Removable devices were historically used mainly in Europe, while fixed devices originate from American research. The clear opposition between these devices has reigned up to recent years, mainly due to habit rather than based on scientific knowledge. When the European and American schools became scientifically closer, in a climate of serious and calm cultural confrontation, the situation modified towards an integration of these devices in daily clinical practice. At present, both fixed and removable devices are used on the basis of the scientific knowledge of their properties and their treatment potential. However, these are not, from a therapeutical point of view, two categories of devices that are equivalent. Each category can supply different solutions. The choice of one or the other, therefore, lies in the knowledge of their possibilities to treat the various types of malocclusions. There are, nonetheless, very few clinical cases that can benefit, indifferently, from one or the other type of device, and the overall treatment of a growing subject may foresee the use of both removable and fixed devices, at alternate or consequent phases. It is thus unthinkable that the patient choose whether to undergo fixed or removable orthodontic treatment according to his liking or desire.

10.2.1 Removable appliances

Removable devices are orthodontic and/or orthopaedic devices that can be inserted and removed from the oral cavity by the patient. In general, they basically consist of acrylic resin, designed according to the problem involved, to which various pieces like arches, clasps, springs or screws can be added or inserted. At present, removable devices are used for tipping, for retention after orthodontic treatment, or to control or correct jaw growth (functional appliances) (Graber and Neumann, 1984).

The most evident advantage offered by removable devices is that they can be taken out of the mouth, which makes them more acceptable to patients, especially at the beginning of treatment. On the other hand, their use must be continuous over the 24 hours and their use only at night is unacceptable.

Another advantage is that they do not interfere with oral hygiene, since they can be removed; teeth and device should be cleaned properly before reinsertion into the oral cavity. Finally, they are easy to manage, since to build them it is sufficient to take a good impression of the dental arches, record the occlusion, where necessary, after which they are made in a laboratory. Operative times for the orthodontist are briefer, both initially and during the sessions dedicated to control and regulation.

At the same time, some disadvantages are also evident. Patient compliance is of primary importance to reach good treatment results. From a biomechanical point of view, these devices only produce tipping movements, as they deliver single forces at the crown level. In other words, they cannot in any way substitute fixed devices, as far as the obtainable biomechanical result is concerned.

In conclusion, removable appliances should be selected when an orthopaedic function is needed, they are useful for retention and rarely for tooth movement. The choice of their use, strictly for orthodontic purposes, that is to say to move teeth, depends on many factors, such as the direction and distance, the number of teeth to be moved, patient compliance, and the general therapeutic program.

Removable appliances are normally made in laboratories, generally using an impression made of irreversible hydrocolloid. When using this type of material, immediate pouring with plaster should be carried out to avoid distorsions. In the case of functional appliances, it is essential to establish an occlusion index or construction bite, to allow all the necessary information to be given to the laboratory so the appliance can be made as desired. This phase can be carried out during the same session for impressions, or at a second stage after asking the laboratory to make a baseplate for recording the construction bite.

In any case, at the latest, the appliance can be given to the patient during a third appointment. Patients must undergo controls on average every three or four weeks, so that any needed modification can be made.

Removable appliances for moving teeth have a main bulk of resin, to which, apart from the active elements, like springs and jackscrews, clasps can be added to increase stability. These clasps may be of various shapes (ball clasp, circumferential clasp, etc.) however, the most widely used takes its name from its inventor: Adams. Labial bows can be inserted into the front section of these appliances to move front teeth lingually or control labial movements that may be generated by same.

As stressed before, from a biomechanical point of view, such devices, also commonly called plates, are only suitable for tipping. Their use, is therefore limited to those cases where one or more teeth are to be tipped. This is the case of movement in the labial direction of one or more teeth, to increase arch diameter or correct a cross bite of one or more teeth. By use of a plate with a section guided through a jackscrew, it is possible to tip teeth. If, on the other hand, the jackscrew is placed in the center of a superior plate, then the activation of the same produces bilateral vestibular movement of the teeth of the upper arch, determining a general expansion of the arch. A great force is generated by the screw, which decays rapidly (intermittent force). In fact, the force is mainly felt as the screws are activated. On average this occurs after a few days. If the patient does not wear the plate correctly (as much as possible over the 24 hours), then it loses stability and dislocates spontaneously. To regain stability means going back with the activation up to when the plate in the mouth is stable, then start activation again. These appliances must be worn as much as possible; if only worn at night they will not guarantee good results in a short time. Removable appliances with the addition of springs can also be used to obtain the repositioning of single teeth. The morphology of the springs varies according to movement required, always bearing in mind that the movement is only a tipping of limited entity. These springs can, contrary to screws, distribute light, constant forces, ideal for dental movement. The entity of the movement is however small and less foreseeable than that obtained with screws. There are also plates that lingually displace anterior teeth of the superior arch, thanks to the use of springs on the labial surface. Removable appliances are widely used as retention devices at the end of active orthodontic treatment. This phase follows active therapy and is an integral part of any orthodontic treatment, especially when using fixed appliances. The type of retention must be planned before starting any type of orthodontic treatment, bearing in mind that the alternatives are: accept relapse or use permanent retention. In any case, retention cannot be abandoned until growth is completed.

There are numerous removable retainers, of which the most commonly used, even today, is the Hawley retainer in its various forms. The concept is always that of stabilizing the position of teeth following active orthodontic treatment. Retaining devices, are also often made with a resin base to which a labial bow and clasps can be attached. Usually the resin does not cover the tooth occlusal surface, but must tightly adhere lingually to prevent undesired movements.

Some devices used in the retaining phase are defined as active (active retainers), since they are able to obtain slight tooth position adjustments. Typical of this are Spring Aligners, which are indicated in cases where there is slight crowding of the lower incisors, occurring at variable times following orthodontic treatment. If stripping is combined to the use of a spring retainer, it is possible to correct such slight malpositioning.

Another indication to the use of removable appliances is that of orthopaedic function. This term means all those therapeutic procedures carried out to control or modify jaw growth. The conditio sine qua non is that the patient be in an active growth phase.

A functional device can vary mandibular posture, holding it open, closed or forward. The pressure reached due to muscle and soft tissue stretching is transmitted to the dento-skeletal structures, the result is tooth movement and possibly growth modification. According to Proffit's classification, functional appliances can be grouped into three major categories: passive tooth-borne, active tooth-borne and tissue borne (Proffit, 2000). Passive tooth-borne appliances have no intrinsic force-generating capacity from springs or screws and depend only on soft tissue stretch and muscular activity to produce treatment effects. Appliances of this type are the Andreasen Activator, the Bionator, the Woodside and the Harvold Activators, the Herbst appliance, removable type, and the Twin-Block.

Active Tooth-borne Appliances are largely modifications of Activator and Bionator designs that include expansion screws or springs to move teeth. For more details regarding screws and springs see previous paragraph.

The Tissue-borne Appliance is the Frankel functional appliance even if it has some contacts with the teeth.

From a biomechanical point of view and for the purpose of this chapter, the category on functional appliances proves less interesting, although they are able to produce tooth movements, especially passive tooth movements, that are not so foreseeable.

10.2.2 Fixed appliances

Fixed appliances consist mainly of brackets and/or bands which have horizontal slots or tubes on the inside of which wires of various materials and sizes are inserted, then ligated by means of metal or elastic ligatures. To this basic system, common to all techniques, springs or elastics can be added (Langlade, 1982; Nanda, 1987; Andrews, 1989; Marcotte, 1990; Graber and Vanarsdall, 1994; Proffit, 2000).

10.2.2.1 Brackets

Actually there is a great variety of brackets available on the market. They differ in construction material, application to teeth, buccal or lingual position, morphology, base size, horizontal slot size, with or without vertical slot, or other structures, and various possibilities of blocking the wires by means of ligatures. It must be borne in mind, despite the type of attachment and therefore the orthodontic technique chosen, that the biomechanical principles are always the same. A good knowledge of the devices is therefore essential in order to biomechanically control tooth movement, no matter the technique proposed. In daily private practice, each orthodontist generally prefers the use of one or two techniques he becomes used to. The choice of one or two techniques originates also from the necessity to contain the costs of materials. Above all, if pre-programmed techniques are chosen, then all the attachments and relative bands would have to have the same pre-programmed characteristics, therefore it would be too costly to consider the simultaneous use of the various techniques available.

Construction material

Generally, brackets are metal (stainless steel alloys, gold, titanium) or aesthetic. The latter have the advantage of being of a color similar to teeth, thus called aesthetic. At present ceramic brackets are used, which only have one advantage compared to metal ones, that is they are aesthetic. These brackets have two objectives, the first is the satisfactory appearance for the patient, the second, they allow the orthodontist to use the same vestibular techniques instead of the lingual, which are more difficult. Clear plastic brackets are obsolete as they do not have sufficient stiffness (unless modified with metal slot) to control tooth movement.

Buccal or lingual application

Fixed orthodontic appliances are more frequently positioned on the labial surface of the teeth. Alternatively, there are techniques that offer the possibility of positioning the brackets in the lingual portion of teeth. The latter have been produced to satisfy the aesthetic needs of patients. Lingual techniques are used more rarely than vestibular, as they prove more difficult to manage, both biomechanically and clinically. Also treatment times are longer and costs are higher. Whereas, the partial lingual application of other supports like cleats and buttons is not unusual, these are useful to control tooth rotation or as a support to inter and intra arch elastics and lingual arch attachments, that are used for two quite different purposes; stabilization of the arch, to reinforce anchorage and tooth movements.

Morphology

Each manufacturer supplies different brackets according to the techniques proposed by various authors. Broadly speaking, the most common techniques used are those of the Edgewise standard, Straight-wire, segmented, and lingual orthodontics.

Some characteristics are common to all brackets, whether buccal or lingual. The bracket is made up of a base that is directly bonded to the tooth or welded to the band as well as a bracket fixed to the base (in some brackets, the two components derive from a single fusion). In the case of direct brackets, the base has a surface that allows the retention of the resin to the base itself, thus increasing the capacity of adhesion of the bracket to the tooth. In the case of brackets for application to the bands, the base is smooth. Above the base, there is a bracket that may have one or two pairs of wings, that allow the ligature of the arch to the bracket (single or twin brackets). The horizontal slot, that can be of various sizes, resulting in a rectangular shape, allows the housing of the wire. The fundamental difference between the brackets lies in their pre-forming. With the Standard Edgewise technique, the brackets have the same angle and thickness, so it is necessary to carry out the in-out bends, the tip bends, and finally the torque bends, in order to reach the correct tooth position in the three space planes. With the other techniques this three dimensional information is already included in the brackets, thus in theory, it is possible to use the arch without bends, hence the term Straight-Wire techniques. In actual fact, it is impossible to totally eliminate the bends, due to the different morphologies teeth present; it is certain however, that bracket pre-planning greatly reduces the need to carry out bends.

Bracket and horizontal slot sizes

Brackets can differ in size: single or twin brackets, as well as in the size of the horizontal slot. The wider the bracket on a tooth, the smaller the inter-bracket distance between adjacent teeth. This decreases the springiness of the archwire and its range of action, but the control of root position mesio-distally, increases. With narrower brackets, a greater inter-bracket distance gives more springiness, even if the rotational and tooth inclination control (due to the smaller counter tip couple created at the bracket) is less effective. The slot size can be 0.022 or 0.018 inch. Although bracket width and slot size interact strongly, the slot size is even more important than the bracket width in determining archwire size and sequence at each stage of treatment.

Vertical slot

In some techniques the bracket has a vertical slot, so a spring can be inserted to give better movement control (for example uprighting springs).

Auxiliary attachments

Some edgewise appliances have headgear tubes, usually positioned on the upper permanent first molars, for the insertion of the inner part of a facebow appliance. The auxiliary Edgewise tubes are used especially in the segmental arch technique and are on bands on the inferior or superior molar bands (see section on bands). Both headgear and auxiliary tubes can be welded to the bands or bonded to the teeth. Auxiliary Labial Hooks are used for the application of interarch elastics and can be on bands of first and second maxillary and mandibular molars. Other hooks can be applied to other teeth, such as canines and premolars (power arms). Lingual arch attachments and lingual cleats and buttons are also available (see above). These can be welded to the bands or bonded directly on the dental surface.

Types of bracket ligatures

The arches can be kept into the brackets by means of stainless steel or elastomeric ligatures. Spring-clip brackets are also available, these foresee wire anchorage, without the use of additional ligatures. The force with which the ligature holds the wire to the brackets, determines frictional resistance, which is the force created by material surface interaction that opposes tooth movement. Spring action of the clip apparently reduces frictional force, enabling teeth to slide more easily. Metal ligatures offer more friction than the elastomeric modules, but both offer more friction than spring-clip brackets. The choice of ligature depends on what is expected of the biomechanical system.

10.2.2.2 Bands

Bands are made up of a metal ring that is cemented to the tooth. Brackets, tubes or other auxiliary attachments are welded to the band, as previously described. Some manufacturers supply bands with single fusion brackets. Preformed bands with a correct anatomic shape for all teeth are available. Although direct bonding of attachments to the tooth surface offers definite advantages, at present, bands are used on both superior and inferior molars, and sometimes on premolar teeth. Vestibular tubes can vary in number from one to three, and in size, to allow the housing of the wires, which in turn, are of different thickness. The tube or tubes can be standard, thus without angles with respect to the bands, or like the brackets they can be pre-planned. In techniques foreseeing pre-planning, the brackets and tubes of the bands usually have the same characteristics and properties.

10.2.2.3 Archwires

Archwires can be made of Stainless Steel (SS), Cobalt-Chromium (CoCr), Nickel-titanium (NiTi), and Beta-Titanium (BetaTi) alloys. The properties of an ideal wire for orthodontic purposes can be described as follows: it should possess high strength, low stiffness and high formability. It should be weldable or solderable and reasonable in cost. Actually, no archwire material meets these requirements. The best results are obtained using specific archwire materials for specific purposes. For each material, the various sizes are available from round to square to rectangular. The choice of alloy and size of wire derives from an accurate assessment, which should bear in mind not only the characteristics of each alloy, but also the size and shape it is made in, as well as bracket sizes in use. The degree of the frictional force depends on the combination of wires with the brackets, relative to the material they are both made of, the reciprocal slot and wire size. Efficiency and reproducibility in orthodontic treatment stay within the modern context of frictional force reduction in archwire/bracket couples. No appliance can be ideal, since no couple exists today whose materials eliminate friction between its opposing load-bearing members. The best that can be done is to minimize frictional forces so the fraction of applied force in moving teeth is higher. The arches can be preformed according to standard archforms found in the population. In any case, in orthodontics, it is always unadvisable to vary the patient's arch shape. The use of preformed arches should be carried out very carefully, as arch adjustment to individual anatomy is nearly always necessary.

10.2.2.4 Elastics and springs

Actually in modern orthodontics, only latex rubber elastics and elastomeric modules are used. With all these materials, the force decays rapidly and in the case of space closure by sliding teeth, it is better to use Nickel-titanium springs that provide nearly constant forces.

10.3 BIOMECHANICS IN ORTHODONTIC CLINICAL PRACTICE

10.3.1 Basic mechanical diagnosis

Orthodontic treatment is a combination of orthodontics (tooth movement) and orthopaedics (relative repositioning of bones), depending on the magnitude, the direction and frequency of applied mechanics.

Orthodontic treatment is based on the principle that if prolonged pressure is applied to a tooth, tooth movement will occur as the bone around the tooth remodels (Proffit, 2000). Biomechanical manipulation of bone is the physiological basis of orthodontics and facial orthopaedics. Orthodontics is bone manipulative therapy (Roberts, 1994). The physiological mediator of orthodontic treatment is the periodontal ligament: the osteogenic bone/tooth interface.

A detailed description of bone physiology and metabolism has not been included as it is not relevant to the aim of this chapter. For further information, see references (Tanne, 1989; Graber and Vanarsdall, 1994; Roberts, 1994; Proffit, 2000).

The tools of an orthodontist are forces and moments to be applied to teeth and facial bony structures. For an appropriate orthodontic diagnosis and treatment planning three are the fundamental premises: a profound knowledge of growth and development is obviously required to allow for a proper treatment timing and for achievable treatment objectives; an understanding of the response of the dental and bony tissues to the application of forces is required; a good grasp of the mechanical principles that guide appliance design, their effects and especially side effects.

Diagnosis is probably the most important step in orthodontic planning. It needs to orderly take into account four main aspects. First of all soft tissues of the patient need to be carefully evaluated. It is not important which type of soft tissue analysis is used by the diagnostician, neither is it fundamental whether he or she utilizes sophisticated computerized tools. It is, though, of the utmost importance to judge the position of the lips, the size of the nose and of the chin and their relationship to the dentition.

A skeletal diagnosis is then carried out. Our main tool in this case remains cephalometry. A lateral and oftentimes a frontal cephalogram, when any type of asymmetry is present, are needed. Again of the utmost importance is the ability to study cephalometry never separating it from clinical appearance. In this regard we suggest the use of natural head position as a reference line, which was demonstrated to be remarkably reproducible (Moorrees and Kean, 1958). Skeletal diagnosis allows for a more accurate assessment of skeletal discrepancies and thereby in growing patients, an approximate growth prediction, and in non growing patients, possible needs for dental compensations or orthognathic surgical needs.

Once these aspects are defined a dental diagnosis is carried out. Dental objectives in treatment need to be listed. Prior to any dental orthodontic treatment planning a careful general dental and periodontal assessment needs to be completed. Periodontal status deeply influences our mechanical plan by radically changing the position of the centre of resistance of a tooth or group of teeth, aside from changing our clinical follow up of the patient. Dental diagnosis uses three main tools. Lateral cephalograms, panoramic radiographs and dental casts. From lateral cephalograms a proper evaluation of lower incisor position is assessed which is, as we will see, a key parameter for the development of a treatment plan. Panoramic radiographs give a reasonably good approximation of root position, which is a fundamental piece of information for a proper mechanical plan. Study models taken in centric relation, if possible mounted casts, give us information about inter-arch relationship, space needed in terms of crowding and curves of Spee (vertical occlusal discrepancy). Bite depth is also well described in study models, but always needs to be integrated by clinical information on the free-space of the patient.

A functional evaluation is needed. Functional criteria might be different in different treatment philosophies and not all functional goals might be met at the end of treatment, though an adequate overjet and overbite and a proper posterior occlusion with no difference between maximum intercuspation and centric relation is usually aimed for. Lip posture and lip strain should also be carefully assessed.

10.3.2 Mechanical treatment planning

Treatment planning has two separate components. First of all the definition of achievable facial and dental treatment objectives. Then the actual mechanical treatment planning is developed.

10.3.2.1 *Visualized treatment objectives*

Initially aesthetic goals are defined, never forgetting the patient's chief complaints and desires. Skeletal objectives are then defined, that is to say, the need for surgical or non surgical treatment, orthopaedic or non orthopaedic treatment phase is decided.

Then the dental objectives are listed. The position of the lower incisors is the basic step. Our diagnostic tools for this purpose, as mentioned, are lateral cephalograms, panoramic radiographs and dental casts. For the definition of the dental objectives we first decide the final position of the lower incisors, vertically, sagittally, and transversally (Figures 10.1 (a), 10.1 (b), 10.2 (a)).

Then the vertical position of the posterior teeth is also chosen, which serves as a treatment guide as to how the curve of Spee is corrected (Figure 10.2 (b)). It is therefore practical to actually draw all of these programmed changes on the lateral tracing (what many authors call VTO, Visualized Treatment Objectives). This will help in subsequently visualizing the mechanical requirements as well.

Sagittal and transverse objectives of the posterior dentition are more easily decided through the use of an occlusogram (Figure 10.3).

An occlusogram, that is to say the tracing of the occlusion, is simply obtained by photocopying the dental casts and tracing the teeth. They allow for a clear calculation of the need for space once the correct incisor position is achieved. It is at this point that a decision is taken on whether there is the need for tooth extractions or stripping. In addition, on the occlusogram it is possible then to define the type of anchorage required. We recall that anchorage is defined as maximum when no posterior mesial movement is allowed. Anchorage requirements are considered medium when up to half of the extraction space may

location of mandibular incisor:
sagittal plane

Φ (MP to LI)

LI to APg

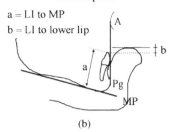

(a)

location of mandibular incisor:
vertical plane

a = LI to MP

b = LI to lower lip

(b)

Figure 10.1 Planning from a lateral cephalogram the desired position of the lower incisors. The angle to the mandibular plane is decided (Φ) and the saggital position of the incisal margin relative to the facial plane (a). Planning of the vertical position of the mandibular incisor, again relative to mandibular plane, but also taking into account lower lip position (b).

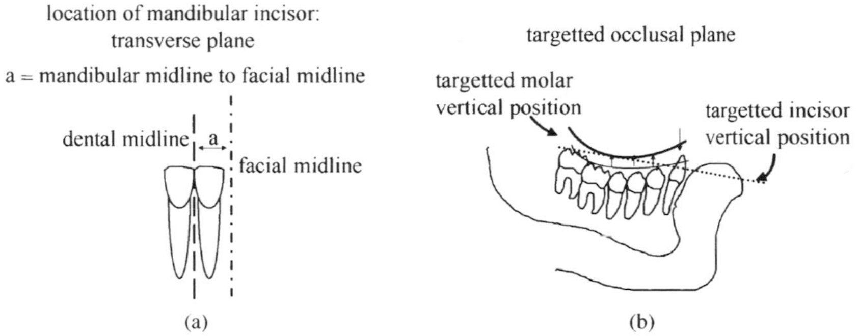

location of mandibular incisor:
transverse plane

a = mandibular midline to facial midline

dental midline ¦→ a ←¦
facial midline

(a)

targetted occlusal plane

targetted molar
vertical position

targetted incisor
vertical position

(b)

Figure 10.2 Planning the desired position of the lower incisors on a transverse plane. Clinical information as to the exact position of the facial midline is fundamental (a). Planning of the vertical position of the mandibular incisor, again relative to mandibular plane, but also taking into account planned position of the mandibular molars and therefore of the targetted occlusal plane (b). This step is fundamental when a curve of Spee is present. Its correction should not be guided by a straight wire, but should be planned ahead, in order not to have unpleasant surprises.

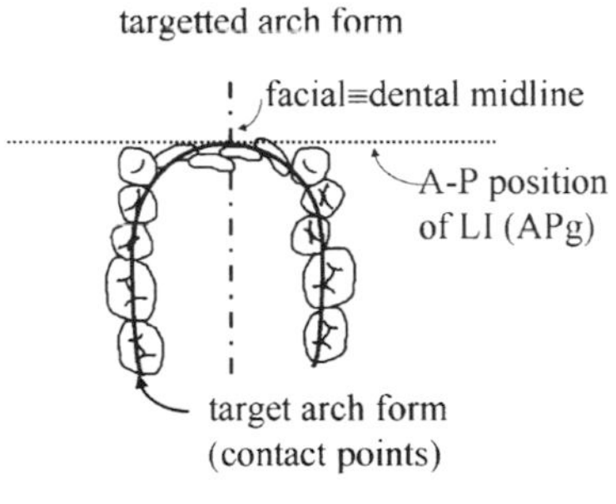

targetted arch form

facial≡dental midline

A-P position
of LI (APg)

target arch form
(contact points)

Figure 10.3 Occlusogram. Tracing of the dental arches. Once the decided position of the lower incisors (transversally and sagittally) is drawn on the tracing, exact measurements of the teeth from the dental casts are reported on the planned arch form. This will allow for an accurate assessment of the space requirements (extractions, stripping, anchorage requirements).

be lost through the mesial movement of the posteriors and minimum when more than half of the space available is desirable to be closed by mesial movement of the posterior teeth.

10.3.2.2 Glossary of orthodontic biomechanics

We will first briefly review some important principles and definitions without which it is impossible to construct a proper mechanical treatment plan.

Center of resistance

A single force applied at the center of resistance produces a translation. In a single tooth it is positioned between the gingival third of the root and the cemento-enamel junction. It is located more apically if there is a loss of bony support and more gingivally in cases of root resorption. In multirooted teeth it is approximately located at the furcation, while for the whole maxillary dental arch it is located at the height of the roots between the two premolars.

Center of rotation

Point around which the actual tooth movement occurs. It depends on the ratio between the applied force and the applied moment.

Equivalent orthodontic force systems

A specific force-moment system can be represented by different combinations of forces and moments. The equivalent force system at the level of the center of resistance can be adopted for determining the type of movement the tooth will be subjected to.

Types of movement (Figure 10.4)

A tooth, a group of teeth or a bony segment, can primarily, as any body, accomplish two types of movements and their combinations: translation and rotation. For clinical purposes these different movements are defined as tipping, controlled or uncontrolled, translation, root movement, intrusion, extrusion, rotation and their various combinations. What defines most accurately the type of movement occurring is the location of the center of rotation around which this movement occurs. Laser holographic studies (Burstone and Pryputniewicz, 1980) and three dimensional finite element method analysis (Tanne, 1988) have shown accurately how the centers of rotation vary with the moment-force ratios. Therefore, by precisely measuring the forces and moments that we apply to a tooth, it is possible to obtain any needed dental or orthopaedic movement.

Uncontrolled tipping

It occurs when a single force is applied to a tooth at the bracket level. The tooth rotates around the center of resistance while moving forward because the equivalent force system at the level of the center of resistance is the force applied plus the moment that this force creates around the center of resistance itself.

This moment is equal to the magnitude of the force multiplied by the distance of the bracket from the center of resistance, which is often by convention considered to be 10 mm.

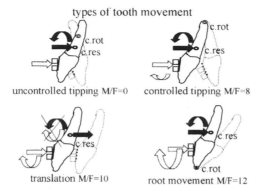

Figure 10.4 Types of tooth movement depend upon the ratio between the applied moment and the applied force, thus the type of movement is defined by the position of the center of rotation. The orthodontist decides where the center of rotation needs to be, not the appliance.

Controlled tipping

It is obtained by adding an anti tip moment which moves the center of rotation down to the root apex.

Translation

This is the type of movement where each point of the tooth or group of teeth moves in the same direction. It is obtained by adding an anti tip moment. More simply, a moment is added at the bracket which is equal and opposite to the moment created by the force applied at the bracket, so that a single force acts at the center of resistance. This type of movement produces a regular stress state in the periodontal ligament, as shown by three-dimensional finite element method applied to stress analysis, less than 30 per cent of that produced by tipping a tooth (Tanne, 1989).

Root movement, or less appropriately torque

It needs a moment-force ratio applied at the bracket capable of moving the center of rotation at the crown level, therefore around 12/1.

10.3.2.3 Mechanical treatment plan

The steps in defining a dental treatment plan require the definition of:

- amount of movement required at the level of the incisors and of the posterior segments.
- direction of movement necessary to achieve a desired goal. Consequently we need to define the center of rotation of the teeth or groups of teeth to be involved, which means, to outline the system of forces and moments to be applied to obtain the correct moment-force ratio which will give us the required center of rotation (= type of movement). Recalling that the two parameters that an orthodontist can influence qualitatively and quantitatively to obtain a planned effect are the forces and the moments applied to the

biologic system (whether one tooth, groups of teeth or bony segments), the different ratio between these two components will give us the desired movement.

Then the diagram of equilibrium needs to be sketched, where we graphically indicate the forces and moments needed to obtain the desired tooth movement, but also the inevitable side effects due to any force system applied. Those side effects may be desirable or may need a further force system to counteract them.

Only after carefully studying the mechanical planning "on paper" is it wise to design the orthodontic appliance.

10.3.3 Appliance configuration

At this point it is clear that, when designing an orthodontic appliance, no matter what the brand of brackets or wires and no matter which technique we have selected in our practice, we have to strive to have at any time a good control of force system we are applying. A good orthodontist should always be able to figure out the forces and moments applied, their side effects, and the methods needed to contrast those side effects. The goal of this chapter, therefore, is not to give any type of clinical recipe to be followed step by step, but simply to analyze the biomechanical properties of many of the tools an orthodontist uses daily, oftentimes forgetting their potential side effects, or believing in miraculous benefits described by the selling companies.

Segmenting arches allows for a simpler evaluation of the force systems, but, as we will see, in many instances techniques utilizing straight wires can be just as valuable, provided that we are aware of most side effects and able to control for them.

We will go through the most common tooth systems, meaning their spatial relationship, and what happens, in terms of side effects when a simple straight wire is placed into the slots. Then the mechanical aspects of a few of the most common auxiliary appliances that can be utilized to avoid side effects or allow for a more efficient result.

10.3.3.1 Two tooth systems

Any time a diagram of equilibrium has to be drawn, for any clinical problem, it is helpful to analyse the geometry of system. The position of teeth or groups of teeth can be more readily understood if schematically visualized as Systems of two teeth (or groups of teeth) and thereafter adding the others. These geometries can be found in many clinical problems or recreated, if they deliver the force system needed, by proper wire bending.

It is obvious that the simpler the system is, the easier it is to calculate the forces and moments applied and their expected side effects.

Charles Burstone (Burstone, 1967), the pioneer in orthodontic biomechanics, has schematized six common two tooth relationships, that he called the "six geometries". Reviewing them rapidly will be very helpful for any practitioner in order to visualize almost any relative position between two teeth or groups of teeth. All of these geometries will apply in different clinical situations, not only in the sagittal plane, but in the transverse and vertical plane as well.

Figure 10.5 (a) shows a common orthodontic situation. Two teeth that have a first order discrepancy, a step with parallel brackets (Burstone geometry 1). What the equilibrium diagram in this geometry tells us is that if we simply insert a straight wire in the two brackets we will obtain an extrusion of the more gingival tooth, an intrusion of the more occlusal one, but also a tipping of both teeth and therefore a tilting of the occlusal plane. The same occurs if we insert a wire with a step in it.

In Figure 10.5 (b) we see yet another common orthodontic situation. Two teeth are tipped reciprocally of the same amount (Burstone geometry six). The equilibrium diagram in this case shows that if we insert a straight wire in the two brackets we will obtain no extrusion or intrusion, but only a tipping of both teeth in opposite directions and therefore an up righting of the two elements or groups of elements. This type of geometry can be recreated easily by bending the wire half way between two teeth, when reciprocal moments are needed without any vertical components. If only mesial root movement and no distal crown movement is desired the two teeth or groups of teeth should be ligated (with metal ligature wires) or the wire should be cinched back both sides.

The ligation creates two medial forces that counteract the lateral forces created at the crown level by the two reciprocal moments. Let us imagine now two teeth or groups of teeth that are tipped towards one another of different degrees (which commonly occurs when a tooth is lost between them) or the situation where one tooth is tipped over the occlusal plane (Burstone geometry four). More specifically in case the two inclinations of the brackets met at around 1/3 of the distance (Figure 10.6 (a)), the equilibrium diagram shows that if we inserted a simple straight wire in the two brackets we would obtain an extrusion of the tipped tooth, an intrusion of the other one, but also an uprighting of the more tipped tooth. The less tipped tooth would feel no moment.

This is a peculiar geometry which can be recreated by putting a Gable bend (Figure 10.6 (b)) between two teeth at 1/3 of the distance. The tooth that is farther from the bend will feel no moment and only an intrusive force, while the other tooth will feel an extrusive force which may be needed or we may wish to counteract, and a large, usually useful tip back moment (see intrusion mechanics). Figure 10.7 (a) shows another peculiar clinical situation. When a tooth is tipped so that its bracket lies on the direction of the bracket of the second

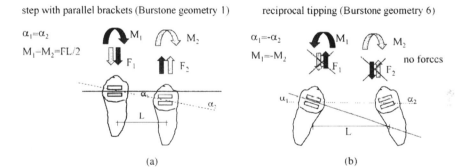

step with parallel brackets (Burstone geometry 1)   reciprocal tipping (Burstone geometry 6)

$\alpha_1 = \alpha_2$

$M_1 - M_2 = FL/2$

M_1 M_2

F_1 F_2

α_1 α_2

L

$\alpha_1 = -\alpha_2$

$M_1 = -M_2$

M_1 M_2

F_1 F_2 no forces

α_1 α_2

L

(a)   (b)

Figure 10.5 Two teeth or groups of teeth with parallel brackets but a vertical step create a specific geometry, where a straight wire inserted will not only reciprocally reduce the step, but in the meantime it will tip the teeth in the direction of the more gingival one or tilt the whole occlusal plane in case of two large segments of teeth (a). The geometry of the system is defined by three parameters, where L is the interbracket distance, α_1 and α_2 are the angles formed by the ideal line connecting the two brackets and the bracket slots inclinations. The black arrows in the figures (these and the subsequent geometries) represent the forces and moments the system feels when the wire is inserted in the slot on the left end brought down to the slot on the right. Vice versa, the white arrows represent what the system feels when the wire is inserted first in the right slot and brought up to height of the bracket on the left. This is very often not a desirable result. Two teeth or groups of teeth with reciprocal equal inclination and no vertical step create another specific geometry, where a straight wire inserted will reciprocally upright the teeth with no vertical side effects (b).

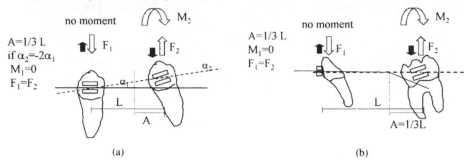

uprighting of an element tipped over the level of the occlusal plane (Burstone geometry 4)

uprighting of an element with a tip back at 1/3 of the distance to the bracket (Burstone geometry 4)

(a)   (b)

Figure 10.6 Two teeth or groups of teeth with brackets positioned so that the their directions meet at 1/3 of the inter-bracket distance. A is the length from the distal bracket to the point where the lines prolonging the two bracket inclinations meet. This creates a specific geometry, where a straight wire inserted will not only correct the vertical discrepancy, but in the meantime it will tip only the most inclined tooth, as no moment is produced on the others, or tilt the whole occlusal plane in case of two large segments of teeth (a). Same geometry reproduced by bending the wire 1/3 of the interbracket distance to obtain a purely intrusive force on the anteriors. The vertical forces are low, enough to intrude single rooted anteriors, but still sufficiently low to be easily counteracted, if extrusion is not desired, in the posterior segment (b).

tooth, if we imagine again placing a straight wire through the brackets we have to know that the effect and side effects of it will be a reciprocal intrusion-extrusion and a very large moment on the tooth that is tipped and a much smaller one in the same direction.

This geometry, and therefore the same force system, can be recreated by placing a tip-back at the bracket (let us suppose the tube of a first molar, Figure 10.7 (b), this will give us a large distal crown tip of the molar, and a small extrusive force (counteracted, even simply by

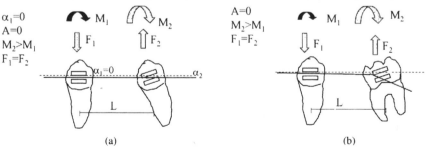

uprighting of an element tipped at the level of the occlusal plane (Burstone geometry 3)

uprighting of an element with a tip back at the bracket (Burstone geometry 3)

(a)   (b)

Figure 10.7 Two teeth or groups of teeth with brackets positioned so that the their directions meet at one of the brackets. This creates a specific geometry, where a straight wire inserted will intrude the least tipped tooth, extrude the other, but in the meantime it will tip both teeth in the same direction, the most inclined one will feel a very large moment (a). Same geometry reproduced by bending the wire in front of one of the two brackets. Useful when distal tipping is desired at the molar and intrusion and some buccal root torque is needed anteriorly (b).

occlusal forces). The other tooth (let us imagine it is a lower incisor) will feel a small lingual crown torque (often desired) and a small intrusive force (all of which can be calculated easily).

The diagram formed by one tooth tipped under the occlusal plane or two teeth tipped in the same direction of different amounts is shown in Figure 10.8 (Burstone geometry 2). The equilibrium diagram in this case shows that if we insert a straight wire in the two brackets we will obtain an extrusion of the more gingival tooth, an intrusion of the more occlusal one, but also a tipping of both teeth. The moments that these teeth will feel can be calculated. It has been calculated that the more inclined one, if its angle to the ideal line uniting the two brackets is the double of the other tooth, will feel a moment in the same direction that is only one 20 per cent higher than the one the less tipped tooth feels. These geometries are obviously useful in all three directions of space while planning the forces and moments that we need to obtain the required movements and especially to be aware of the side effects of our mechanics, whereby designing an appropriate appliance to counteract them.

Again foreseeing on "paper" all of these clinical situations allows for proper calculations prior to the actual banding and bonding, wire selection and auxiliary appliances selection. Orthodontics is really not just a matter of placing a wire into brackets and straightening teeth.

10.3.3.2 Intrusion mechanics

Incisor intrusion is a very important step in many treatment plans. It can be accomplished in many ways and with different timing. It is the tool through which a deep overbite is corrected in patients with a vertical growth pattern. In patients with periodontal problems it can increase gingival attachment and bony support (Melsen, 1988). No matter what appliance is chosen a constant force delivery is required. The magnitudes required per tooth arc of 10–15 grams per tooth for maxillary incisors, 5–10 grams for mandibular incisors, 15–25 grams for canines (Dermault, 1986).

First of all it is important to be aware of the type of intrusion needed (Figure 10.9).

Intrusion with proclination can be obtained applying the forces anterior to the center of resistance of the incisors or of the anterior group of teeth. If pure intrusion is needed with no axial inclination changes, the mechanics needs to be changed, either positioning the point of application of the force more posteriorly (for example lengthening the base arch ligated to the incisors) or adding an equal and opposite moment (not very easy to measure)

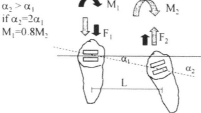

Figure 10.8 Two teeth or groups of teeth with brackets positioned so that the their angle to the occlusal plane (or to the ideal line connecting the brackets) is one double than the other. They both feel an uprighting moment that in the case of the most tipped tooth is only 20 per cent larger than the one felt by the other tooth.

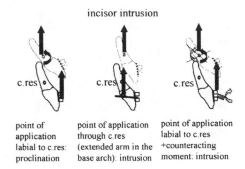

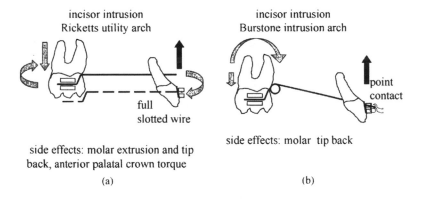

Figure 10.9 An intrusive force on an incisor can produce different types of movements depending on its point of application relative to the center of resistance of the tooth. When the force is applied at the bracket and the tooth has a normal inclination (not retro-clined), the line of action of the force will pass anterior to the center of resistance inducing an additional proclining moment. Extreme care has to be taken, especially in case of periodontal damage, where as seen before, the center of resistance is positioned more apically and icisors are usually pathologically proclined. In order to obtain a purely intrusive force an extension arm has to be bent distally to the teeth to be intruded. Alternatively a counter-tip moment has to be added at the bracket.

in case we were using a full slotted wire (Figure 10.9), such as a Ricketts Utility arch (Figure 10.10 (a)).

Again the importance of visualizing the treatment objectives prior to deciding the mechanics is evident. Figures 10.10 (a) and 10.10 (b) show the effects and side effects of two different common types of intrusion arches. The obvious advantage of the Burstone Intrusion arch (Burstone, 1977) is that using a point contact anteriorly, it acts as a simple

Figure 10.10 Ricketts utility arch (a). The rectangular arch is inserted into the posterior tubes and the anterior brackets. A large tip back moment is felt at the molar, but also a large extrusive force. A large buccal root torque moment is felt at the incisors, and depends on the wire/bracket relationship (careful for root resorption). Burstone intrusion arch (b). The arch is not inserted into the anterior brackets. A large tip back moment is felt at the molar, with a small extrusive force. The single anterior point contact allows for precise calculation of the force delivery and it can be applied at the desired level relative to the position of the center of resistance of the anterior segment.

lever, and forces can be easily measured, while moments can be precisely calculated. Both arches deliver an extrusive force on the molars, which is usually counteracted with either a high pull headgear, a posterior bite plate or naturally by the forces of occlusion in a brachycephalic musculature.

10.3.3.3 Transpalatal bars and lingual arches

These two types of auxiliary arches are extremely useful during treatment both to obtain specific movements, such as molar rotations, but especially to avoid dangerous side effects caused by active wires and springs. As usual schemes are particularly helpful in understanding the mechanics of an appliance. Figure 10.11 shows the diagram of equilibrium of a symmetrically activated transpalatal bar. The same mechanics is valid for lingual arches. We obtain a symmetric rotation of the molars, with no forces applied. This leads us to a very important consideration as it is a very common mistake in clinical practice, explained in Figure 10.12 (a): a trans palatal arch is not an anchorage tool, it cannot provide any distal forces when symmetrically activated. The mesial forces felt by each molar are simply added up and felt by both teeth together as if they were a lage multirooted tooth.

If a rotation is needed only on one side it is fundamental to remember that a mesial force will be produced on the same side and a distal force on the controlateral side

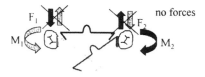

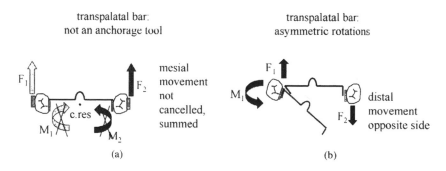

Figure 10.11 Symmetrically activated transpalatal bar. Its insertion creates on each side a unilateral distal force while on each opposite side a mesial force and a moment which tends to rotate the controlateral molar. All the mesio-distal forces on the molars cancel out, and only the two moments on the molars are felt.

Figure 10.12 A transpalatal bar is not an anchorage tool. When mesial forces are applied on the molars it can control for rotational and arch width problems (moments are cancelled), but not for mesial drift (a). A trans palatal arch used asymmetrically can produce a unilateral distal force, but a mesial force is felt on the opposite side together with a moment which tends to readily rotate the controlateral molar (b).

(Figure 10.12 (b)). If unwanted, these forces need to be contrasted by consolidating the whole posterior segment on the opposite side, for example from second premolar to second molar with a stiff rectangular wire.

Differential root torque can also be delivered with a transpalatal arch, but again an extrusive force is created on the opposite side (Figure 10.13), which might be highly undesired in case of long face patients. Extrusion occurs much faster than root torque as it does not imply as much bone resorption and it is therefore a much more dangerous side effect.

10.3.3.4 Headgear

Headgears are one of the most dated and still efficient tools in an orthodontist armamentarium. They can be used for orthodontic or orthopaedic purposes.

In terms of orthopaedics the best action is delivered in the pre adolescent age. The center of resistance of the maxilla is positioned at a point over the roots of the first and second premolar. It can be used to inhibit or redirect growth.

When applied to the posterior teeth as a segment it can steepen or flatten the occlusal plane. Dentally it can tip or translate molars distally.

There are three different types of headgear depending on the position of the strap. A cervical headgear, an occipital headgear and a high pull headgear. The outer bow can be long or short, and can be bent at different heights in order to obtain different type of movements. It is fundamental to be well aware of the effects and side effects of each type.

Figures 10.14 and 10.15 describe clearly the different effect on the molar of a cervical and a high pull headgear utilizing long or short outer bows bent at different heights. It is simple and useful for any practitioner to draw a little scheme and devise the position giving the desired combination.

High pull headgear, delivering forces on the buccal of the teeth tend to expand the molars. In case this were not desired a trans palatal bar should be inserted (Figure 10.16).

Although rarely, headgears can also be used asymmetrically, cutting one arm shorter, which is the one side where less distal movement is needed. The biomechanics of it is shown in Figure 10.17. The longer arm will deliver three times more force than on the side where the outer bow is cut short, but it will also have a palatal component which will tend to create a cross bite (Hershey, 1981).

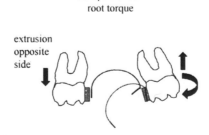

transpalatal bar:
root torque

extrusion
opposite
side

Figure 10.13 A transpalatal bar can be used for transverse problems, for example it can deliver buccal root torque. Side effects in the vertical plane should be carefully considered. A desired buccal root torque on one molar gives an extrusive force on the contralateral molar which occurs much more readily than the root torque. This side effect might be quite dangerous in dolichocephalic patients.

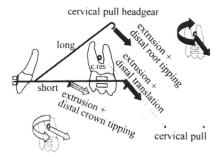

Figure 10.14 Different effects of a headgear with a cervical pull. The line of action of the distalizing force can be varied by bending or cutting the outer bow, whereby varying the vertical extrusive component and by adding a distal crown tip moment (short outer bow or bent low, under the center of resistance of the molar) or a distal root tip moment (long outer bow or bent high, over the center of resistance of the molar).

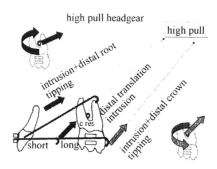

Figure 10.15 Different effects of a headgear with a high pull. The line of action of the distalizing force can be varied by bending or cutting the outer bow, whereby varying the vertical intrusive component and by adding a distal crown tip moment (long outer bow or bent low, under the center of resistance of the molar) or a distal root tip moment (short outer bow or bent high, over the center of resistance of the molar).

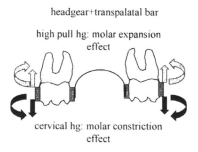

Figure 10.16 Different transverse side effects of a headgear with a cervical pull or a high pull. The extrusive vertical component of a cervical headgear constricts the molars and needs to be counteracted if not desired with a trans palatal arch or expanding the inner bow. The intrusive vertical component of a high pull headgear expands the molars and needs to be counteracted if not desired with a trans palatal arch or constricting the inner bow.

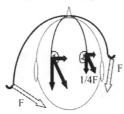

Figure 10.17 Asymmetric headgear: Outer bow cut short on the side where less distal force is needed. Note the palatal force (quite large on the molar to be distalized) could give an undesired cross bite if not carefully controlled for.

10.3.3.5 The mechanics of space closure

When a treatment plan includes tooth extractions a fundamental step is having a proper mechanical design for space closure. As seen in paragraph 5.2 the occlusogram tells us how much of the space needs to be closed by the posterior teeth moving mesially and how much by the anterior group coming distally, which means classifying the anchorage requirements.

Anchorage is partially controlled by consolidating teeth together, but especially by controlling differential moment to force ratio. Another way by which clinicians used to try to control for anchorage was by utilizing canine retraction and then incisor retraction instead of en masse retraction. In reality what seems to be the case is that en masse retraction is simply the addition of single cuspid retraction plus incisor retraction anchorage requirements. Therefore the major significance of single cuspid retraction is related to the fact that it allows to relieve anterior crowding without proclining the incisors.

Space closure can be attained by two main types of orthodontic methods. By sectional non frictional mechanics, or by sliding mechanics, where the main problem lies in the frictional forces created at the wire-bracket interface. Friction is defined as the force that resists movement and it is proportional to the coefficient of friction, which is an index of how rough two materials are between each other. The highest frictional coefficients are created by the relation of any wire with ceramic or by any bracket with Nickel Titanium wires. The least friction is attained by sliding stainless steel wires into stainless steel brackets.

Sliding mechanics can allow for adequate space closure as long as side effects are well controlled and the physical characteristics of the materials used for wires and brackets are well known.

First of all when applying a single force to a bracket to retract a tooth, whether an elastic chain or a closed coil spring the tooth tips and rotates. Bodily movement can be obtained only by applying the force at the center of resistance of the tooth. The closest way to do this is using a power arm gingival to the bracket (Figure 10.18). Alternatively the typical sequence in tooth movement is tipping and subsequently tooth uprighting due to the forces created by the bracket engaging the wire (Figure 10.18). These forces create a countertip moment that induces root uprighting.

Sectional mechanics allows for a more precise control of the moments and forces and therefore for a more accurate anchorage control. As mentioned the best way to control anchorage is by varying the difference between anterior and posterior moments and therefore applying differential moment to force ratios (Figure 10.19) (Burstone, 1982). In order to reduce movement of a group of teeth we have to introduce a high moment-force ratio.

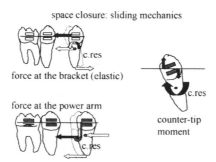

Figure 10.18 Forces applied at the bracket produce a tipping moment. Once the tooth (the bracket) tips enough to engage in the wire a countertip moment is created, (Figure 10.18 on the right, the two contact forces create a couple which gives a counter-tip moment around the center of resistance) but also a frictional force is felt.

A high moment-force ratio (12/1) means root movement and therefore a much slower and more biologically difficult type of movement. To increase moment-force ratio one can obviously either increase the moment applied (larger angle of tip back in the wire) or by decreasing the force applied (applying a headgear or a Nance button if the aim is reducing a mesial force on the posteriors).

Both with sliding mechanics and segmental mechanics one major side effect of anterior retraction is deepening of the anterior overbite. Regarding sectional mechanics the reason is the extrusive force created by the differential moments (in posterior protraction anchorage) as reported in Figure 10.19.

The group of teeth that should more readily move needs a low moment-force ratio (7/1, tipping movement). In case medium anchorage is required equal and opposite moments need to be introduced in the system.

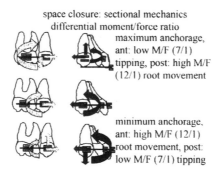

Figure 10.19 Segmental mechanics allows for anchorage control through the use of differential moment to force ratios applied at the different tooth segments. If maximum posterior anchorage is required a large moment is applied so that root movement, which is much slower, is initiated while crown tipping of the anteriors is required through a low moment to force ratio. An intrusive component allows for bite deepening control.

canine retraction

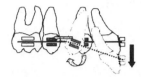

side effects: bite deepening

Figure 10.20 Sliding mechanics has one major side effect during canine retraction, which is anterior bite deepening . The mechanism by which this occurs is evident from this scheme.

molar uprighting: open coil spring

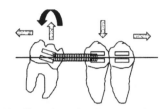

side effects: loss of anchorage, molar
rotation, extrusion and distal movement

Figure 10.21 Side effects of the use of an open coil spring to upright a molar.

In sliding mechanics, as clear from Figure 10.20, the tipping of the cuspid causes a deflection in the wire, thus the importance of a rigid wire with a counteracting tip.

10.3.3.6 Uprighting mechanics

An other very important chapter in orthodontic clinical practice is uprighting mechanics. It is most often utilized in the posterior segments in pre-prosthetic orthodontics to restore molar axial inclination which will eventually become an abutment tooth for a fixed pros- thesis and thus provide an optimal periodontal environment for the molar itself, but the same biomechanical principles apply to any tooth uprighting.

Three types of common approaches are schematized in Figures 10.21, 10.22 (a) and 10.22 (b).

A large number of orthodontists would simply utilize an open coil spring. This method though has a series of side effects such as the extrusion and the mesio-buccal rotation of the molar, as well as a loss of anchorage anteriorly which needs to be contrasted.

Figures 10.22 (a) and 10.22 (b) on the other hand, show two different types of uprighting springs. Both allow the practitioner to accurately measure the forces and therefore better control moment to force ratios in order to produce the desired molar uprighting movement. With the so called root uprighting spring, two equal and opposite moments can be obtained without any extrusive forces. When only mesial root movement of the molar is desired the wire distal to the molar tube needs to be cinched back. Advantages of this approach involve also the precision and ease of activation and a favorable load/deflection rate control (Roberts, 1982).

molar uprighting: uprighting spring   molar uprighting: root uprighting spring

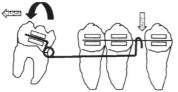 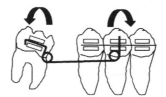

side effects: molar distal movement,   no vertical components, molar crown distal
anterior intrusive force   movement can be avoided with a stop in the

(a)   (b)

Figure 10.22 Uprighting spring (a). The lever arm functions like a Burstone intrusion arch, with an intrusive force on the anterior segment which can be dispersed on a large number of teeth. There is a small extrusive component on the molar that occlusal forces can usually counteract. The distal movement due to the large distal crown tipping moment can be controlled by cinching or ligating the tooth. Better vertical control is obtained using a root uprighting spring, which as in Burstone's geometry six allows for equal and opposite moments with no vertical component (b).

10.4 CONCLUSIONS

In this chapter the clinician will be guided through an orderly method in patient approach. Starting from a clinical inspection, leading to an accuratetreatment plan.

Diagnosis is the most important step in treatment. Both clinical and radiological data are required. These data can be analyzed with the help of treatment planning tools such as the occlusogram and the cephalometric Visualized Treatment Objectives. We have attempted to schematized for the clinical orthodontist, and not only for the researcher, the force systems delivered by the most commonly utilized orthodontic tools.

Modern orthodontics has righteously reached the level of a science thanks to the advances in two main fields. Bone biology, on one hand, and biomechanics on the other hand. An understanding of the biologic response of the dental and bony tissues to the application of forces is required together with a profound knowledge of the mechanical principles that guide appliance design, their effects and especially side effects. Therefore, the goal of this chapter has been mainly to warn the clinician against the numerous, often forgotten, side effects of most of the orthodontic appliances. The clinician should never forget that being aware of the unwanted effects of a therapy allows for a more efficient treatment, both in terms of time and results.

REFERENCES

L.F. Andrews, Straight Wire: The Concept and Appliance, L.A. Wells Co 2025 Chatsworth Boulevard San Diego, CA, 1989.

C.J. Burstone, Deep overbite correction by intrusion, Am J Orthod Jul, Vol. 72, Issue 1, pp. 1–22, 1977.

C.J. Burstone, R.J. Pryputniewicz, Holographic determination of centers of rotation produced by orthodontic forces, Am J Orthod Apr, Vol. 77, Issue 4, pp. 396–409, 1980.

C.J. Burstone, The segmented arch approach to space closure, Am J Orthod Nov, Vol. 82, Issue 5, pp. 361–378, 1982.

I.R. Dermault, Evaluation of intrusive mechanicson macerated human skull using laser reflection technique, Am J Orthod, Vol. 89, Issue 3, pp. 251–263, 1986.

T.M. Graber, B. Neumann, Removable Orthodontic Appliances, second edition W.B. Saunders Company, 1984.

T.M. Graber, R.L. Vanarsdall Jr, Orthodontics Current principles and Techniques, second edition Mosby-Year Book, Inc., 1994.

H.G. Hershey, C.W. Houghton, C.J. Burston, Unilateral face-bows: a theoretical and laboratory analysis, Am J Orthod Mar, Vol. 79, Issue 3, pp. 229–249, 1981.

M. Langlade, Terapia Ortodontia, Scienza e Tecnica Dentistica Edizioni Internazionali s.n.c. Milano, 1982.

M.R. Marcotte, Biomechanics in Orthodontics, B.C. Decker Inc. Mosby-Year Book, Inc. St. Louis, Missouri, USA, 1990.

B. Melsen, New attachment through periodontal treatment and orthodontic intrusion, Am J Orthod Dentofacial Orthop Aug, Vol. 94, Issue 2, pp. 104–116, 1998.

C. Moorrees, M. Kean, Natural head position, Am J Phys Anthropol, 6, pp. 213–234, 1958.

R. Nanda, Biomechanics in Clinical Orthodontics, W.B. Saunders Company, 1997.

W.R. Proffit, R.P. White Jr., Surgical Orthodontic treatment, Mosby-Year Book, Inc., 1991.

W.R. Proffit, Contemporary Orthodontics, third edition Mosby, Inc., 2000.

W.W. Roberts 3rd, F.M. Chacker, C.J. Burstone, A segmental approach to mandibular molar uprighting, Am J Orthod Mar, Vol. 81, Issue 3, pp. 177–184, 1982.

W.E. Roberts, Bone physiology, Metabolism, and Biomechanics in Orthodontic Practice in T.M. Graber, R.L. Vanarsdall Jr., Orthodontics Current principles and Techniques second edition Mosby-Year Book, Inc. pp. 193–234, 1994.

K. Tanne, H.A. Koenig, C.J. Burstone, Moment to force ratios and the center of rotation, Am J Orthod Dentofacial Orthop Nov, Vol. 94, Issue 5, pp. 426–431, 1988.

K. Tanne, H.A. Koenig, C.J. Burstone, M. Sakuda, Effect of moment to force ratios on stress patterns and levels in the PDL, J Osaka Univ Dent Sch Dec, Vol. 29, pp. 9–16, 1989.

11 Numerical approach to dental biomechanics

AN Natali, PG Pavan

11.1 INTRODUCTION

The chapter intends to outline the contribution offered by numerical techniques, in particular by the finite element method for the investigation of biomechanical problems in the dental area. The chapter does not claim to show all the activities developed in this field, rather, to show only the potentiality of the numerical approach. To do this, attention is focused on two specific fields: the numerical analysis of the response of dental implants and the numerical analysis of the response of natural teeth to the application of different types of loading. The research activity developed within classical fields of material mechanics can give bio-engineers and clinicians a powerful tool for investigating the problems pertaining to dental implants and natural tooth response.

The behaviour of endosseus dental implants can be studied by means of numerical techniques, using different approaches aimed at interpreting the functional responses of dental implants in different conditions. This can be considered mainly as a structural problem, where stress and strain states on bone and the stiffness of implant devices and jawbone (Natali and Meroi, 1989; Cowin, 2001) play an essential role, as they do in more traditional structural problems.

The problem of bone-implant interaction regards, in particular, the effects induced by the implant on the surrounding bone tissue under the application of functional loading (Natali, 1999). The evaluation of strain and/or stress in bone can be the basis of an analysis of the efficiency and reliability of the shape or dimension of endosseus implants. This is a crucial aspect in determining the possible risk of implant failure. Numerical analyses can also give important information to develop a more appropriate configuration for multi-implant systems, with regard to the number and placement of the implants. The thickness, shape, and material of implants and the framework for their connection can be considered, by keeping in mind not only fundamental clinical and biological requirements but also their biomechanical function.

The second topic considered in this chapter pertains to the mobility of natural teeth (Ross, 1976; Berkovitz and Moxham, 1995). This involves complex biological structures such as the periodontal ligament. The study of the behaviour of a tooth under loading has usually been treated making use of approximate schemes of the soft tissues, which are suitable only for an initial description of their functional response. At present, refined numerical models of soft tissues can give not only qualitative but also quantitative representations of a tooth and its response to loading. These activities will probably, and hopefully, offer clinicians valid information to help them better understand the problem of tooth mobility under short time loading and the effects of orthodontic forces on natural dentition, i.e. long lasting loads. The results obtained in this field are the first step toward the possibility of studying complex phenomena such as the correlation between the strain state induced in the periodontal ligament by orthodontic appliances and the stimulus to bone remodelling (Yamamoto, 1998).

11.2 INTERACTION BETWEEN IMPLANT AND BONE

To understand the biomechanics of dental implants, it is very important to evaluate the displacement, strain and stress fields induced on bone by an implant under loading, in a wide range of conditions related to each patient-specific situation. The variability of the bone-implant system, as quality of bone, shape of implant, etc. can be taken into account in numerical models, which, for this purpose, represent an effective and versatile tool.

In order to evaluate the system's biomechanical response, the stress acting on the different components of the implant are analysed and the implant effects on the periimplant tissue estimated. This is particularly important for design optimisation for a better configuration of the implant in terms of length or shape. The loading considered is represented by forces directly applied to the single implant or by the forces resulting from the distribution among the different implants through the bridgework in a multi-implant configuration. In both cases the analysis allows an estimation of the mechanical response with regard to the implant and surrounding portion of the jawbone, mostly at the bone-implant interface.

Figures 11.1 and 11.2 show a preliminary view of two typical models adopted for the analysis of threaded and smooth cylindrical implants. The geometrical configuration of numerical models, as far as the anatomical site is concerned, is defined by gathering data from a tomographic survey and elaborating them with specific software. The result is a precise virtual model of the anatomy. Parametric analysis gives important information regarding the mechanical response obtained for different types of implants or for different dimensions of similar shape implants.

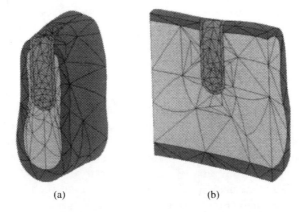

(a)   (b)

Figure 11.1 Three-dimensional model of a portion of jawbone with detail of the site for a smooth implant: transversal (a) and longitudinal (b) sections.

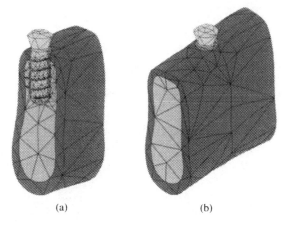

(a)   (b)

Figure 11.2 Three-dimensional model of a threaded implant inserted in a portion of jawbone: transversal (a) and longitudinal (b) sections.

11.2.1 Mechanical characterisation of bone tissue

A relevant problem for developing numerical models of dental implants is the definition of bone properties. Different configurations of the mechanical properties of both cortical and trabecular bone should be considered. The scheme frequently adopted is usually isotropic, but a more realistic representation should involve transversally isotropic or orthotropic schemes (Cowin, 2001).

Since numerical analysis can be used to verify the interaction between an implant and bone under different conditions of the periimplant tissue, the evolutionary trend of the tissue must be taken into account, for example during the healing process, after the implant insertion. Therefore, a variation in the elastic moduli of the periimplant tissue can be adopted to verify the displacement field of the implant and the distribution of strain and stress in the bone to simulate the osseointegration process. During the initial recovery period following implantation, the portion of the bone tissue close to the implant has poor mechanical properties and is usually represented by means of an isotropic scheme. This assumption can be made for both cortical and trabecular bone. The trabecular portion, in particular, is also heavily disturbed by the typical actions of surgical procedure, which create the hole for implant insertion. When bone rearrangement occurs, a thin cortical portion forms around the implant; this portion tends to assume an anisotropic configuration. It is difficult to define the orthotropic properties of this region. The use of micro-tomography techniques to estimate the structural configuration of the bone tissue can give information about this problem. By using a numerical simulation of the process, as later described, the material axes can be defined by evaluating the principal strain directions, starting from the initial situation of isotropic material under the application of the loading corresponding to the functional activity of a patient. The results obtained represent a valid information for a preliminary estimation of the level of deformability and load bearing capacity as a function of the tissue conditions.

It is important to recall the effects induced by the specific characteristics of the surfaces of the implant, given by treatments made on the titanium surface or by coatings, on the osseointegration process. Moreover, valid results have been obtained using specific biochemical treatments, adopting peptide mimicry techniques that determine a better adhesion of the implant to the surrounding tissue and lead to a relevant grow of the tissue.

11.2.2 Implant loading

Loading on implants is related to different functional activities, for example swelling, chewing and occlusal activity. It is difficult to precisely define the forces acting on a single implant or on an implant as part of a multiple system, in which a bar provides mutual connections. In the latter case, the forces acting on a single implant can only be evaluated by taking into account the configuration of the framework and its stiffness. In fact, the superposed structures and loading diffusion through influence the overall response of the system.

The definition of loads is almost always based on experimental tests (Paphangkorakit and Osborn, 1998; Brunski, 1992; Mericske-Stern, 1992). Since *in vivo* results show a wide variability, a suitable range of values should be taken into account in order to estimate the behaviour of the system for a reasonable set of conditions.

The type of analysis to be performed depends on the result to be obtained. If the focus is on the behaviour of the bone-implant system with regard to its strength limit, the maximum values of loading that can act on the implant will be used. On the contrary, if the bone remodelling is the aim of the analysis, the interest will be focused on medium or low values of cyclical loading. This second case is particularly important in the evaluation of the possible loss of marginal bone that can even lead to the failure of the system.

11.2.3 Boundary conditions

In some cases the numerical analyses can be developed with reference to limited portions of an anatomical site, i.e. focusing only on the regions where the single implants or multi-implant configurations have the most significant effects. In order to have reliable numerical simulations, the definition of the actual conditions at the boundaries of the anatomical region plays a key role. For the analysis of a single implant, the definition of the boundary conditions pertains to the evaluation of the effects of the constraint imposed on the end zones of the numerical model. To represent the real mechanical response, the boundary conditions at the ends of the region, of the upper or lower jaw, should be assumed to be elastic constraints. This makes it possible to take into account the deformation of the adjacent portions and, for the entire jawbone, the final constraint of the temporo-mandibular joint. The boundary condition assumptions depend on the accuracy requirements of the specific analysis. This aspect should be considered mostly with regard to the configuration of multiple implant systems, according to a much more complex configuration due to the presence of a framework.

11.3 MECHANICS OF SINGLE IMPLANTS

A preliminary investigation of the interaction between single implants and surrounding bone tissue can be based on the use of axial-symmetric models. The resulting models have a limited applicability since the actual possible loading configurations are very generic while, with the axial symmetrical model, only axial loads acting along the axis of the implant can be considered. The adoption of three-dimensional models seems in any case necessary because of the asymmetry characterising both the morphometry of the anatomical site and the loading configuration. Nonetheless, preliminary analyses carried out using axialsymmetrical models are suitable for verifying the influence of the main parameters governing the biomechanical response and can also give useful indications for specific tasks, such as the optimisation of the screw thread.

Figures 11.3 and 11.4 show a comparison of the different responses of the bone surrounding a threaded cylindrical implant as a function of the cortical thickness around the coronal part of the implant; the intrusive force applied is 200 N. Figure 11.3 presents the displacement field, while in Figure 11.4 the distribution of the maximum principal stress is shown, with particular reference to the bone region in proximity of the implant surface. The comparison among different results shows a distinct effect on the resulting displacement, as well as on the distribution of stress in the coronal region of the bone.

Other parameters of bone tissue can also be taken into account, such as the values of the elastic moduli. The magnitude displacement fields are shown in Figures 11.5 and 11.6 respectively, again for the application of an intrusive force of 200 N on a threaded cylindrical implant, as a function of the Young modulus of the periimplant bone tissue. The transition region is here divided into two parts, one for the cortical bone-implant transition and one for the trabecular bone-implant transition. Two couples of values are proposed for a comparative analysis. The case depicted in Figure 11.5 is related to a Young modulus E_{ic} = 15000 MPa for the transition region between the implant and cortical bone and a Young modulus E_{it} = 1500 MPa for the transition region between the implant and trabecular bone. The case of Figure 11.6 refers to values E_{ic} = 600 MPa and E_{it} = 600 MPa of the Young modulus. The aim of this type of analysis is to highlight the effects of periimplant bone mechanical properties as a result of the healing process that follows the insertion of the implant. The deformability of the bone-implant system can be evaluated in a wide range of conditions identifying which limits are also admitted from a clinical point of view.

Particular attention should be paid to the modelling of the interaction phenomena which occur between the implant and bone. Conditions at the bone-implant interface depend on the

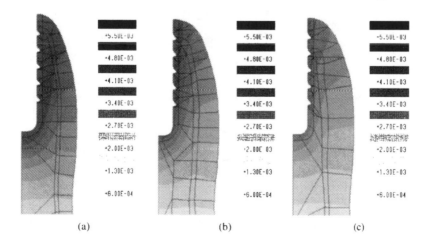

Figure 11.3 Effects of the cortical thickness s_{cb} on displacements induced in the bone region surrounding a threaded implant: magnitude displacement fields for s_{cb} = 1 mm (a) s_{cb} = 1.5 mm (b) and s_{cb} = 2.6 mm (c) due to an intrusive force of 200 N.

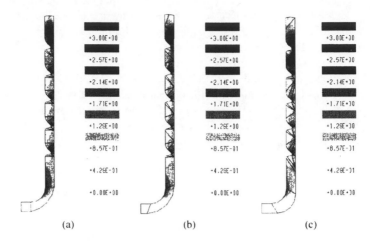

(a)   (b)   (c)

Figure 11.4 Effects of the cortical thickens s_{cb} induced in the periimplant bone tissue of a threaded implant: maximum principal stress for s_{cb} = 1 mm (a) s_{cb} = 1.5 mm (b) and s_{cb} = 2.6 mm (c) due to an intrusive force of 200 N.

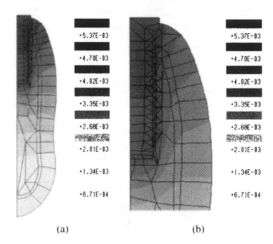

(a)   (b)

Figure 11.5 Effects of the elastic properties of periimplant bone on deformability: magnitude displacement fields on the entire section (a) and detail around the implant (b) for E_{ic} = 15000 MPa and E_{it} = 1500 MPa.

osseo-integration process that leads to the continuity between the implant and bone. In the numerical modelling this condition is simulated by providing continuity between the elements used for the discretisation of the bone-implant interface. On the other hand, a lack of osseo-integration of the implant is described as a detachment between the sets of elements representing implant and bone. The contact surfaces between the implant and bone are represented in the numerical model; they correspond to the areas of non-integration. Friction phenomena can be introduced in order to describe the bone-implant interaction, in different configurations, from total integration to the discontinuity condition at the bone-implant interface. From a numerical point of view, the problem is solved by a contact analysis that implies a non-linear procedure.

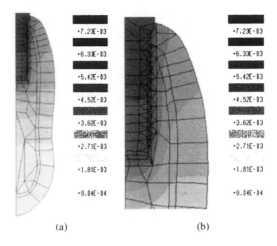

Figure 11.6 Magnitude displacement fields on the entire section (a) and detail around the implant (b) for E_{ic} = 600 MPa and E_{it} = 600 MPa.

The detachment between the implant and bone is always accompanied by a suitable definition of the elastic properties of the bone tissue. In other words, in the case of osseo-integration, good mechanical properties can be estimated for the bone around the implant, while a detachment is usually related to low quality bone tissue. Figures 11.7 to 11.10 offer a preliminary representation of the different behaviour between an integrated implant and the same implant when detachment occurs at the bone-implant interface, assuming a theoretical limit condition of full detachment. The analyses are carried out assuming an intrusive force of 200 N. Figures 11.7 and 11.8 refer to the case of bone-implant integration, showing the effects in terms of magnitude displacements and maximum and minimum principal stresses. The same load is considered in the case of bone-implant

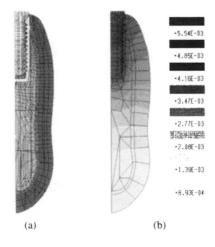

Figure 11.7 Axial-symmetrical model of a threaded implant and portion of a jawbone (a) Magnitude displacement field (b) for the application of a 200 N intrusive force in an osseo-integrated condition.

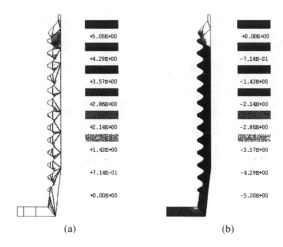

Figure 11.8 Maximum (a) and minimum (b) principal stress fields found in periimplant bone tissue for the application of a 200 N intrusive force in an osseo-integrated condition.

detachment, represented in Figures 11.9 and 11.10. A comparison of the two cases shows the amount of deformability and presence of concentrated stress in the periimplant tissue for the case of bone-implant detachment.

The comparison of different behaviours related to the specific level of integration at the bone-implant interface is proposed for smooth and threaded cylindrical implants by using three-dimensional models. Therefore, it is possible to take more realistic loading conditions into account, e.g. an intrusive force of 200 N and a transversal force of 20 N applied in a lingual-labial direction at the top of the implant.

The loading condition adopted here represents a situation often considered as representative of the actual load acting on single implants because of functional activity. A negligible friction between the implant and bone is considered as a limit condition of their interaction. Numerical

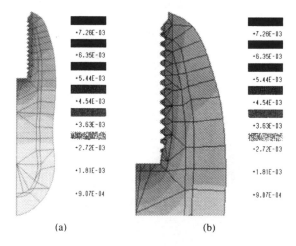

Figure 11.9 Magnitude displacement field (a) in case of bone-implant detachment and detail in the bone region around the implant (b) for the application of an intrusive force of 200 N.

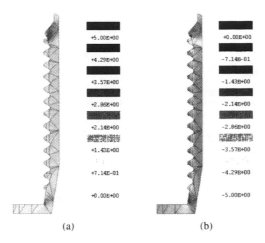

Figure. 11.10 Maximum (a) and minimum (b) principal stress fields found in periimplant bone tissue for the application of a 200 N intrusive load in the case of bone-implant detachment.

results show the significant differences between bone-implant integration and detachment. In fact, in the latter case, there is a localisation of the displacement gradient and a consequent localisation of the stress and strain states on the bone. The difference between the two limit conditions is particularly evident for the case of a smooth implant (Figure 11.11) while the thread acts efficiently to give the implant a larger load bearing capacity with limited localised effects compared to the case of osseo-integration represented in Figure 11.12.

Advanced evaluations of the stress state acting on the bone tissue surrounding an implant can be performed on the basis of a more precise definition of the mechanical characteristics of the tissue, regarding its structural configuration and the consequent anisotropic response. The material axes configuration should be considered as a result of the evolutionary process

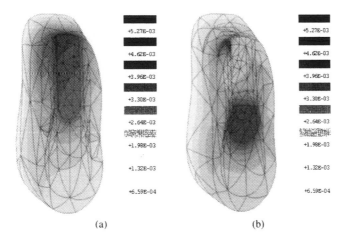

Figure 11.11 Magnitude displacements in the bone region around a smooth implant in integration (a) and detachment (b) conditions, for the application of an intrusive force of 200 N and a transversal force of 20 N.

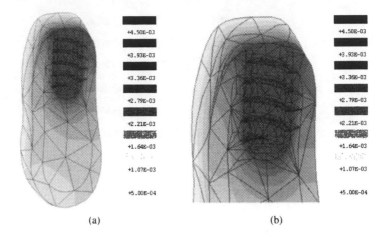

(a)   (b)

Figure 11.12 Magnitude displacement field (a) and detail around the thread of the implant (b) in an osseo-integrated condition, due to an intrusive force of 200 N and a transversal force of 20 N.

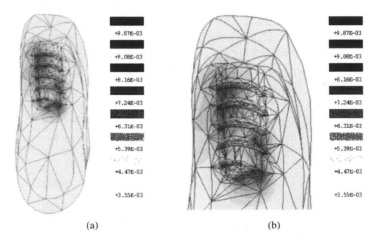

(a)   (b)

Figure 11.13 Magnitude displacement field (a) and detail around the thread of the implant (b) in the case of implant detachment, for the application of an intrusive force of 200 N and a transversal force of 20 N.

induced by the significant effects of the loads acting on the implant and transmitted to the periimplant bone tissue.

Different schemes of adaptive elasticity can be taken into account in order to define material equilibrium configurations (Cowin and Hegedus, 1976; Hart, 2001). A procedure to define the material configuration is to evaluate, step by step, the distribution of the principal stresses and their principal directions depending on the different loading combinations, which are representative of the possible functional activity (Natali et al., 2001a; Natali and Pavan, 2002). Orthotropic schemes are defined assuming that the material axes are oriented according to the principal directions related to the principal stresses with the most significant magnitudes. This leads to a final configuration of the material, which is then used to analyse the deformability of the system and the limit strength with regards to the bone tissue.

To that end, anisotropic yield surfaces are considered as the limit condition of the bone for multi-axial states (see chapter one). Figure 11.14 shows the definition of the material axes in a limited region of the bone around a threaded cylindrical implant. The initial configuration is isotropic, representing the initial state of trabecular bone around the implant. Details of the material axes are shown in Figure 11.14 (b) for the application of an intrusive force, considered as the main part of the forces applied to the implant in a generic loading history. Adaptive elasticity is a reasonable model of the evolutionary process of the bone tissue around the implant; however, it represents an idealised scheme that cannot fully take into account the real situation at the implant-bone interface, where a lot of heterogeneity affects the general and local response of the system. Furthermore, it is not well known how to properly define the elastic parameters and strength limits along the directions of orthotropy as a function of time, since several factors, over the process induced by the loading, can affect the final result. This represents another difficulty in the application of the general approach here presented. Figure 11.15 shows the values of the Tsai-Wu function $f_{TW}(\sigma_{ij})$ (Tsai and Wu, 1971) in the

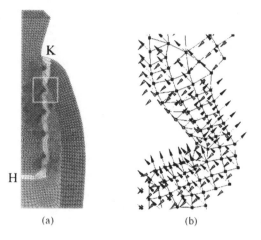

(a)   (b)

Figure 11.14 Axialsymmetrical model (a) and configuration of the material axes defined according to the orientation of the principal directions of the stress in a specific region around the implant (b).

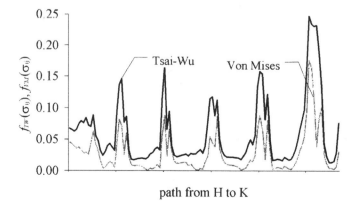

path from H to K

Figure 11.15 Tsai-Wu function value (black line) around the implant for an intrusive force of 200 N. The function is evaluated along the path of figure 11.14 from H to K. The Tsai-Wu function is compared with the Von Mises criterion (grey line).

transition region of the bone around the implant. An intrusive force of 200 N is assumed. The value of the function is a measure of the stress state that is compared to the limit condition of the bone; it represents an indication of the possible risk of failure of the system (Hayes, 1991). The Tsai-Wu function is compared, in the same chart, to another strength criterion, and related function $f_{VM}(\sigma_{ij})$, based on an isotropic configuration of the periimplant tissue, and using the Von Mises stress as representative of the stress state. The failure limit corresponds to the unit value of the different stress functions. The comparison of the two criteria shows how the use of isotropic or anisotropic schemes for the periimplant bone tissue leads to different evaluations of the limit strength in bone, hence to different estimated load bearing capacities of the system. In the specific case here represented, the use of an isotropic strength criterion is less precautionary with respect to the choice of the Tsai-Wu criterion.

11.4 MECHANICS OF MULTIPLE IMPLANT SYSTEMS

The design of multiple implant frameworks is aimed at obtaining suitable structures from the biomechanical, clinical and manufacturing points of view. In particular, with regard to the biomechanical response, the device must be designed according to adequate requirements in terms of shape and stiffness, in order to ensure an adequate response in conjunction with bone tissue.

The possibility to evaluate the behaviour of different implant-bar systems, using numerical methods, represents a useful tool for helping clinical practice find the most reliable solutions. The placement, dimension and number of implants, stiffness of their connection by means of a coupling bar, etc. can be evaluated by considering different conditions of loading or bone properties. Other aspects that can be taken into account are related to the effects induced by defects, such as gaps or mis-fittings between the framework and implants. In fact, to force the coupling of the bar with the implants can induce stress states on the jawbone as well as on the prosthetic structures, which are summed to the stresses related to functional activity. Therefore, the evaluation of these aspects is also the basis for defining the possible precision requirements that clinicians must take into account.

11.4.1 Geometrical configuration

The techniques to define the numerical models are the same as those presented above. The difference with respect to the case of a single implant consists only in a more time-consuming activity since the entire lower and/or upper jaw must be modelled. Again, a precise distinction of the different regions of bone, such as cortical and trabecular portions, is important in order to reach a realistic representation of the anatomical site.

The numerical model in Figures 11.16 and 11.17 represents a partial view of a four-implant system on a lower jawbone. First a virtual solid model is defined on the basis of computer tomography data. The numerical model is then carried out starting from a geometric model, the choice of which depends on the specific analysis to be performed.

The function of the titanium bar connecting the implant is to offer a fixed base to the superposed structure and to distribute loading related to the functional activity of the patient among the implants. In the definition of the numerical model, the boundary conditions should represent the complex structure of the temporal articulation of the jawbone. The system of muscle constraints can be modelled in a suitable way by introducing elastic constraints at the end of the ramus.

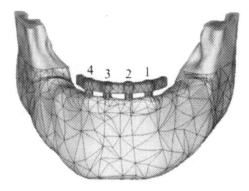

Figure 11.16 Numerical three-dimensional model of a multi-implant system inserted in a human jawbone.

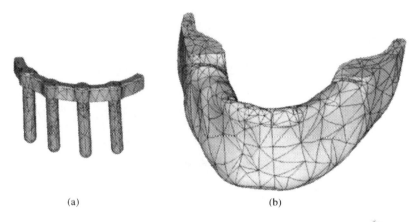

(a)   (b)

Figure 11.17 Numerical three-dimensional model of framework (a) and jawbone (b).

11.4.2 Loading conditions

Loading condition can be represented by vertical and transversal forces acting on the framework. When superposition of effects is possible, i.e. in the case of geometric and material linearity, the linear combination of the basic load conditions is a valid method to explore a wide range of loading with limited computational efforts.

The sequence of Figures from 11.18 to 11.21 proposes the magnitude displacement field in the jawbone corpus, implants and framework pertaining to different loading cases for the osseo-integration of all the implants. Two loading combinations are defined, on the basis of the numeration of figure 11.16.

The first loading case, related to the solution represented in Figure 11.18, is defined by a 100 N intrusive force applied on the top of the second implant and two 50 N intrusive forces acting on the first and third implants. Transversal forces, equal to ten per cent of the intrusive loads, are also applied to the three implants. The second loading case is defined by an intrusive force of 200 N and a transversal force of 20 N, applied at the end of the cantilever on the first implant side. For the second loading case, details of the magnitude displacement fields around the second and third implants are depicted in Figures 11.20 and 11.21, respectively. Results show the effects of the bar in distributing the loads among the different implants. When the morphometry of the jawbone

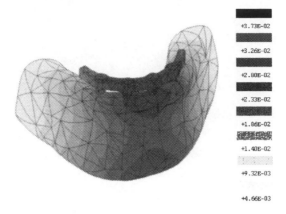

Figure 11.18 Magnitude displacement field for the first loading configuration in the case of osseo-integration of all the implants.

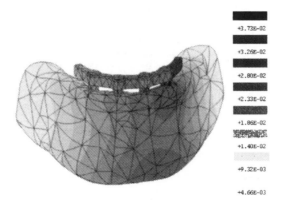

Figure 11.19 Magnitude displacement field for the second loading configuration in the case of osseo-integration of all the implants.

and configuration of the implants are defined, the distribution of the loads depends on the stiffness of the bar: the stiffer the bar, the more relevant is generally the effect of distribution among the implants. The load distribution effect provided by the bar is particularly evident if the analysis is performed with regards to a possible lack of osseo-integration of an implant.

Results regarding the lack of osseo-integration are shown in Figures 11.22 and 11.23. The second loading case is considered for a detachment of the first implant, while the other three implants are assumed as perfectly integrated with the bone tissue. The magnitude displacement field shows greater peak values with respect to the case of the osseo-integration of all the implants. Concentrated effects are found in the bone tissue around the tip of the detached implant.

Numerical analyses of multi-implant systems also give interesting information about the behaviour of the bar, as a function of the implant configuration and loading condition

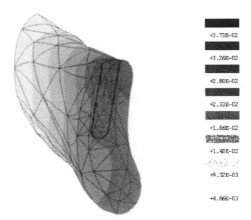

Figure 11.20 Magnitude displacement field for the second loading configuration in the case of osseo-integration of all the implants. Transversal section is performed at the level of the first implant.

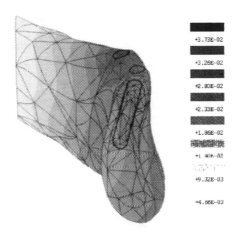

Figure 11.21 Magnitude displacement field for loading configuration 2 in the case of osseo-integration of all the implants. Section at the third implant.

considered. Figure 11.24 shows the magnitude displacement field of the bar for the load applied to the extremity of the cantilever.

The Von Mises stress acting on the bar and implants is depicted in Figure 11.25 for the same loading combination. The maximum stress on the bar is localised at the level of the detached implant, while the other portions of the bar are slightly stressed.

The stress states acting on the bar are evaluated with reference to the mechanical characteristics of the material and can also be directly related to the aspects pertaining to the casting process and its influence on the limit strength or fatigue strength of titanium (Bonollo et al., 2002). An estimation of the parameters necessary for fatigue analyses also depends on the definition of a suitable loading spectrum, i.e. the amplitude and number of stress cycles corresponding to variable loading.

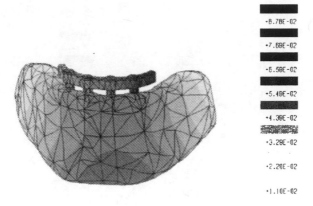

Figure 11.22 Magnitude displacement field for the second loading configuration in the case of detachment of the first implant.

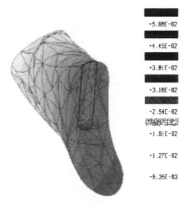

Figure 11.23 Magnitude displacement field for the second loading configuration in the case of detachment of the first implant. Section at the first implant.

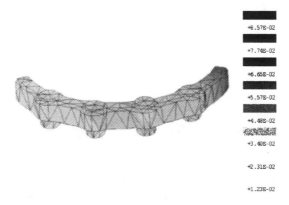

Figure 11.24 Magnitude displacement field on the bar for loading configuration 2, in the case of detachment of the first implant.

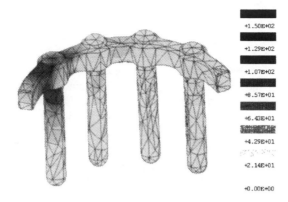

▬	+1.50E+02
▬	+1.29E+02
▬	+1.07E+02
▬	+8.57E+01
▬	+6.43E+01
▬	+4.29E+01
	+2.14E+01
	+0.00E+00

Figure 11.25 Von Mises stress field on the bar and implants for the second loading configuration, in the case of detachment of the first implant.

11.5 THE MOBILITY OF NATURAL DENTITION

Numerical methods, in particular the finite element method, have many possible applications in the study of tooth mobility. Many efforts have been spent on defining models capable of describing the mechanical response of natural dentition under the application of different types of loading. There has been particular focus on understanding the complex phenomena affecting the mobility of teeth in orthodontic treatments (Provatidis and Toutountzakis, 1998). The use of numerical techniques has made it possible to generalise the initial results obtained by means of analytical methods (Nikolai, 1974), e.g. in the definition of the centre of rotation and centre of resistance of a tooth (Provatidis, 2000). In particular, the ability to account for non-linear material behaviour and accurately define the actual geometry of the system is the key factor in properly simulating the response of a tooth, which greatly depends on the mechanical behaviour of the periodontal ligament. The mechanism of the tooth support offered by the periodontium can be better understood by comparing different functional schemes of this connective tissue (Berkovitz and Moxham, 1995). It is important to formulate some hypotheses about a suitable relationship between the level of strain in the periodontal ligament and the subsequent cellular activity. These phenomena lead to the appearance of a remodelling of the alveolar bone; this then leads to the movement of a tooth during orthodontic treatment (Sato et al., 1998). Numerical methods can also be used to simulate the movement of a tooth, due to the effects of an orthodontic appliance (Bourael et al., 1999; Soncini and Pietrabissa, 2001). This is a reliable tool to help the clinicians who operate in this field carry out pre-operational planning and predict the orthodontic treatment needed.

It is not superfluous to underline how the use of numerical techniques strongly depends on the need to provide for a lot of experimental activity, aimed at setting up of models that require the definition of several parameters. In the following paragraphs, attention is mainly focused on the modelling of the periodontal ligament, since this is the key topic of advanced numerical activity in the field of tooth mobility.

11.5.1 Geometric configuration of the periodontium

The general notes presented in the previous sections, with regard to the definition of numerical models in implantology, can be extended to the problem of the definition of natural tooth geometry. The morphometry of the tooth and periodontium (Figure 11.26) is extremely variable from patient to patient and largely affects the mechanical response of the system. It is therefore clear that a numerical model must be related to a very specific anatomical site. Nonetheless, the results and information taken from the analysis of a specific model can be appropriately used to identify the general principles that govern the behaviour of the phenomena under investigation. The definition of the correct geometry of the model is even more complicated than in the problem of bone-implant modelling, because of the presence of soft tissues.

Whether or not the alveolar bone region surrounding the tooth is to be included in the finite element model strictly depends on the specific aim of the analysis at hand. In the simulation of the movement of dentition in orthodontic treatments, the presence of the alveolar bone, and its evolution in time, must be considered. On the other hand, if the analysis regards short-term loads, the model can include only the tooth and the periodontal ligament. In fact, in the latter case, the strain in the periodontal ligament and the deformability of the whole system can be considered independent from the deformation of the alveolar bone. Furthermore, the periodontal ligament can be bound on its external surface, apart from the apical and coronal portions.

11.5.2 Loading configurations

A basic distinction must be made with regards to the loading induced on teeth, taking into account chewing or orthodontic forces. The former are forces limited in time and characterised by significant intensity, while the latter are related to long lasting loads of low intensity. These two different configurations of loading lead to very specific formulations of the model, because of the different processes of the biological tissues involved. In fact, while functional loading involves only the deformation of the periodontal ligament, orthodontic loads, and any other long-term load, stimulate cellular activity within the periodontal ligament and a consequent remodelling of the alveolar bone.

It is not easy to define the loads acting on a tooth during chewing since there is a sensitive variability regarding their magnitude, direction and region of application. Specific experimental

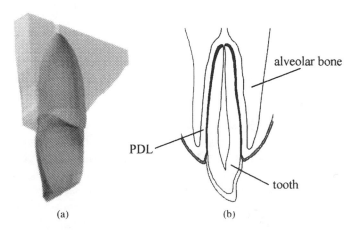

(a)   (b)

Figure 11.26 Geometric model of the anatomical site (a) and indication of the main constituents (b).

activity in this field has been carried out (Parfitt, 1960; Pincton et al., 1978; Korioth et al., 1997), in spite of the objective difficulty in providing for a suitable measurement system.

Orthodontic loads are better defined in magnitude, direction and region of application, since they are the result of a specifically planned treatment. Since the mechanics of the orthodontic appliance are known, for example superelastic alloy wires, it is easier to precisely define the loads in this case than it is in the case of the loading related to functional activity.

11.5.3 Constitutive models

The definition of a constitutive model for the different regions of the tooth, as dentin, enamel, etc., is a relatively simple problem, since the materials can be considered as linear elastic and isotropic. Anisotropic properties have also been considered for the enamel (Rees and Jacobsen, 1997). However, it is clear that the mechanical response of the periodontium to the loading transmitted by a tooth is tremendously dependent on the behaviour of the periodontal ligament and, sometimes, the surrounding portion of the alveolar bone. The components of the tooth are much stiffer than the periodontal ligament. The need to include the alveolar bone in the model is justified if the loading application time induces a remodelling process; this is a typical situation in orthodontic treatments (Morikawa et al., 1998). Even though the remodelling of alveolar bone is beyond the aims of this analysis, the model can either include the alveolar bone, considered as linear elastic material, or be limited only to the tooth and periodontal ligament. This is justified by the fact that the elastic modulus of the alveolar bone is largely greater than the elastic modulus of the periodontal ligament.

Many details on the constitutive models for the periodontal ligament and on the relative mathematical frameworks are given in chapter two. Here the problem is mentioned in order to point out the relationship between the type of analysis and the constitutive model adopted. The choice of an appropriate constitutive model for the periodontal ligament is essential to making the model reliable. Numerical simulations have often been based on the strong simplification of the constitutive models of the periodontal ligament. This is also due to difficulties in getting data from experimental tests, as well as in formulating the numerical problem.

Many contributions have been made in the field of numerical simulation of tooth mobility with regard to the immediate or long term response for the application of orthodontic forces (Middleton et al., 1990; Andersen et al., 1991).

The usual approach to the modelling of the periodontal ligament tends to consider a linear elastic model, with a Young modulus varying in a wide range as a function of the rate of loading considered. More refined constitutive models of the periodontal ligament have been considered in order to try to simulate its mechanical behaviour in a more general way, i.e. under a wide range of conditions (Pini, 1999; Natali et al., 2000).

There are significant difficulties in defining numerical models from both the theoretical and operational points of view because of the need to include the ground substance, which is reinforced by highly oriented collagen fibres. This leads to an anisotropic behaviour. In addition, the wavy configuration of collagen fibres implies a null stiffness in compression and a non-linear behaviour for evaluation of tensile states. An appropriate constitutive model can be defined as shown in chapter two, separating the influence of the ground matrix, which is isotropic, from the effect of the fibres as a function of their spatial disposition. It is useful to point out that, because of the above-mentioned wavy initial disposition of collagen fibres, the anisotropy of the tissue is more significant for large values of the strain. It is reasonable to maintain that isotropic models are able to simulate the response of the tissue if the strains attained by the periodontal ligament are limited.

The periodontal ligament, as many other soft tissues, shows a visco-elastic behaviour, which can be significant depending on the type of loading (Dorow et al., 2001; Krstin et al., 2001). A suitable model to describe the periodontal ligament in these conditions can be made by coupling hyperelastic constitutive models with viscosity models. This approach does not take into account the actual micro-structure of the periodontal ligament; it uses viscosity as a macro modelling of the complex behaviour related to the presence and movement of the liquid content in the tissue. In spite of a limited micro-structural consistency, this approach can give interesting results, as shown below. A numerical model with more micro-mechanical coherence can be achieved using a porous media approach (van Driel et al., 1998; Natali et al., 2001b) as an extension of consolidated multi-phase approaches used in the numerical simulation of other soft tissues (Mow et al., 1980; Spilker et al., 1992; Meroi et al., 1999). The simulation of the periodontal ligament as a porous media with the presence of liquid phases can give a more precise description of the strain evolution in time and a better explanation of the differences found for compressive and tensile states.

The actual behaviour of this connective tissue should probably be properly represented by coupling multi-phase material and the visco-elastic behaviour of the solid matrix, in order to capture the viscous response of the latter, which can be caused by, for example, the relative movement of the collagen fibres. This approach could be more suitable to account for all the conditions in which the relative velocity of the different phases is low (Miller, 1998).

The structure of the periodontal ligament is very difficult to represent using a numerical model and more efforts will certainly be needed to reach a complete definition of the problem. The complexity of the fitting of all the parameters defining non-linear constitutive models and the difficulty of the experimental testing are the main problems to be overcome in order to achieve reliable results.

11.5.4 Numerical analysis of *in vivo* response

The numerical results presented in this section pertain to the model shown in Figure 11.27. A thin layer representing the periodontal ligament, having mean thickness of 0.2 mm, surrounds an upper incisor with a total length of about 30 mm and a radicular length of about 17 mm. This model can be adopted to show the outcomes of different approaches in

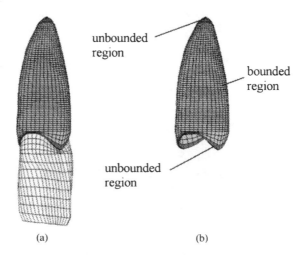

(a)   (b)

Figure 11.27 Finite element model adopted (a) and details of the periodontal ligament (b).

the simulations of the response of a tooth under the application of different types of loading. In all the cases presented, the alveolar bone is not modelled and the nodes belonging to the external surface of the periodontal ligament are bound. This last factor is related to the short-term loading considered; therefore, the bone has no appreciable influence on the global deformation of the system, as was explained in the previous section.

11.5.4.1 Non-linear elastic response

The example reported on non-linear numerical analysis refers to the well known experimental tests carried out by Parfitt, (Parfitt, 1960). The tests consisted in the application of a vertical intrusive force, with a maximum magnitude of 0.03 N, on the upper incisor of human adults (Figure 11.28) and in the evaluation of the corresponding vertical displacement.

Parfitt's experimental data, represented by open circles in the chart in Figure 11.29, show a strongly non-linear behaviour, with a very low initial stiffness and a hardening response, as the force increases. It is reasonable to attribute this response to a non-linear mechanical

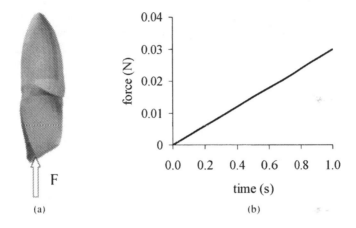

(a)   (b)

Figure 11.28 Application of the intrusive force (a) and loading history (b) according to the experimental procedure of Parfitt.

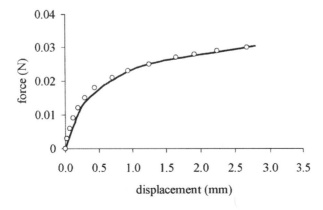

Figure 11.29 Comparison of experimental data from Parfitt's experiments and numerical results. Open circles represent experimental data, while a continuous line is adopted to represent numerical results.

response of the periodontal ligament. In this regard, the adoption of a linear elastic constitutive model gives unsatisfactory results and can describe, at most, the response of the system for a specific magnitude of the load by choosing a suitable value of the elastic modulus. The numerical analysis is performed here by choosing an isotropic, compressible, hyperelastic constitutive model. An intrusive force with a maximum magnitude of 0.03 N is applied to the tooth. Figure 11.29 shows a comparison of the experimental data and the numerical results of this analysis, reported by a continuous line. The vertical displacement of the load application point versus the vertical force is very close to the experimental values, showing the suitability of the model used here.

Parametric analyses can be performed in order to evaluate the influence of the periodontal ligament's bulk and shear modulus on the response of the system. Even though a definite answer to the problem cannot be given, it is nonetheless clear that a finite value of the bulk modulus should be adopted.

In the past, the periodontal ligament was generally considered to be incompressible or almost-incompressible, according to the general schemes proposed for other soft biological tissues, while in this analysis a compressible form was chosen. At present, both *in vitro* analyses and the comparison of numerical results with *in vivo* tests (Pini, 1999; Natali et al., 2000) show that the periodontal ligament has an appreciable volumetric deformability. This conclusion is also consistent with intuitive schemes of the possible deformational behaviour of the system.

11.5.4.2 *Time-dependent behaviour*

When a load, even of low magnitude, is applied to a tooth, the mechanical response of the system shows a time-dependent behaviour, with a deformation that can increase over time with the application of constant loads. In addition, the apparent stiffness of the periodontal ligament clearly depends on the rate of the applied load. These facts limit the possibility of applying simple elastic schemes for the simulation of the periodontal ligament and show the need for models capable of describing the mechanical response of the tissue over time. In this section, reference is made to the experimental activity of Ross et al. (1976), who applied transversal forces on the upper incisors of different patients, monitoring the mobility of the teeth over time. Low magnitude forces with a square-wave shape, as shown in Figure 11.30, were applied in the labial-lingual direction. The maximum value of the forces was in the range of 0.05 N to

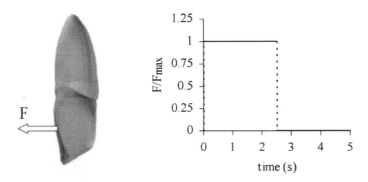

Figure 11.30 Horizontal force on the upper incisor and loading history according to the experimental tests of Ross et al..

0.1 N. The loading time was limited to the first 2.5 s of the loading history. A typical response of the system is shown in Figure 11.31, where the transversal displacement of the load application point is plotted versus time. The chart shows the case of a loading history with a maximum force of 0.05 N, reporting numerical results by the continuos curve.

The sudden application of the load at time zero induces an elastic response, followed by an increase in displacement over time, moving towards an asymptotic value. The rapid unloading at 2.5 s causes an initial elastic recovery of the deformation, with a subsequent asymptotic tendency back to the unloaded configuration.

Figure 11.32 shows the results obtained from a numerical simulation of the movement of the incisor for the application of the load in Figure 11.30, with a maximum magnitude of 0.1 N, if a visco-elastic model (see chapter 12) is adopted for the periodontal ligament. It can be noted that the numerical curve fits the experimental curve very well.

The time-dependent behaviour is described using an alternative approach, by adopting a bi-phase and fully saturated model (see chapter 12) for the periodontal ligament.

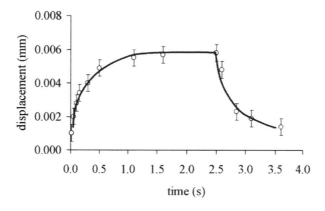

Figure 11.31 Typical time-dependent response of the tooth from the experimental results of Ross et al. The transversal displacement of the point of application of a 0.05 N force is plotted versus time.

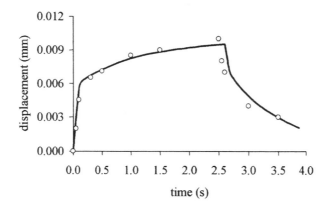

Figure 11.32 Visco-elastic model: horizontal displacement vs. time for the application of a 0.1 N transversal force. Open circles represent experimental data, while a continuous line is adopted to represent numerical results.

In particular, the constitutive model is defined using a non-linear elastic constitutive model for the solid matrix and a constant value for the permeability, which was set at 100 m²/s. A porosity of 0.7 was chosen on the basis of the estimated liquid content in the periodontal ligament (Berkovitz and Moxham, 1995). The results for the application of a loading history with a maximum force of 0.0.5 N can be seen in Figures 11.33 to 11.35. The transversal displacement of the load application point versus time is depicted in Figure 11.33, showing excellent agreement with experimental data. The magnitude and transversal displacement fields are described in Figure 11.34, where the centre of rotation of the tooth can also be located. The variation of the overpressure within a point of the PDL region compressed in the loading phase, is finally shown in Figure 11.35.

The use of numerical models is extremely interesting if additional information is needed to identify the mechanical properties of a biological tissue, especially when experimental activity appears difficult. The possibility of proposing different assumptions about the

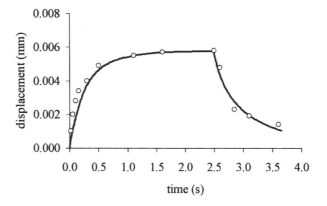

Figure 11.33 Bi-phase constitutive model: displacement vs. time for the application of a 0.0.5 N transversal force. Open circles represent experimental data, while a continuous line is adopted to represent numerical results.

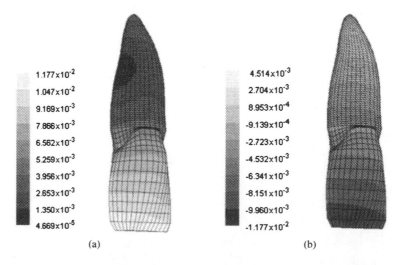

Figure 11.34 Bi-phase constitutive model: magnitude (a) and transversal (b) displacement fields at the end of the loading phase for the application of 0.05 N transversal force.

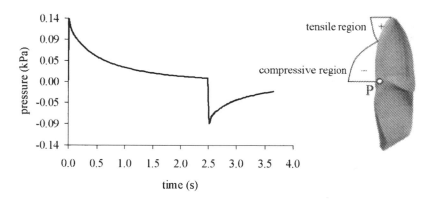

Figure 11.35 Bi-phase constitutive model: magnitude displacement in the PDL a) and contour of volumetric strain b) at the end of the loading phase.

behaviour of the tissue can help guide the experimental tests, showing the more or less significant effect of different parameters on the behaviour of the system.

For example, the chart in Figure 11.36 shows the results obtained from the numerical simulation of the experimental tests of Ross et al., adopting a bi-phase constitutive model of the periodontal ligament with a linear elastic solid matrix and constant permeability. A parametric analysis was developed considering different values of permeability, in order to fit the experimental data as well as possible. The chart shows that a linear model is not capable of correctly describing the entire phenomenon, neither in the loading phase nor in the unloading phase. This fact leads one to think that the hypothesis of linearity should be excluded, as has also been confirmed by the numerical results shown above.

11.5.5 Pseudo-elasticity

Another typical behaviour of the periodontal ligament, emerging from *in vitro* experimental tests is defined as pseudo-elasticity and can be represented and simulated by using damage

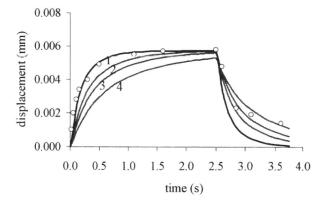

Figure 11.36 Bi-phase constitutive model with linear elastic solid matrix: displacement vs. time for the application of a 0.05 N transversal force plotted for different values of permeability: k = 55 m²/s (curve 1), k = 80 m²/s (curve 2), k = 110 m²/s (curve 3), k = 200 m²/s (curve 4). Open circles represent experimental data, while a continuous line is adopted to represent numerical results.

models (see chapter 12). The response for a periodontal ligament tissue specimen taken from cows (Pini, 1999) is shown in Figures 11.37 to 11.39 for a cyclical application of tensile strain with increasing amplitude. During the unloading phase (Figure 11.38) the stress-strain curve is located below the curve of the first loading phase (Figure 11.37), revealing degradation in the elastic properties of the sample.

The subsequent loading phase (Figure 11.39) coincides with the unloading phase up to the maximum strain attained during the first loading phase. The following phases, for cycles with larger amplitudes of strain, show similar behaviour, with degradation in the elastic properties in every new strain path. The numerical simulation is performed by adopting elasto-damage models, with a non-increasing damage function that depends on the maximum strain attained during the history of the material. This represents the 'memory' of the tissue from a numerical point of view.

Obviously this representation refers to *in vitro* tests and cannot be entirely extended to *in vivo* periodontal ligament tissue. The first reason is due to the fact that the material probably does not experience strains large enough to degrade its elastic properties. The second reason is related to the complex phenomena of cellular activity, which are antagonist to the

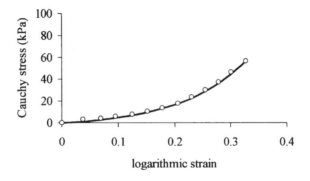

Figure 11.37 Tensile strain tests on a periodontal ligament tissue sample. Open circles represents experimental data during the first loading phase. The black continuous line represents the numerical solution.

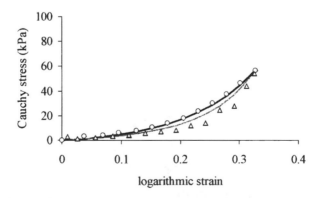

Figure 11.38 Tensile strain tests on a periodontal ligament tissue sample. The open triangles represents experimental data during the unloading phase. The continuous grey line represents the numerical solution.

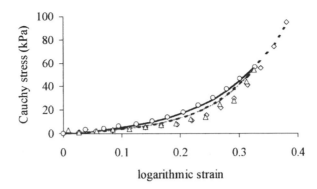

Figure. 11.39 Tensile strain tests on a periodontal ligament tissue sample. The open squares are experimental data during the re-loading phase and new loading phase over the maximum strain attained during the previous cycle. The numerical solution is represented by a dotted black line.

degradation of living tissues. Nonetheless, the use of inelastic constitutive models can be useful in order to identify the actual response of a biological tissue and to correctly interpret the results coming from experimental activity.

11.6 CONCLUSIONS

The overview presented in this chapter, as part of a large research activity developed, is aimed at showing how numerical methods can represent a useful contribution in the field of dental biomechanics. These methods can lead to a deeper understanding of complex phenomena, related, for example, to the bone-implant interaction, as well as to the mechanical response of natural dentition under different types of loading. Numerical methods can be aimed at the investigation of biological systems, in order to explain some phenomena from a mechanical point of view. Numerical techniques can also be used to create specific tools to help clinicians in their pre-operational planning and for a general evaluation of the effectiveness of their methods in operational practice.

The characteristic of biological systems shown in the present chapter is their complexity, due both to geometry and material aspects. This complexity limits the possibility of describing the behaviour of such systems with simple schemes. The complexity of geometry, non-linear behaviour of material and the strong variability of mechanical properties reinforce the idea that numerical methods may be the most suitable tool for realistically describing the mechanical response of biological structures.

Since the procedure to set all the parameters of a model is a very demanding task, it is fundamental to have many data from experimental tests in order to be able to continuously compare results obtained using numerical analysis. In fact, experimental and numerical analyses must reciprocally contribute to the investigation performed. Only in this way the reliability of the models and results from numerical analysis can be evaluated.

REFERENCES

K.L. Andersen, H.T. Mortensen, E.H. Pedersen, B. Melsen, Determination of stress levels and profiles in the periodontal ligaments by means of an improved three-dimensional finite element model for variuos types of orthodontic and natural force system, Journal Biomedical Engineering, Vol. 13, Issue 14, pp. 293–303, 1991.

B.K.B. Berkovitz, B.J. Moxham, H.N. Newman, The periodontal ligament in health and disease, Mosby-Wolfe, 1995.

F. Bonollo, N. Gramegna, A. Natali, P. Pavan, Numerical analysis of titanium cast devices for dental implantology, Computer Methods in Biomechanics and Biomedical Engineering, Vol. 5, Issue 2, pp. 615–623, 2002.

C. Bourael, D. Freudenreich, D. Vollmer, D. Kobe, D. Drescher, A. Jäger, Simulation of orthodontic tooth movements. A comparison of numerical models, J. Orofac. Orthop., Vol. 60, pp. 136–151, 1999.

J.B. Brunski, Biomechanical forces affecting the bone-dental implant interface, Dent. Mats., Vol. 10, pp. 153–201,1992.

S.C. Cowin, D.H. Hegedus, Bone Remodeling I: Theory of Adaptive Elasticity, Journal of Elasticity, Vol. 6, pp. 313–326, 1976.

S.C. Cowin, Bone Mechanics Handbook, CRC Press, Boca Raton, 2001.

B. Dorow, N. Krstin, F.G. Sander, Examination of the viscoelastic material properties of the peri-odontal ligament 'in vivo', 5th International Symposium on Computer Methods in Biomechanics and Biomedical Engineering, Roma, 2001.

R.T. Hart, Bone Modeling and Remodeling: Theories and Computation. In Bone Mechanics Handbook (Edited by S. C. Cowin), CRC Press, Boca Raton, Ch. 31, pp. 1–42, 2001.

W.C. Hayes, Biomechanics of cortical and trabecular bone: implication for assessment of fracture risk, Basic Orthopaedic Biomechanics, Reven Press, New York, 1991.

T.W. Korioth, T.W. Waldron, J.K. Schulte, Forces and moments generated at the dental incisor during forceful biting in humans, Journal of Biomechanics, Vol. 6, pp. 631–633, 1997.

N. Krstin, R.P. Franke, F.G. Sander, Experimental investigation of visco-elastic material behaviour of the periodontal ligament of human specimen 'in vitro', 5th International Symposium in Computer Methods in Biomechanics and Biomechanical Engineering, Roma, Italy, 2001.

R. Mericske-Stern, A. Geering, W. Bürgin, H. Graf, Three-dimensional force measurements on mandibular implants supporting overdentures, International Journal of Oral and Maxillofacial Implants, Vol. 7, pp. 185–194, 1992.

E.A. Meroi, A.N. Natali, B.A. Schrefler, A porous media approach to finite deformation behaviour in soft tissues, Comp. Meth. Biomech. Biomed. Eng., Vol. 2, pp. 157–170, 1999.

J. Middleton, M.L. Jones, A.N. Wilson, Three-dimensional analysis of orthodontic tooth movement, Journal Biomedical Engineering, pp. 319–327, 1990.

K. Miller, Modelling soft tissue using biphasic theory – A word of caution, Comp. Meth. Biomech. Biomed. Eng., Vol. 1, Issue 3, pp. 261–263, 1998.

H. Morikawa, K. Yamamoto, M. Nishihira, Y. Sato, H. Ishikawa, S. Nakamura, Elastic properties of the periodontal ligament and optimal stress for osteoclast appearance, 5th Japan-USA-Singapore-China Conference of Biomechanics, Miyagi, Japan, 1998.

V.C. Mow, S.C. Kuei, W.M. Lai, C.G. Armstrong, Biphasic creep and stress relaxation of articular car-tilage in compression: theory and experiments, J. Biomech. Engng., Vol. 102, pp. 73–84, 1980.

A.N. Natali, E.A. Meroi, A review of the biomechanical properties of bone as a material, J. Biomed. Eng., pp. 266–276, 1989.

A.N. Natali, The simulation of load bearing capacity of dental implants, Computer Technology in Biomaterials Science and Engineering, pp. 132–148, J. Wiley and Sons, 1999.

A. Natali, P. Pavan, M. Pini, R. Ronchi, Numerical analysis of short time response of periodontal ligament, ESB Conference, Dublin (Ireland), 2000.

A.N. Natali, P.G. Pavan, E. Schileo, Evaluation of biomechanical response of dental implants assuming anisotropic configuration of bone tissue, Ceramics, Cells and Tissue, CNR, pp. 18–25, 2001a.

A. Natali, P. Pavan, S. Secchi, The study of tooth mobility by means of finite element models: definition of a multi-phase constitutive model of the periodontal ligament, 5th International Symposium on Computer Methods in Biomechanics and Biomedical Engineering, Roma (Italy), 2001b.

A.N. Natali, P.G. Pavan, A comparative analysis based on different strength criteria for evaluation of risk factor for dental implants, Computer Methods in Biomechanics and Biomedical Engineering, Vol. 5, Issue 1, pp. 511–523, 2002.

R.J. Nikolai, Periodontal ligament reaction and displacements of maxillary central incisor subjected to transverse crown loading, J. Biomechanics, Vol. 7, pp. 93–99, 1974.

J. Paphangkorakit, J.W. Osborn, Effects on human maximum bite force of biting on a softer or harder object, Archives or Oral Biology, Vol. 43, pp. 833–839, 1998.

G.J. Parfitt, Measurement of the physiological mobility of individual teeth in an axial direction, Journal of Dental Research, Vol. 39, pp. 608–618, 1960.

D.C.A. Pincton, D.J. Wills, W.T.R. Davies, The intrusion of the tooth for different loading rates, Journal of Biomechanics, Vol. 4, pp. 429–434, 1978.

M. Pini, Mechanical characterization and modeling of the periodontal ligament, Ph.D. Thesis, Trento (Italy), 1999.

C.G. Provatidis, N.E. Toutountzakis, A critical review of older and contemporary applications of biomechanical methods in orthodontics, Hellenic Orthodontic Review, Vol. 1, pp. 27–49, 1998.

C.G. Provatidis, A comparative FEM-study of tooth mobility using isotropy and anisotropic models of the periodontal ligament, Medical Engineering and Physics, Vol. 22, pp. 359–370, 2000.

J.S. Rees, P.H. Jacobsen, Elastic modulus of the periodontal ligament, Biomaterials, Vol. 18, pp. 995–999, 1997.

G.R. Ross, C.S. Lear, R. DeCou, Modelling the lateral movement of teeth, Journal of Biomechanics, Vol. 9, pp. 723–734, 1976.

M. Soncini, P. Pietrabissa, Computational simulation of the tooth movement during the orthodontic treatment, Computer Methods in Biomechanics & Biomedical Engineering – 3, Gordon and Breach Science Publishers, 2001.

R.L. Spilker, J.K. Suh, V.C. Mow, A finite element analysis of the indentation stress-relaxation response of linear biphasic articular cartilage, J. Biomech. Eng., Vol. 114, pp. 191–201, 1992.

S.W. Tsai, E.M. Wu, A general theory of strength for anisotropic materials, J. of Composite Materials, Vol. 5, pp. 58–60, 1971.

W.D. van Driel, F.J. van Leeuwen, L. Blankevoort, J.W. Von de Hoff, J.C. Maltha, Time dependent displacement of the tooth in response to orthodontic forces, 11th Conference of the ESB, Tolouse, France, 1998.

K. Yamamoto, M. Wakita, H. Morikawa, The relationships between tissue response and stress distribution in the periodontal ligament during orthodontic tooth movement, 11th Conference of the ESB, Tolouse (France), 1998.

12 Mechanics of materials

AN Natali, PG Pavan, EM Meroi

12.1 INTRODUCTION

This chapter deals with the basic concepts of continuum mechanics (Malvern, 1969; Marsden and Hughes, 1980). The presence of a specific chapter on this topic is motivated by its use in the wide application of numerical techniques in the field of biomechanics. In particular, the application of the finite element method (Hughes, 1996; Zienkiewicz and Taylor, 1996; Crisfield, 1997) represents a powerful approach to the qualitative and quantitative estimation of the complex mechanical behaviour of both hard and soft tissues, as well as of the interaction between implants and biological tissues. The following topics are given particular attention: anisotropy (Spencer, 1990), finite elasticity (Ogden, 1984) and visco-elasticity (Simo and Hughes, 2000), damage (Kachanov, 1986; Lemaitre, 1996) and poroelasticity (Lewis and Schrefler, 1998). Anisotropic behaviour must be generally taken into account in the modelling of bone tissue (Cowin, 2001), particularly for its cortical portion and it can also regard soft tissues. The concept of finite elasticity is fundamental in describing the mechanical response of soft tissues such as ligaments, intervertebral discs and skin (Maurel et al., 1998). The visco-elastic approach (Christensen, 1982) can provide a sophisticated modelling for a direct formulation of the time dependent behaviour of living tissues. Damage models are also presented since they are commonly adopted to describe inelastic effects on bone (Lee et al., 2000) and, in addition, offer possible approaches to defining a bone remodelling theory (Prendergast and Taylor, 1994; Ramtani and Zidi, 2001). Finally, multi-phase media formulations probably represent the most advanced approach in the analysis of biological tissue mechanics because it is consistent with the micro-mechanical structure of the tissue, including the description of the behaviour of fluid phases and their effects (Mow et al., 1980; Almeida and Spilker, 1998; Cowin, 1999).

12.2 MATERIAL MODELS

The mechanical characterisation of a material, including biological tissues, can be based on the use of mathematical models that make it possible to describe the response of the material itself to loading. The aim of this approach is mainly to evaluate the deformability of the structure or its load bearing capacity.

As an introduction to the problem, a simple structure, such as a homogeneous bar subjected to an axial force, will be considered (Figure 12.1). Defining the mechanical response of the bar means saying how the structure is deformed, i.e. how its initial length is changed, when a force is applied at one end. The most simple relationship between the

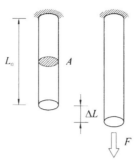

Figure 12.1 Elongation of a bar with initial length L_0, constant section A and applied force F.

elongation of the bar and the value of the force acting on it is depicted in Figure 12.2, where the elongation is proportional to the force applied. If this condition holds, the material is said to be linear elastic. When the load is removed, the bar recovers its initial length and the unloading path matches the loading curve. Many materials show this linear response, at least in the initial phase of loading.

If the elongation of the bar is not proportional to the applied force, as depicted in Figure 12.3, the material is said to be non-linear elastic. Non-linear elasticity is found in biological tissues, especially in soft connective tissues, but is also typical of rubber-like materials. As for linear-elastic material, the loading and unloading paths are coincident and the initial length is recovered if the force is removed.

When the force on the bar is significant, inelastic phenomena can occur due to the degradation of the internal structure of the bar, such as the formation of cracks or permanent strains. The presence of permanent strain is evident in the typical loading-unloading curve in Figure 12.4. After an initial elastic phase, the bar is permanently stretched. The initial length is not recovered with the unloading phase and the residual stretch is a measure of the inelastic process that has occurred. A material showing such a mechanical response is described as elasto-plastic.

The term damage refers to the formation of cracks or other defects, which are usually small with respect to the dimension of the structure. The presence of cracks degrades the elastic properties of the structure. A loading-unloading cycle for an elasto-damaged material is depicted in Figure 12.5. With the unloading, the bar recovers the initial length but is less stiff.

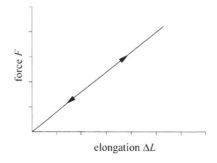

Figure 12.2 Loading-unloading path for a linear elastic material.

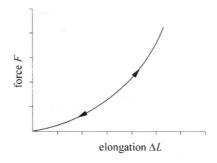

Figure 12.3 Loading-unloading path for a non-linear elastic material.

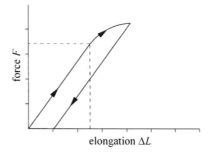

Figure 12.4 Loading-unloading path for elasto-plastic material.

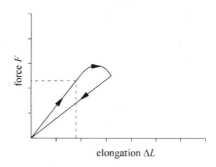

Figure 12.5 Loading-unloading path of an elasto-damaged material.

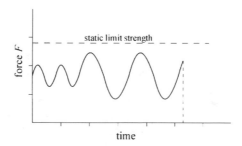

Figure 12.6 Fatigue failure due to cyclic loading.

Damage effects can also be given by recurrent applications of low magnitude loads, in which case, the damage is due to a progressive accumulation of inelastic phenomena in the loading history of the structure. This phenomenon is called fatigue. Fatigue phenomena can be particularly dangerous since they can also induce an abrupt failure of the structure, without evident warning signs.

A time-dependent behaviour can be found as a consequence of the internal re-arrangements of the material, as shown in Figures 12.7 and 12.8. This mechanical response is typical of polymeric materials, but is often found in almost all biological tissues as well. These materials are described as visco-elastic.

Figure 12.7 shows the behaviour of the bar under the action of a force, constant in time, and then removed. After an initial instantaneous elongation, due to the sudden application of the force, the bar is progressively stretched. This phenomenon is called creep. When the force is removed, the bar shows an elastic response, vertical portion of the curve, followed by a creeping recovery back to the initial length.

A different effect, due to visco-elasticity is depicted in Figure 12.8. A constant stretch of the bar is imposed by applying a displacement at one of the ends. The initial reaction force, depending on the initial value of the elongation, shows a decrease in time, toward an asymptotic value. This effect is known as a relaxation process.

The ideal schemes presented above are usually combined, e.g. a material can show an elasto-plastic behaviour coupled with viscous effect. The global behaviour of the material also depends on the type of loading or on environmental factors such as temperature, and the resulting force–elongation laws are obviously more complex.

The interest is usually in knowing what the behaviour of structures with generic shapes is. For this purpose, it is useful to introduce the concepts of stress and strain, which make it possible to represent the behaviour of a small portion of the bar or, in other words, of the

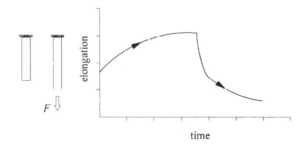

Figure 12.7 Visco-elastic material: creep process.

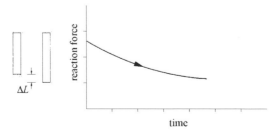

Figure 12.8 Visco-elastic material: relaxation process.

material itself. Stress is the force acting on an infinitesimal area surrounding a generic point of the cross section, and strain is the elongation of a fibre of the bar, having unit undeformed length. For the case at hand, the stress is represented by the ratio between the force F acting at the tip and the area A of its transversal section, which is assumed to be constant for simplicity's sake:

$$\sigma = \frac{F}{A}$$

The strain is defined as the ratio between the elongation and the undeformed length of the bar:

$$\varepsilon = \frac{\Delta L}{L_0}$$

The force vs. displacement curves can be replaced by analogous curves showing the relationships between stress and strain and representing the mechanical behaviour of a generic portion of the material. One can note how the measures of stress and strain are, in some ways, not dependent on the geometric dimensions of the structures. Therefore, they offer the possibility of generalising the relationships established between elongation and force. The mathematical framework, needed to extend the concepts presented in this section, for a simple uni-axial problem to the three-dimensional case, is explained in detail in the following sections.

12.3 DEFORMATION OF CONTINUUM

12.3.1 Kinematics

A body in the three dimensional space $\mathbb{R}^3$ is defined as an open set $\mathcal{B}_0 \subseteq \mathbb{R}^3$ with boundary $\partial\mathcal{B}_0$. A configuration of the body is given by a one to one mapping $\varphi:\mathcal{B}_0 \rightarrow \mathcal{B} \subseteq \mathbb{R}^3$. The body motion is defined as the set of configurations assumed by the body in time $\mathcal{B} = \varphi(\mathcal{B}_0, t)$. The reference configuration is the body configuration assumed at time zero. A material point $\mathbf{X}$ is a point in its reference configuration $\mathcal{B}_0$, while a spatial point is the place occupied by the material point at time t and is denoted $\mathbf{x} = \varphi_t(\mathbf{X})$ where the function φ_t is called deformation.

The motion is defined as regular if integrity of body is ensured at any time t, i.e. if the motion maps every material point of the body with one and only one point of the current

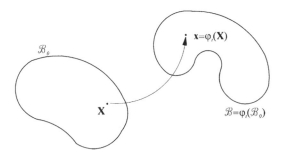

Figure 12.9 Motion of a body: reference (undeformed) and current (deformed) configuration.

(deformed) configuration at time *t*. In other words, the motion is regular if the map φ_t has inverse φ_t^{-1}. Once the deformation gradient is defined:

$$\mathbf{F}(\mathbf{X},t) = \partial \varphi(\mathbf{X},t)/\partial \mathbf{X} \tag{1}$$

its determinant *J* is the Jacobian deformation and measures the ratio of the current and reference volumes in the neighbourhood of the material point considered. The only class of deformations of physical interest is the one which fulfils the inequality $J > 0$, which is equivalent to saying that no penetration of different parts of the body occurs.

The trajectory of a material point **X** is the set of points $\varphi(\mathbf{X},t) = \varphi_x(t)$. The velocity of material point **X** is defined as the derivative of the trajectory with respect to time:

$$\mathbf{V} = \partial \varphi_x(t)/\partial t \tag{2}$$

The second derivative of the trajectory with respect to time is called material acceleration:

$$\mathbf{A}(\mathbf{X},t) = \partial \mathbf{V}/\partial t = \partial^2 \varphi_x(t)/\partial t^2 \tag{3}$$

and it is the rate of change of velocity with time. This description of the body and its motion is called lagrangian or material description, since it refers to the undeformed configuration of the body. The time derivative, with the material coordinates held constant, is the material time derivative. Velocity and acceleration can also be expressed with reference to the current configuration of the body. In this case the description of the motion is called eulerian or spatial description. The velocity of material point **X** is a vector emanating by point **x** and thus $\mathbf{V}(\mathbf{X},t) = \mathbf{v}(\mathbf{x},t) = \mathbf{v}(\varphi(\mathbf{X},t),t)$. The spatial acceleration is given as a function of $(\mathbf{x},t)$ by the chain rule:

$$\mathbf{a} = \frac{\partial \mathbf{v}}{\partial t} + \mathbf{v} \cdot \frac{\partial \mathbf{v}}{\partial \mathbf{x}} \tag{4}$$

12.3.2 Strain and its measures

A deformation is said homogeneous if **F** is constant. In the neighbourhood of a point, deformation behaves like a homogeneous deformation. The simplest case of homogeneous deformation of a body is pure translation where the deformation gradient is the second order unit tensor **I**. If a rigid body motion is applied, the relative distance between particles does not change and the deformation gradient becomes a proper orthogonal tensor, i.e. $\mathbf{F} = \mathbf{R}$ with $\mathbf{R}^{-1} = \mathbf{R}^T$ and det $\mathbf{R} = 1$.

The application of a deformation gradient **F** gives the following transformation of a unit vector **A**, pertaining to the body and starting from a point **X** of its reference configuration:

$$\lambda \mathbf{a} = \mathbf{F}(\mathbf{X},t) \cdot \mathbf{A} \tag{5}$$

where **a** is a unit vector in the current configuration and the scalar λ is the stretch of the initial vector **A**. Since the deformation gradient has a positive determinant, the polar decomposition theorem holds and **F** can be split in multiplicative way:

$$\mathbf{F} = \mathbf{RU} = \mathbf{VR} \tag{6}$$

R being the unique orthogonal tensor giving the rigid rotation of the motion. Figure 12.10 partially explains this concept: the deformation of the neighbourhood of a point can be obtained by applying the right stretch tensor **U**, followed by the rigid rotation **R** or by applying the rigid rotation followed by the left stretch tensor **V**. Tensors **U** and **V** are related to the deformation gradients by the following relationships:

$$\mathbf{U}^2 = \mathbf{C} = \mathbf{F}^T\mathbf{F}, \quad \mathbf{V}^2 = \mathbf{b} = \mathbf{F}\mathbf{F}^T \tag{7}$$

where tensors **b** and **C** are respectively left and right Cauchy tensors. Tensors **U** and **V** become the unit tensor for pure rigid motion, i.e. when **F** is an orthogonal tensor. This property shows how they are related to the pure stretch of the body. This is also why they are the basis for the definition of the strain measures.

The right and left Cauchy tensors are symmetric and positive defined, hence they have real eigenvalues and orthogonal eigenvectors. The eigenvalues are the square of the principal stretches, while the eigenvectors represent the principal directions of the strain, in the undeformed configuration for **C** and current configuration for **b**. The eigenvectors are also a function of the principal invariants given by:

$$I_1 = \operatorname{tr}\mathbf{C}, \quad I_2 = \frac{1}{2}(I_1^2 - \operatorname{tr}\mathbf{C}^2), \quad I_3 = \det\mathbf{C} \tag{8}$$

and are deduced as solutions of the polynomial form:

$$\lambda^6 - I_1\lambda^4 + I_2\lambda^2 - I_3 = 0 \tag{9}$$

It is useful, especially for numerical applications to incompressible or almost-incompressible materials, to separate the deformation into its volumetric and volume-preserving parts. Such a distinction can be carried out considering the equivalence:

$$\mathbf{F} = \tilde{\mathbf{F}}(J^{\frac{1}{3}}\mathbf{I}) \tag{10}$$

The determinant of the volume-preserving deformation gradient is the unit, i.e. the correlated part of the deformation leaves the volume unchanged.

The definition of deformation in the neighbourhood of a particle of the body can be based on the lagrangian (material) description or on the eulerian (spatial) description. Following

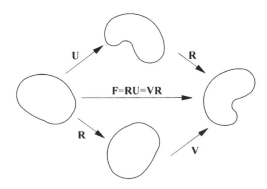

Figure 12.10 Decomposition of the deformation gradient in finite rotation and pure stretch tensors.

the lagrangian description the strain can be described in terms of the Green-Lagrange strain tensor:

$$\mathbf{E} = \frac{1}{2}(\mathbf{C} - \mathbf{I}) \tag{11}$$

resulting $\mathbf{E} = \mathbf{0}$ for a body in the undeformed state. By taking into account the displacement vector, defined as $\mathbf{u} = \mathbf{x} - \mathbf{X}$, the deformation gradient can be re-written as:

$$\mathbf{F} = \frac{\partial \mathbf{x}}{\partial \mathbf{X}} = \frac{\partial(\mathbf{X} + \mathbf{u})}{\partial \mathbf{X}} = \mathbf{I} + \frac{\partial \mathbf{u}}{\partial \mathbf{X}} = \mathbf{I} + \nabla \mathbf{u} \tag{12}$$

and the expression of the Green-Lagrange strain tensor depends on the gradient of displacement up to its second order terms:

$$\mathbf{E} = \frac{1}{2}(\nabla \mathbf{u} + \nabla^T \mathbf{u} + \nabla \mathbf{u} \nabla^T \mathbf{u}) \tag{13}$$

For a uni-dimensional problem in which a body with an initial length L is stretched up to a length l, the unique non-zero component of the Green-Lagrange strain tensor is given by:

$$E = \frac{1}{2} \frac{l^2 - L^2}{L^2} \tag{14}$$

Decomposition in volumetric and volume-preserving deformation can also be used for measuring strains. In particular, the volume-preserving components of the right Cauchy and Green-Lagrange strain tensors are respectively:

$$\tilde{\mathbf{C}} = J^{-\frac{2}{3}}\mathbf{C}, \quad \tilde{\mathbf{E}} = \frac{1}{2}(\tilde{\mathbf{C}} - \mathbf{I}) \tag{15}$$

Given a generic scalar function of the volume-preserving right Cauchy tensor: $f = f(\tilde{\mathbf{C}})$, its derivative with respect to $\mathbf{C}$ is then (chain rule):

$$\frac{\partial f}{\partial \mathbf{C}} = J^{-\frac{2}{3}}\mathrm{Dev}\left[\frac{\partial f}{\partial \tilde{\mathbf{C}}}\right] = J^{-\frac{2}{3}}\left[\frac{\partial f}{\partial \tilde{\mathbf{C}}} - \frac{1}{3}\left(\mathbf{C}:\frac{\partial f}{\partial \tilde{\mathbf{C}}}\right)\mathbf{C}^{-1}\right] \tag{16}$$

obtaining the definition for the volume-preserving operator in the material description.

Expression (16) is commonly applied in cases of hyperelasticity, when the stress tensor is deduced by starting with the definition of the stored energy function. These concepts will be reverted to in greater depth in the following pages. The spatial form of relation (16) is carried out by a push forward to the deformed configuration:

$$\mathbf{F}\frac{\partial f}{\partial \mathbf{C}}\mathbf{F}^T = J^{-\frac{2}{3}}\mathrm{dev}\left(\mathbf{F}\frac{\partial f}{\partial \mathbf{C}}\mathbf{F}^T\right) = J^{-\frac{2}{3}}\left[\tilde{\mathbf{F}}\frac{\partial f}{\partial \tilde{\mathbf{C}}}\tilde{\mathbf{F}}^T - \frac{1}{3}\mathrm{tr}\left(\frac{\partial f}{\partial \tilde{\mathbf{C}}}\right)\mathbf{I}\right] \tag{17}$$

finding the more familiar form for the volume-preserving operator in the current configuration.

The material derivative of deformation is taken by deriving the deformation gradient with respect to time. It can be expressed with simple considerations in the equivalent forms:

$$\dot{\mathbf{F}} = \frac{\partial \mathbf{F}}{\partial t} = \frac{\partial}{\partial t}\left[\frac{\partial \varphi(\mathbf{X}, t)}{\partial \mathbf{X}}\right] = \frac{\partial}{\partial \mathbf{X}}\left[\frac{\partial \varphi(\mathbf{X}, t)}{\partial t}\right] = \frac{\partial \mathbf{V}}{\partial \mathbf{X}} \tag{18}$$

The gradient of material velocity can be related to the gradient of spatial velocity:

$$\frac{\partial \mathbf{V}}{\partial \mathbf{X}} = \frac{\partial \mathbf{v}}{\partial \mathbf{x}} \frac{\partial \mathbf{x}}{\partial \mathbf{X}} = \frac{\partial \mathbf{v}}{\partial \mathbf{x}} \mathbf{F} \tag{19}$$

and, by comparison with the previous relationship, the following equation holds:

$$\frac{\partial \mathbf{v}}{\partial \mathbf{x}} = \dot{\mathbf{F}} \mathbf{F}^{-1} \tag{20}$$

The gradient of spatial velocity allows for an additive decomposition of (20) in a symmetric tensor, usually called deformation rate tensor **d**, and an anti-symmetric tensor, the spin or vorticity tensor **w**:

$$\frac{\partial \mathbf{v}}{\partial \mathbf{x}} = \frac{1}{2}\left[\left(\frac{\partial \mathbf{v}}{\partial \mathbf{x}}\right) + \left(\frac{\partial \mathbf{v}}{\partial \mathbf{x}}\right)^T\right] + \frac{1}{2}\left[\left(\frac{\partial \mathbf{v}}{\partial \mathbf{x}}\right) - \left(\frac{\partial \mathbf{v}}{\partial \mathbf{x}}\right)^T\right] = \mathbf{d} + \mathbf{w} \tag{21}$$

The rate of deformation tensor **d** is related to the ratio of the stretch of the body, while the spin tensor is associated to a rigid body rotation rate. Relation (21) explains the usual form assumed for the measure of strains in infinitesimal deformation problems; the time derivative of small strain tensor **ε** is approximately equal to tensor **d** when derivation with respect to material and spatial coordinates can be confused, namely when displacements and displacements gradients are very small:

$$\dot{\boldsymbol{\varepsilon}} = \frac{1}{2}\left[\left(\frac{\partial \mathbf{v}}{\partial \mathbf{x}}\right) + \left(\frac{\partial \mathbf{v}}{\partial \mathbf{x}}\right)^T\right] \tag{22}$$

An alternative way of defining the infinitesimal strain tensor **ε** is to consider the case of infinitesimal components:

$$\left|\frac{\partial u_i}{\partial X_j}\right| \ll 1 \ \ (i, j = 1,2,3) \tag{23}$$

Taking into account that the binomial expansion of the spatial derivative of the displacement field up to the first order term assumes the form:

$$\frac{\partial \mathbf{u}}{\partial \mathbf{x}} = \nabla \mathbf{u} \mathbf{F}^{-1} = \mathbf{I} - \mathbf{F}^{-1} \cong \mathbf{F} - \mathbf{I} \tag{24}$$

in terms of components and on the basis of (23) one obtains:

$$\frac{\partial u_i}{\partial x_j} = \frac{\partial u_i}{\partial X_j} \ \ (i, j = 1,2,3) \tag{25}$$

This shows how the gradient does not depend on the differentiation with respect to material or spatial coordinates. The tensor of infinitesimal strains can be written in an equivalent form as:

$$\boldsymbol{\varepsilon} = \frac{1}{2}(\nabla \mathbf{u} + \nabla^T \mathbf{u}) = \frac{1}{2}(\mathbf{F} + \mathbf{F}^T) - \mathbf{I} \tag{26}$$

An explicit form of the infinitesimal strain tensor (26) is given below with respect to the small displacement vector $\mathbf{u} = (u,v,w)$ which refers to an orthogonal coordinate system x, y, z:

$$\boldsymbol{\varepsilon} = \begin{bmatrix} \dfrac{\partial u}{\partial x} & \dfrac{\partial u/\partial y + \partial v/\partial x}{2} & \dfrac{\partial u/\partial z + \partial w/\partial x}{2} \\[3mm] \dfrac{\partial v/\partial x + \partial u/\partial y}{2} & \dfrac{\partial v}{\partial y} & \dfrac{\partial v/\partial z + \partial w/\partial y}{2} \\[3mm] \dfrac{\partial w/\partial x + \partial v/\partial z}{2} & \dfrac{\partial w/\partial y + \partial v/\partial z}{2} & \dfrac{\partial w}{\partial z} \end{bmatrix} \tag{27}$$

12.4 THE CONCEPT OF STRESS AND ITS MEASURES

Let $\mathcal{B}_0$ be the reference configuration of a body in a three-dimensional space (Figure 12.11), constrained on a portion $\partial_u \mathcal{B}_0$ of its boundary and subjected to surface traction in the other part $\partial_\sigma \mathcal{B}_0$. In the following, sets $\partial_u \mathcal{B}_0$ and $\partial_\sigma \mathcal{B}_0$ are assumed to be distinct and their sum gives the whole boundary surface. A deformation map is considered, which takes the body to the current configuration $\mathcal{B} = \varphi(\mathcal{B}_0)$. Traction on the deformed boundary surface is defined as the external forces $d\,\mathbf{F}_s^{ext}$ acting on an element with infinitesimal area dA:

$$\mathbf{f} = \lim_{dA \to 0} \frac{d\mathbf{F}_s^{ext}}{dA} \tag{28}$$

In similar way, assuming that volume forces act on the body as well, it can be defined:

$$\mathbf{b} = \lim_{dV \to 0} \frac{d\mathbf{F}_V^{ext}}{dV} \tag{29}$$

where dV is the infinitesimal volume of the neighbourhood of a point of the body. The volume forces depend on the mass of the body.

12.4.1 Stress vector

Any surface within a continuous medium separates two portions of the medium, each exerting a traction on the other. If a portion with area dA containing the point P is identified

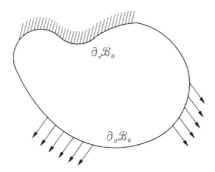

Figure 12.11 Boundary conditions acting on a body.

on this surface, forces acting on it are equivalent to a resultant force $d\mathbf{F}$ and a resultant moment $d\mathbf{M}$ and approach a definite limit on the surface dA at the point P:

$$\mathbf{t} = \lim_{dA \to 0} \frac{d\mathbf{T}}{dA} \qquad \mathbf{m} = \lim_{dA \to 0} \frac{d\mathbf{M}}{dA} \tag{30}$$

with $\mathbf{t}$ and $\mathbf{m}$ respectively the force and moment per unit area.

The condition $\mathbf{m} = \mathbf{0}$ identifies a particular class of continua, known as Cauchy continua. The traction vector $\mathbf{t}$ is usually not parallel to the normal $\mathbf{n}$ to the surface dA, admitting also a component acting in the plane of the surface itself. The normal component of the traction vector to the surface is indicated with the symbol σ while the tangential or shear component with τ (see Figure 12.12).

If the stress vector is parallel to the normal $\mathbf{n}$, the latter defines a principal direction of stress. The corresponding scalar value of the normal stress defines the related principal stress, while the shear component vanishes. It can be demonstrated that, at least, three principal directions, one orthogonal to the other, exist. If the related principal stresses are all non-zero, the stress state acting on the point considered is said three-axial. If one of the principal stresses is zero the stress state is said bi-axial, while if two of the principal stresses are zero, the stress state is uni-axial. If two of the principal stresses are equal, every direction lying in the plane defined by the related principal directions is also principal. Finally, a particular stress state is found if all the principal stresses are equal. In this case, every direction is principal and the stress state is said hydrostatic. The unique value of the principal stresses defines the hydrostatic pressure p.

12.4.2 Cauchy stress tensor

The traction vector at a given point and for an arbitrary plane can be expressed as a function of the traction vectors on three planes perpendicular to a Cartesian coordinate system x, y, z. The Cauchy stress tensor $\boldsymbol{\sigma}$ is introduced (see Figure 12.13) by taking the components of normal and shear tractions relative to the coordinate axes:

$$\boldsymbol{\sigma} = \begin{bmatrix} \sigma_{xx} & \tau_{xy} & \tau_{xz} \\ \tau_{yx} & \sigma_{yy} & \tau_{yz} \\ \tau_{zx} & \tau_{zy} & \sigma_{zz} \end{bmatrix} \tag{31}$$

The traction vector at a given point is then given by:

$$\mathbf{t} = \boldsymbol{\sigma} \cdot \mathbf{n} \tag{32}$$

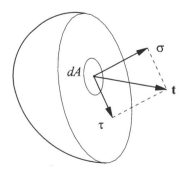

Figure 12.12 Decomposition of the stress vector in normal and shear components.

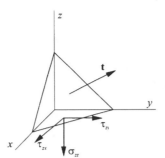

Figure 12.13 Definition of the special components of the stress tensor.

12.4.2.1 The symmetry of the Cauchy stress tensor

Taking into account a static problem and imposing the balance of forces for the element of Figure 12.13, the local form of momentum balance is obtained as:

$$\frac{\partial \sigma_x}{\partial x} + \frac{\partial \tau_{xy}}{\partial y} + \frac{\partial \tau_{xz}}{\partial z} + \rho b_x = 0 \tag{33}$$

$$\frac{\partial \tau_{yx}}{\partial x} + \frac{\partial \sigma_y}{\partial y} + \frac{\partial \tau_{yz}}{\partial z} + \rho b_y = 0$$

$$\frac{\partial \tau_{zx}}{\partial x} + \frac{\partial \tau_{zy}}{\partial y} + \frac{\partial \sigma_z}{\partial z} + \rho b_z = 0$$

having indicated the volume forces of the current configuration with the vector $\mathbf{b} = (b_x, b_y, b_z)$. Equation (33) can be written in compact form by making use of the divergence operator:

$$\text{div}(\boldsymbol{\sigma}) + \rho \mathbf{b} = \mathbf{0} \tag{34}$$

Since the Cauchy continuum does not transfer moments per unit area, the rotation equilibrium of the element in Figure 12.12 simply leads to the symmetry of the Cauchy stress tensor, i.e.: $\tau_{xy} = \tau_{yx}$, $\tau_{yz} = \tau_{zy}$ and $\tau_{xz} = \tau_{zx}$.

Equation (34) must hold for every point of the body and can be considered as the local form of the balance of momentum with respect to the current configuration of the body. At the boundary $\partial_\sigma \mathcal{B}$ the conditions are given as:

$$\sigma_x n_x + \tau_{xy} n_y + \tau_{xz} n_z = f_x \tag{35}$$

$$\tau_{yz} n_x + \sigma_y n_y + \tau_{yz} n_z = f_y$$

$$\tau_{zx} n_x + \tau_{zy} n_y + \sigma_z n_z = f_z$$

or, in compact form:

$$\boldsymbol{\sigma} \cdot \mathbf{n} = \mathbf{f} \tag{36}$$

12.4.3 Different stress measures

The Cauchy stress tensor is defined on the deformed configuration of the body. If small strains and displacements problems are considered, deformed and undeformed configurations of the body can be superposed and the Cauchy stress can be thought of as acting on the undeformed body. In finite deformation problems, deformed and undeformed configurations are clearly distinct and the above assumption does not hold. If the balance equations are given with reference to the undeformed configuration, as usual approach to many problems, new stress measures should be adopted, namely the first Piola-Kirchhoff stress tensor $\mathbf{P}$ and the second Piola-Kirchhoff stress tensor $\mathbf{S}$:

$$\mathbf{P} = J\boldsymbol{\sigma}\mathbf{F}^{-T} = \mathbf{FS} \tag{37}$$

$$\mathbf{S} = J\mathbf{F}^{-1}\boldsymbol{\sigma}\mathbf{F}^{-T} = \mathbf{F}^{-1}\mathbf{P} \tag{38}$$

The physical meaning of the first Piola-Kirchhoff stress tensor is represented in Figure 12.14 for uniaxial problems.

It is important to note that the first Piola-Kirchhoff is not symmetric. Since this is a disadvantage in numerical applications, the symmetric second Piola-Kirchhoff stress tensor is often preferred. It is associated with the rate of the Green-Lagrange strain tensor in the energetic sense since the following stress-strain couples give the same internal power:

$$\mathbf{S}{:}\dot{\mathbf{E}} = \mathbf{P}{:}\dot{\mathbf{F}} = J\boldsymbol{\sigma}{:}\mathbf{d} \tag{39}$$

where $\mathbf{d}$ is the strain rate and $\dot{\mathbf{F}}$ the rate of the deformation gradient. Equivalence (39) is commonly used in numerical approaches to continuum mechanics such as the finite element method.

A relation between the first Piola-Kirchhoff tensor and the Cauchy stress tensor can be established by observing that the traction vector does not change if the undeformed or deformed configurations are referred to, hence one can write:

$$\mathbf{t} = \int_{\partial\mathscr{B}} \boldsymbol{\sigma} \cdot \mathbf{n}dA = \int_{\partial\mathscr{B}_0} \mathbf{P} \cdot \mathbf{N}dA_0 = \mathbf{T} \tag{40}$$

Since equation (40) holds for any region of the body, relation (37) follows straight.

12.5 BALANCE LAWS

Continuum mechanics is based on some balance laws, among which the conservation of momentum and mass are fundamental. These balance laws theoretically have general validity and are not restricted by class of materials or bodies to which they are applied. The validity of these principles is a concept that can be applied both with reference to a point of the body, and its infinitesimal neighbourhood, and to the whole body itself. As in the

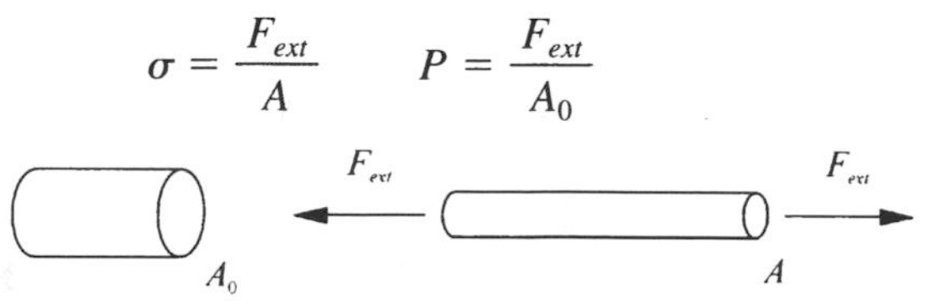

$$\sigma = \frac{F_{ext}}{A} \qquad P = \frac{F_{ext}}{A_0}$$

Figure 12.14 Definition of Cauchy stress and first Piola-Kirchhoff stress for a uni-axial case.

description of the kinematics of a body, balance laws can be expressed by adopting a lagrangian description or an eulerian description of continuum.

12.5.1 Conservation of mass

A first simple law of conservation is the mass balance law or continuity equation. The density in reference and current configuration is defined as the scalar function given by the ratio between the mass dm of a neighbourhood of a point X and its infinitesimal volume, undeformed dV_0 and deformed dV, when it tends to zero:

$$\rho_0(\mathbf{X}) = \lim_{dV_0 \to 0} \frac{dm}{dV_0} \qquad \rho(\mathbf{X}, t) = \lim_{dV \to 0} \frac{dm}{dV} \tag{41}$$

For a neighbourhood of point $\mathbf{X}$ the conservation of mass is written as:

$$\rho_0 dV_0 = \rho dV \tag{42}$$

By recalling the definition of the jacobian of deformation, the previous equation can trivially be transformed in:

$$\frac{\rho_0}{\rho} = \frac{dV}{dV_0} = J \tag{43}$$

The same law can be expressed from an eulerian point of view. Considering an arbitrary region of a body $\mathcal{B}$ with boundary $\partial\mathcal{B}$, conservation of mass is ensured if the time rate of mass in its whole volume is equal to the flux of mass through the boundary surface:

$$\int_{\mathcal{B}} \frac{\partial \rho}{\partial t} dV = -\int_{\partial\mathcal{B}} \rho\mathbf{v} \cdot \mathbf{n} dA \tag{44}$$

$\mathbf{n}$ being the outward normal to the surface $\partial\mathcal{B}$ on every point. By applying the divergence theorem, with surface integral supposed differentiable, the previous equation is transformed involving volume integrals only:

$$\int_{\mathcal{B}} \frac{\partial \rho}{\partial t} dV + \int_{\mathcal{B}} \text{div}\,(\rho\mathbf{v})\, dV \tag{45}$$

Since the region considered is arbitrary, from (45) the so-called continuity equation can be trivially deduced as follows:

$$\frac{\partial \rho}{\partial t} + \text{div}\,(\rho\mathbf{v}) = 0 \tag{46}$$

12.5.2 Weak form of momenta balance

The balance of linear and angular momenta in the current configuration and in local form has already been exposed in section 3.2. The local form of momenta balance can be written upon the reference (undeformed) configuration having:

$$\text{Div}\,\mathbf{P} + \rho_0\mathbf{B} = \mathbf{0} \qquad \mathbf{PF}^T = \mathbf{FP}^T \tag{47}$$

with the boundary conditions:

$$\mathbf{T} = \mathbf{P} \cdot \mathbf{N} \tag{48}$$

$\mathbf{T}$ representing the traction forces acting on $\partial_\sigma \mathcal{B}_0$.

The momentum balance can be written in a weak form, particularly suitable to developing numerical approaches, as the finite element method. The weak form is obtained considering the equilibrium of the whole body. Again one can refer either to the undeformed configuration or to the deformed one. If the traction vector is imposed on the boundary $\partial_\sigma \mathscr{B}_0$ and the body is fixed on $\partial_u \mathscr{B}_0$, admissible variations in the configuration of the body can be defined as the displacement set respecting the prescribed boundary conditions:

$$\mathscr{S}_0 = \left\{ \eta_0 \; : \; \mathscr{B}_0 \to \mathbb{R}^3 \quad J > 0 \text{ on } \mathscr{B}_0 \text{ and } \eta_0 = \mathbf{0} \text{ on } \partial_u \mathscr{B}_0 \right\} \tag{49}$$

The set of admissible variations of configurations can also be defined with respect to the current configuration of the body. By taking the dot product of equations (47) with any element of the set $\mathscr{S}_0$, integrating over the volume of the body and applying the divergence theorem one obtains:

$$\int_{\mathscr{B}_0} \mathbf{P} : \mathrm{Grad}\, \eta_0 \, dV_0 - \int_{\partial \mathscr{B}_0} \mathbf{PN} \cdot \eta_0 dA_0 - \int_{\mathscr{B}_0} \rho_0 \mathbf{B} \cdot \eta_0 \, dV_0 = 0 \tag{50}$$

which is the weak form of balance of momentum. The operator $\mathrm{Grad}(\cdot)$ is the gradient applied with respect to the reference configuration. The eulerian formulation leads to an equivalent form, but in the current configuration of the body, of the previous equation, leading to:

$$\int_{\mathscr{B}} \sigma : \mathrm{grad}\, \eta \, dV - \int_{\partial \mathscr{B}} \sigma \mathbf{n} \cdot \eta \, dA - \int_{\mathscr{B}} \rho \mathbf{b} \cdot \eta \, dV = 0 \tag{51}$$

The vectors η are elements of the space of admissible variations in the current configuration.

12.6 CONSTITUTIVE MODELS

The mechanical response of materials is defined by specifying the relation between stress and strain, stress and strain rates, or other internal variables. Mechanical response can also depend on other parameters such as temperature. In the following, only isothermal problems will be considered. Some constitutive schemes typically adopted in continuum mechanics are presented below. They are linear elasticity, non-linear elasticity and visco-elasticity, damage models and poroelastic models. Non-linear elasticity, visco-elasticity and poroelasticity, in particular, are often used to describe the mechanical response of soft biological tissues. Elasto-damage models are presented as possible approaches to defining a theory of bone remodelling. Constitutive equations must respect the fundamental principles of a purely mechanical theory: principles of determinism and local action for stress and the principle of material frame indifference, also called the principle of material objectivity. The latter is particularly significant in finite strain or finite rotation problems since, in these cases, constitutive theories must be defined which are independent of rigid body motion.

12.6.1 Linear elasticity

Almost all materials show a mechanical response that is characterised by a linear relationship between stress and strain, as they approach their undeformed configuration. This approximation is valid if body deformation is limited to an infinitesimal strain range. The most general relationship between stress and strain can be written as:

$$\sigma_{ij} = D_{ijkl}\varepsilon_{kl} \quad (i, j, k, l = 1, 2, 3) \tag{52}$$

where D_{ijkl} are the 81 coefficients of the fourth order constitutive tensor, ε_{ij} the components of the infinitesimal strain tensor and σ_{ij} the elements of the Cauchy stress tensor. Not all 81 elastic constants D_{ijkl} are independent since equation (52) must fulfil some basic requirements. Because of the symmetry of strain and stress tensors, the following symmetries hold:

$$D_{ijkl} = D_{jikl} = D_{ijlk} \quad (i, j, k, l = 1, 2, 3) \tag{53}$$

Further symmetries are due to the existence of a stored energy function defined as follows (summation convention for repeated index is adopted):

$$W = \frac{1}{2} D_{ijkl}\, \varepsilon_{ij}\, \varepsilon_{kl} \tag{54}$$

The stored energy function defined by the previous quadratic form is the density of energy accumulated by a body because of its deformed state. The existence of a stored energy function means that for a closed deformation path the work done is zero, i.e. energy is not dissipated. These symmetry relationships are:

$$D_{ijkl} = D_{klij} \quad (i, j, k, l = 1, 2, 3) \tag{55}$$

reducing the independent constants to 36. Any symmetry in the mechanical response of a material simplifies the form of the constitutive tensor. If a material shows the same response for every direction considered, it is said to be isotropic. In this case, it can be demonstrated that there are 2 independent constants and relationship (52) can be rewritten as:

$$\boldsymbol{\sigma} = (2\mu\mathbf{I}_1 + \lambda\mathbf{I} \otimes \mathbf{I})\boldsymbol{\varepsilon} \tag{56}$$

where the terms μ and λ are Lamè's elastic constants, related to the Young modulus E and to the Poisson ratio v by the formulas:

$$\mu = \frac{E}{2(1 + v)} \qquad \lambda = \frac{vE}{(1 + v)(1 - 2v)} \tag{57}$$

Isotropic models identify a very simple class of materials. Especially in the field of biological tissues, materials show a mechanical response related to their particular fabric, depending on the orientation of some components. Two particular types of anisotropic materials are presented here: orthotropic materials and transversally isotropic materials. Orthotropic materials are characterised by a symmetry of behaviour with respect to three orthogonal axes (material axes). This symmetry introduces some restrictions in relationship

(52). Since direct and shear components are orthogonal from an energetic point of view, the relation between stress and strain components for an orthotropic material can be written in the two following explicit forms:

$$
\begin{bmatrix} \varepsilon_{11} \\ \varepsilon_{22} \\ \varepsilon_{33} \end{bmatrix} = \begin{bmatrix} \dfrac{1}{E_1} & -\dfrac{v_{21}}{E_2} & -\dfrac{v_{31}}{E_3} \\[2mm] -\dfrac{v_{12}}{E_1} & \dfrac{1}{E_2} & -\dfrac{v_{32}}{E_3} \\[2mm] -\dfrac{v_{13}}{E_1} & -\dfrac{v_{23}}{E_2} & \dfrac{1}{E_3} \end{bmatrix} \begin{bmatrix} \sigma_{11} \\ \sigma_{22} \\ \sigma_{33} \end{bmatrix} \text{ with } \dfrac{v_{ij}}{E_i} = \dfrac{v_{ji}}{E_j} \tag{58}
$$

$$
\begin{bmatrix} \varepsilon_{12} \\ \varepsilon_{13} \\ \varepsilon_{23} \end{bmatrix} = \begin{bmatrix} \dfrac{1}{2G_{12}} & 0 & 0 \\[2mm] 0 & \dfrac{1}{2G_{13}} & 0 \\[2mm] 0 & 0 & \dfrac{1}{2G_{23}} \end{bmatrix} \begin{bmatrix} \sigma_{12} \\ \sigma_{13} \\ \sigma_{23} \end{bmatrix} \tag{59}
$$

where $G_{ij} = E_i/2(1 + v_{ij})$ type relationships hold, with $i, j = 1, 2, 3$ and $i \neq j$.

Transversally isotropic materials are characterised by the symmetry with respect to a specific direction, thus defining the plane of transversal symmetry. Under the hypothesis that direction 1 is normal to this plane of symmetry, the stress-strain relationship is simplified with respect to (58) and (59), taking on the form:

$$
\begin{bmatrix} \varepsilon_{11} \\ \varepsilon_{22} \\ \varepsilon_{33} \end{bmatrix} = \begin{bmatrix} \dfrac{1}{E_1} & -\dfrac{v_{21}}{E_2} & -\dfrac{v_{21}}{E_2} \\[2mm] -\dfrac{v_{12}}{E_1} & \dfrac{1}{E_2} & -\dfrac{v}{E_2} \\[2mm] -\dfrac{v_{12}}{E_1} & -\dfrac{v}{E_2} & \dfrac{1}{E_2} \end{bmatrix} \begin{bmatrix} \sigma_{11} \\ \sigma_{22} \\ \sigma_{33} \end{bmatrix} \text{ with } \dfrac{v_{ij}}{E_i} = \dfrac{v_{ji}}{E_j} \tag{60}
$$

$$
\begin{bmatrix} \varepsilon_{12} \\ \varepsilon_{13} \\ \varepsilon_{23} \end{bmatrix} = \begin{bmatrix} \dfrac{1}{2G_{12}} & 0 & 0 \\[2mm] 0 & \dfrac{1}{2G_{12}} & 0 \\[2mm] 0 & 0 & \dfrac{1+v}{E_2} \end{bmatrix} \begin{bmatrix} \sigma_{12} \\ \sigma_{13} \\ \sigma_{23} \end{bmatrix} \tag{61}
$$

Transversal isotropy is a typical scheme for the mechanical characterisation of long bones, as femur, tibia, etc.

The thermodynamic consistency of constitutive laws restricts the values of the different elastic constants for orthotropic, transversally isotropic and isotropic materials.

12.6.1.1 Extension to finite displacements

If finite displacements and, above all, finite rotations must be taken into account, relations (52) and (54) are written in terms of the Green-Lagrange strain tensor and the second

Piola-Kirchhoff stress tensor. This is done in order to avoid a rigid body motion giving non-zero stress states, thus maintaining objectivity:

$$S_{ij} = C_{ijkl} E_{kl} \quad (i, j, k, l = 1, 2, 3) \tag{62}$$

$$W = \frac{1}{2} C_{ijkl} E_{ij} E_{kl} \tag{63}$$

If finite rotations are excluded and only small strain states are reached in the body, equations (62) and (63) coincide with relations (52) and (54), respectively.

12.6.2 Non-linear elasticity

Materials usually show a linear response only in the neighbourhood of their undeformed configuration. This is especially the case of biological soft tissues such as ligaments or tendons. Non-linear relations between stress and strain can be generally written as:

$$\sigma = f(\varepsilon) \tag{64}$$

where the function f can take on different forms. For example, it can be an exponential function or a polynomial function of the strain tensor. Non-linear stress-strain behaviours tend to happen when materials go under a large strain. In fact, in the following, non-linear elasticity will be formulated in terms of finite measures, namely $\mathbf{E}$ (or $\mathbf{C}$) and $\mathbf{S}$, in order to ensure the objectivity of stress:

$$\mathbf{S} = f(\mathbf{E}) = g(\mathbf{C}) \tag{65}$$

For isotropic materials, the previous relationship can be formulated as follows:

$$\mathbf{S} = \mu_0 \mathbf{I} + \mu_1 \mathbf{C} + \dots + \mu_n \mathbf{C}^n \tag{66}$$

where the scalar coefficients play the role of elastic constants, set on the basis of testing results to fit the numerical stress-strain curves to the experimental ones. It is important to note how relation (65) must fulfil the basic requirement of having null stress in the undeformed configuration:

$$\mathbf{S} = f(\mathbf{0}) = g(\mathbf{I}) = \mathbf{0} \tag{67}$$

12.6.2.1 Hyperelasticity

A special class of non-linear elastic models are represented by the so-called hyperlastic constitutive models, defined by a stored energy function W. The stored energy function depends on $\mathbf{C}$ or $\mathbf{E}$ (homogeneity is assumed here) and with the property:

$$\mathbf{S} = 2 \frac{\partial W(\mathbf{C})}{\partial \mathbf{C}} = \frac{\partial \hat{W}(\mathbf{E})}{\partial \mathbf{E}} \tag{68}$$

It's worth noting how the linear elastic model (62) is hyperelastic as well, according to the existence of the function (63). Further restrictions are usually introduced in order to ensure the convexity of the stored energy function, which can be related to the idea that stress increases with strain. If the material is assumed to be isotropic, the stored energy function depends on $\mathbf{C}$ through the principal invariants or, in an equivalent form, through the principal stretches:

$$W = W(I_1, I_2, I_3) = \hat{W}(\lambda_1, \lambda_2, \lambda_3) \tag{69}$$

When materials show an almost incompressible behaviour, from a numerical point of view, it is better to split the stored energy function into two additive terms, depending on the volume-preserving and volumetric part of strain respectively. Hence, with reference to (69), one obtains:

$$W = \tilde{W}\left(\tilde{I}_1, \tilde{I}_2\right) + U(J) \tag{70}$$

Following the latter approach, the second Piola-Kirchhoff stress tensor is given by:

$$\mathbf{S} = 2J^{-\frac{2}{3}} \mathrm{Dev}\left[\frac{\partial \tilde{W}(\tilde{\mathbf{C}})}{\partial \tilde{\mathbf{C}}}\right] + \frac{\partial U(J)}{\partial J} J\mathbf{C}^{-1} \tag{71}$$

where the second term of the right-hand side represents the hydrostatic term of stress with respect to the reference configuration of the body. If perfect incompressibility is assumed, the term U in equation (70) vanishes and the hydrostatic term of stress is in general undetermined and can be evaluated by introducing a kinematic constraint.

The definition of the stored energy function depends on the characteristics of the mechanical properties of the material. On this basis, several forms have been proposed in the past. Only a few models are reported here as examples for possible approaches. One of the simplest isotropic hyperelastic constitutive models is known as the Mooney-Rivlin model which, in the case of incompressibility, is written as:

$$W = C_1(I_1 - 3) + C_2(I_2 - 3) \tag{72}$$

The Piola-Kirchhoff stress tensor is given by the derivative of the stored energy function with respect to the Green-Lagrange strain tensor plus a term related to the is the hydrostatic pressure p:

$$\mathbf{S} = 2C_1\mathbf{I} + 2C_2(I_2\mathbf{I} - \mathbf{C}) + p\mathbf{C}^{-1} \tag{73}$$

The coefficients C_1 and C_2 depend on the shear modulus of the material and are chosen to fit experimental tests. The Mooney-Rivlin constitutive model is suitable to describe materials under reasonably large strain and showing modest non-linearity in the first phase of deformation. To describe materials with strong non-linear behaviour, the Ogden constitutive model is more appropriate:

$$W = \sum_{r=1}^{N} \frac{\mu_r}{\alpha_r^2}\left(\lambda_1^{\alpha_r} + \lambda_2^{\alpha_r} + \lambda_3^{\alpha_r} - 3\right) \tag{74}$$

where the terms μ_r are related to the shear modulus and the coefficients α_r affects the non-linearity of the stress-strain curves.

Other approaches, especially in numerical modelling of soft biological tissues, take into account the stored energy function as an exponential function of the principal invariants.

12.6.3 Linear visco-elasticity

The simple application of stress states can lead to a mechanical response that cannot be described by pure elastic schemes. Experimental tests show that the application of constant stress may lead some materials to have an increase in strain in time. This phenomenon is known as creep. Other materials reveal a dependence on the mechanical response on the applied strain rate. Moreover, if a constant strain is imposed, stress tends to vanish in time. These mechanical behaviours can be described by assuming visco-elastic models.

These models can be thought of as a combination of elastic elements with viscous dampers in which the stress depends on the strain rate. Figure 12.15 shows the typical combination of elements adopted to construct a standard uni-dimensional linear visco-elastic model. The terms G_∞ and G_1 are the elastic constants of the springs and η_1 is the viscosity of the dashpot, i.e. the ratio between the rate of stress and the rate of its strain γ. Terms ε and σ represent the strain and stress of the whole element while the term q is the (non-equilibrated) stress of the viscous branch. Stress and strain measures are all functions of time t. The stress–strain relation with time is deduced by taking the equilibrium of the system into account. From the global balance of the element, the following relation is obtained:

$$\sigma = G_\infty \varepsilon + G_1 (\varepsilon - \gamma) \qquad (75)$$

The equilibrium of the viscous branch is given by the differential equation:

$$q = G_1 (\varepsilon - \gamma) = \eta_1 \dot{\gamma}, \ \gamma(0) = 0 \qquad (76)$$

After a simple manipulation of the previous equations and integrating in time from the initial instant to the current one, the expression for the stress σ is:

$$\sigma(t) = E_\infty \varepsilon + q_0 e^{-t/\alpha_1} + \int_{\tau=0}^{t} \left[E_1 \frac{d\varepsilon}{d\tau} e^{(\tau - t)/\alpha_1} \right] d\tau \qquad (77)$$

where the parameter α_1 is given by the ratio η_1/G_1.

Figures 12.16 and 12.17 show the response with time of the element represented in Figure 12.15 for two typical situations: constant stress applied (Figure 12.16) and constant strain applied (Figure 12.17). In the first case, the strain at time zero is related to the initial stiffness of the system, given by $G_\infty + G_1$. The strain increases with time up

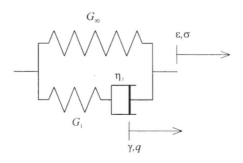

Figure 12.15 Combination of elastic (spring) and viscous (dashpot) elements.

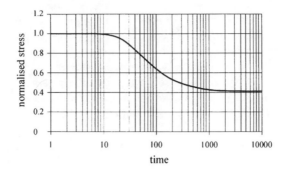

Figure 12.16 Qualitative representation of the mechanical response of a viscoelastic material under an imposed constant strain state (relaxation): stress normalised to the initial value vs. time.

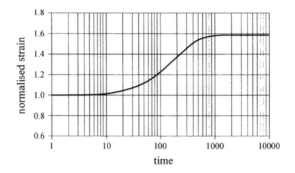

Figure 12.17 Qualitative representation of the mechanical response of a viscoelastic material under an imposed constant stress state: strain normalised to the initial value vs. time.

to the final equilibrium state for $t = \infty$, characterised by a reduced elastic constant G_∞. The case of imposed constant strain is characterised by an initial stress state, which is proportional to the initial elastic modulus $G_\infty + G_1$. The system shows a relaxation of the stress with time, which reaches the final equilibrium with a stress proportional to the final elastic modulus G_∞.

The model represented in Figure 12.15 and described by the previous relations is suitable for a generalisation, accounting for three-dimensional states. This is obtained in a straight way by substituting the variables ε, σ, γ, and q with the corresponding second order tensors. It is also possible to provide for more sophisticated relaxation functions or for elastic elements with a non-linear response.

12.6.4 Elasto-damage models

Elasto-damage constitutive models are adopted in order to describe the degradation of the elastic properties of materials. The degradation of materials can be represented, for example, by the initiation and growth of microvoids or microcracks in the material's structure.

The basic idea in the assumption of these constitutive models is to describe the degradation from a macroscopic point of view, through the use of a homogenisation concept. Under the elastic response hypothesis, the stress is a function of the strain state only, through the elastic constants. If one takes into account the presence of defects on a microscale level, which are given by the same strain condition, their macroscopic effect will be a lower stress state than in the undamaged material. The stress acting on the body will be defined as a function not only of the current strain but also of the stress-strain history of the material, taken into account through a damage function. This damage function is scalar if the damage does not depend on the orientation of micro-defects. On the other hand, a tensorial variable is needed if damage introduces anisotropy. The initiation and growth of defects is usually an irreversible process, hence the damage function is monotonic, except in the case of bio-logical tissues where regeneration process can be antagonist to the damage itself.

The general dependence for the stress can be given by:

$$\boldsymbol{\sigma} = \boldsymbol{\sigma}(\varepsilon, d, \boldsymbol{D}) \tag{78}$$

where d and $\boldsymbol{D}$ are respectively scalar and tensorial damage functions. A scalar damage can be introduced by using a multiplicative function $(1-d)$, thus defining the stress function:

$$\boldsymbol{\sigma} = (1-d)(2\mu\boldsymbol{I}_1 + \lambda\boldsymbol{I}\otimes\boldsymbol{I})\varepsilon \tag{79}$$

The multiplicative term is equal to unit for undamaged material ($d = 0$) while a total failure is reached for $d = 1$. One can assume, for example, the following damage function:

$$
\begin{aligned}
d &= 0 & \text{if} \quad \Pi \le \Pi_0 \\
d &= 1 - \frac{1 - e^{-\Pi/a}}{\Pi/a} & \text{if} \quad \Pi > \Pi_0
\end{aligned}
\tag{80}
$$

where the scalar Π is an equivalent strain depending on the maximum value of the stored energy function W attained during the strain history of the material:

$$\Pi = \max_{\tau\in(-\infty,t)} \sqrt{2W(\tau)} \tag{81}$$

and Π_0 is its threshold value. Obviously, the damage model presented here can include finite strains and be generalised in order to describe more complex effects of degradation of the elastic properties of the materials.

The definition of the terms affecting the value of the damage is related to the type of structure and the type of loading. For example, the use of the damage concept in the mechanics of biological tissues is applied, in particular, to the modelling of the degradation of bone due to application of loading cycles. At that aim, the damage can also be related to the number and amplitude of the loading cycles, with a consequent modification in relationships (80).

12.6.5 Multi-phase media

A hydrated biological tissue cannot always be homogenized to a continuous single phase medium. The presence of filling liquid phases, in fact, can deeply affect the mechanical response of tissues, leading to a delayed response to loading or increasing their bearing capacity. Some aspects can be studied by introducing an equivalent visco-elastic constitutive models, but the response of hydrated tissue response to mechanical loading can be better investigated by using multiphase models. They are better suited to this case because they take into account the coupling effects of a fluid phase, totally or almost incompressible, partially or fully saturating the pores of a solid matrix, even when undergoing finite deformations.

It has just been shown as balance laws and material relationships are stated in classical mechanics for a single component medium, with the assumption that it is continuously distributed. A multiphase medium can be defined as the superposition of different phases: the solid matrix and fluid phases, liquid and/or gaseous, which occupy the remaining part of the domain, i.e. the void space. Each phase is a chemically homogeneous portion of the system and occupies a distinct part of the void space, limited by a physical boundary. The description of multiphase media is scale dependent. The real non-homogeneous structure of the porous medium domain is considered at a microscopic level where the behavior of a mathematical point within each phase is studied in terms of the field variables which describe the status of that phase. The real multiphase system is modeled by overlapping continua since each phase is assumed to continuously fill the entire domain. This macroscopic description of porous media, as interpenetrating continuous bodies, is based either on the mixture theory integrated by the concept of volume fractions or on averaging theories. Since averaging theories link the microscopic level with the macroscopic one through averaging procedures, they allow for a better understanding of the relation between the microscopic and macroscopic domain, which is the natural one for all continuum mechanical models.

The motion of any π phase particle is described as introduced in paragraph two. The deformation process of a porous medium regards its solid matrix, while the motion of fluid phases is usually given in terms of mass averaged velocities relative to the moving solid: $\mathbf{v}^{fs}$ is the relative velocity of the fluid phase particle referred to the corresponding point of the solid skeleton.

Fluid acceleration is given as:

$$\mathbf{a}^{f} = \mathbf{a}^{s} + \mathbf{a}^{fs} + \mathbf{v}^{fs} \cdot \mathrm{grad}\,(\mathbf{v}^{s} + \mathbf{v}^{fs}) \tag{82}$$

where $\mathbf{a}^{fs}$ is the relative acceleration of the fluid phase particle referred to the corresponding point of the solid matrix. Derivatives are taken in the current configuration.

12.6.5.1 Balance conditions

The classical equations of continuum mechanics must hold at a microscopic level for any π phase while step discontinuities of material properties and thermodynamic quantities may arise at the interfaces to other constituents.

The averaged macroscopic mass balance equations are given in the case of immiscible and chemically not reacting constituents, absence of phase change and when all fluids are in contact with the solid phase.

The eulerian forms of the mass conservation equation of solid and fluid phases are:

$$\frac{D^{s}[(1 - \phi)\rho^{s}]}{Dt} + \rho^{s}(1 - \phi)\,\mathrm{div}\,\mathbf{v}^{s} = 0 \tag{83}$$

$$\frac{D^{f}(\phi S^{f}\rho^{f})}{Dt} + \phi S^{f}\rho^{f}\mathrm{div}\,\mathbf{v}^{f} = 0 \tag{84}$$

where ϕ is porosity and S^{f} fluid saturation.

The linear momentum balance equations for solid and fluid phases are respectively:

$$\text{grad } \boldsymbol{\sigma}^s + \rho^s (\mathbf{b}^s - \mathbf{a}^s) + \rho^s \hat{\mathbf{t}}^s = 0 \tag{85}$$

$$\text{grad } \boldsymbol{\sigma}^f + \rho^f (\mathbf{b}^f - \mathbf{a}^f) + \rho^f \hat{\mathbf{t}}^f = 0 \tag{86}$$

where $\rho^\pi \mathbf{b}^\pi$ is the external momentum supply, $\rho^\pi \mathbf{a}^\pi$ is the volume density of the inertia force and $\rho^\pi \hat{\mathbf{t}}^\pi$ accounts for the exchange of momentum due to mechanical interaction with other phases.

12.6.5.2 Constitutive laws

Constitutive laws describe the solid skeleton behavior and the momentum exchange between different phases. They are based on quantities currently measurable in experiments and extensively validated. When dealing with large deformation effects, care must be taken in the material frame invariancy of the constitutive laws. This is obtained by expressing these relationships as functions of objective fields.

Reference can be given to paragraph five for constitutive law, with the solid matrix relationship given in terms of effective stress σ'':

$$\boldsymbol{\sigma}'' = \boldsymbol{\sigma} - \mathbf{I} \, \alpha \, S^f p^f \tag{87}$$

Deviatoric stress components are not considered for fluids, even if their dissipative effects are taken into account in linear momentum balance equations through momentum exchange terms:

$$\rho^f \hat{\mathbf{t}}^f = -\Xi^f \phi S^f \mathbf{v}^{fs} + p^f \, \text{grad} \, (\phi S^f) \tag{88}$$

where Ξ^f is the resistivity tensor, related to the permeability tensor $\mathbf{K}^f$, through $(\Xi^f)^{-1} = \mathbf{K}^f/(\phi S^f)$. $\mathbf{K}^f$ can be expressed as a function of the dynamic viscosity μ^f, the intrinsic permeability $\mathbf{k}$, the relative permeability k^{rf}, function of the degree of saturation:

$$\mathbf{K}^f = \frac{k^{rf} \mathbf{k}}{\mu^f} \tag{89}$$

The constitutive laws are then introduced into the balance conditions to obtain the general field equations, which are then rearranged in weak form for numerical applications.

12.7 CONCLUSIONS

In this chapter the basic concepts of continuum mechanics were presented with the aim of introducing the reader to the formulation adopted within numerical approach to biomechanics and, in particular, to dental biomechanics.

Attention was given to the definition of constitutive models, which can be used in the modelling of both hard and soft biological tissues. The reliability of numerical models is closely related to the affinity between the effective stress-strain response shown by biological materials and the mathematical stress-strains relationships. Because biological materials show complex behaviour, with inelastic effects, such as viscosity or damage, the mathematical framework that must be adopted for an appropriate modelling of the tissues reflects this complexity. An additional complexity is due to the fact that soft tissues undergo large strains.

In spite of the difficulty that can arise in an initial approach to these topics, they must be carefully defined and acquired. They represent the basis for the development of software tools, such as finite element method programs, for the simulation and prediction of the mechanical behaviour of biological tissues.

REFERENCES

E.S. Almeida, R.L. Spilker, Finite element formulations for hyperelastic transversely isotropic biphasic soft tissues, Comput. Methods Appl. Mech. Engrg., Vol. 151, pp. 513–538, 1998.

K.J. Bathe, Finite Element Procedures, Prentice-Hall, New Jersey, 1996.

R.M. Christensen, Theory of Viscoelasticity: an introduction, 2nd Edition, Academic Press, New York, 1982.

S.C. Cowin, Bone poroelasticity, J. Biomechanics, Vol. 32, pp. 217–238, 1999.

S.C. Cowin, Bone mechanics, 2nd Edition, CRC Press Inc., 2001.

M.A. Crisfield, Non-linear Finite Element Analysis of Solid and Structures, John Wiley & Son, 1997.

T.J.R. Hughes, The Finite Element Method, Prentice-Hall, Inc., Englewood Cliffs, New Jersey, 1987.

L.M. Kachanov, Introduction to Continuum Damage Mechanics, Martinus Nijhoff, Dordrecht, The Netherlands, 1986.

T.C. Lee, F.J. O'Brien, D. Taylor, The nature of fatigue damage in bone, International Journal of Fatigue, Vol. 22, pp. 847–853, 2000.

J.A. Lemaitre, Course in Damage Mechanics, 2nd Edition, Springer-Verlag, Berlin, 1996.

R.W. Lewis, B.A. Schrefler, The Finite Element Method in the Static and Dynamic Deformation and Consolidation of Porous Media, J. Wiley, Chichester, 1998.

L.E. Malvern, Introduction to the Mechanics of Continuos Media, Prentice-Hall, New Jersey, 1969.

J.E. Marsden, T.J.R. Hughes, Mathematical Foundations of Elasticity, Prentice-Hall, Inc., Englewood Cliffs, New Jersey, 1983.

W. Maurel, Y. Wu, N. Magnenat Thalmann, D. Thalmann, Biomechanical Models for Soft Tissue Simulation, Springer, 1998.

V.C. Mow, S.C. Kuei, W.M. Lai, C.G. Armstrong, Biphasic creep and stress relaxation of articular cartilage in compression: theory and experiments, J. Biomech. Engng., Vol. 102, pp. 73–84, 1980.

R.W. Ogden, Non-Linear Elastic Deformation, Ellis Horwood, Chichester, U.K., 1984.

P.J. Prendergast, D. Taylor, Prediction of bone adaptation using damage accumulation, Journal of Biomechanics, Vol. 27, Issue 8, pp. 1067–1076, 1994.

S. Ramtani, M. Zidi, A theoretical model of the effect of continuum damage on a bone adaptation model, Journal of Biomechanics, Vol. 34, Issue 4, pp. 471–479, 2001.

A.J.M. Spencer, Continuum Mechanics, Longman Scientific and Technical, New York, 1990.

J.C. Simo, T.J.R. Hughes, Computational inelasticity, Springer, 2000.

O.C. Zienkiewicz, R.L. Taylor, The Finite Element Method, 4th edition, 1996.

Index